Cardiovascular Complications of Chronic Rheumatic Diseases

Editors

GEORGE A. KARPOUZAS
M. ELAINE HUSNI

RHEUMATIC DISEASE CLINICS OF NORTH AMERICA

www.rheumatic.theclinics.com

Consulting Editor
MICHAEL H. WEISMAN

February 2023 • Volume 49 • Number 1

ELSEVIER

1600 John F. Kennedy Boulevard • Suite 1800 • Philadelphia, Pennsylvania, 19103-2899
http://www.theclinics.com

RHEUMATIC DISEASE CLINICS OF NORTH AMERICA Volume 49, Number 1
February 2023 ISSN 0889-857X, ISBN 13: 978-0-323-84928-9

Editor: Joanna Gascoine
Developmental Editor: Karen Solomon

Rheumatic Disease Clinics of North America (ISSN 0889-857X) is published quarterly by Elsevier Inc., 360 Park Avenue South, New York, NY 10010-1710. Months of issue are February, May, August, and November. Business and editorial offices: 1600 John F. Kennedy Boulevard, Suite 1800, Philadelphia, PA 19103-2899. Periodicals postage paid at New York, NY and additional mailing offices. Subscription prices are USD 377.00 per year for US individuals, USD 865.00 per year for US institutions, USD 100.00 per year for US students and residents, USD 444.00 per year for Canadian individuals, USD 1081.00 per year for Canadian institutions, USD 100.00 per year for Canadian students/residents, USD 484.00 per year for international individuals, USD 1081.00 per year for international institutions, and USD 230.00 per year for foreign students/residents. To receive student/ resident rate, orders must be accompanied by name of affiliated institution, date of term, and the *signature* of program/residency coordinator on institution letterhead. Orders will be billed at individual rate until proof of status received. Foreign air speed delivery is included in all *Clinics* subscription prices. All prices are subject to change without notice. **POSTMASTER:** Send address changes to *Rheumatic Disease Clinics of North America,* Elsevier Health Sciences Division, Subscription Customer Service, 3251 Riverport Lane, Maryland Heights, MO 63043. **Customer Service: 1-800-654-2452 (US and Canada). From outside of the US and Canada: 314-447-8871. Fax: 314-447-8029. For print support, e-mail: JournalsCustomerService-usa@elsevier.com. For online support, e-mail: JournalsOnlineSupport-usa@elsevier.com.**

Reprints. For copies of 100 or more of articles in this publication, please contact the Commercial Reprints Department, Elsevier Inc., 360 Park Avenue South, New York, New York, 10010-1710; Tel.: +1-212-633-3874, Fax: +1-212-633-3820, and E-mail: reprints@elsevier.com.

Rheumatic Disease Clinics of North America is covered in MEDLINE/PubMed (Index Medicus), Current Contents/Clinical Medicine, Science Citation Index, ISI/BIOMED, and EMBASE/Excerpta Medica.

Contributors

CONSULTING EDITOR

MICHAEL H. WEISMAN, MD
Adjunct Professor of Medicine, Stanford University, Distinguished Professor of Medicine
Emeritus, David Geffen School of Medicine at UCLA, Professor of Medicine Emeritus,
Cedars-Sinai Medical Center, Los Angeles, California, USA

EDITORS

GEORGE A. KARPOUZAS, MD
Professor of Medicine, David Geffen School of Medicine at UCLA, Chief, Division of
Rheumatology, Harbor-UCLA Medical Center, The Lundquist Institute of Biomedical
Innovation, Torrance, California, USA

M. ELAINE HUSNI, MD, MPH
Vice Chair, Department of Rheumatic and Immunologic Diseases, Director, Arthritis and
Musculoskeletal Center, Cleveland Clinic, Cleveland, Ohio, USA

AUTHORS

MARIA PIA ADORNI, PhD
Department of Medicine and Surgery, Unit of Neuroscience, University of Parma, Parma,
Italy

VIKAS AGARWAL, DM, FRCP(Edin)
Professor, Department of Clinical Immunology and Rheumatology, Sanjay Gandhi
Postgraduate Institute of Medical Sciences (SGPGIMS), Lucknow, India

SAKIR AHMED, DM
Associate Professor, Department of Clinical Immunology and Rheumatology, Kalinga
Institute of Medical Sciences (KIMS), Bhubaneswar, India

FRANCO BERNINI, PhD
Department of Food and Drug, University of Parma, Parma, Italy

ALISON H. CLIFFORD, MD
Associate Professor, Department of Medicine, Division of Rheumatology, University of
Alberta, Edmonton, Alberta, Canada

CYNTHIA S. CROWSON, PhD
Department of Quantitative Health Sciences, Division of Rheumatology, Mayo Clinic,
Rochester, Minnesota, USA

MOHIT GOYAL, MD, FRCP(Edin)
Consultant, Department of Rheumatology and Clinical Immunology, CARE Pain and
Arthritis Centre, Udaipur, Rajasthan, India

ELLEN M. HAUGE, MD, PhD
Division of Rheumatology, Aarhus University Hospital, Aarhus, Denmark

IVANA HOLLAN, MD, PhD
Associate Professor, Norwegian University of Science and Technology, Gjøvik, Norway

M. ELAINE HUSNI, MD, MPH
Vice Chair, Department of Rheumatic and Immunologic Diseases, Director, Arthritis and Musculoskeletal Center, Cleveland Clinic, Cleveland, Ohio, USA

GEORGE A. KARPOUZAS, MD
Professor of Medicine, David Geffen School of Medicine at UCLA, Chief, Division of Rheumatology, Harbor-UCLA Medical Center, The Lundquist Institute of Biomedical Innovation, Torrance, California, USA

GEORGE D. KITAS, MD, PhD
Dudley Group NHS Foundation Trust, United Kingdom

BRIAN BRIDAL LØGSTRUP, MD, PhD, DMSc
Associate Professor, Department of Cardiology, Institute of Clinical Medicine, Aarhus University Hospital, Aarhus, Denmark

KATHERINE P. LIAO, MD, MPH
Division of Rheumatology, Inflammation, and Immunity, Brigham and Women's Hospital, Harvard Medical School, Boston, Massachusetts, USA

LOTTA LJUNG, MD, PhD
Department of Public Health and Clinical Medicine/Rheumatology, Umeå University, Umeå, Sweden; Center for Rheumatology, Academic Specialist Center, Stockholm Health Services, Stockholm, Sweden

DEEBA MINHAS, MD
Clinical Assistant Professor, Department of Internal Medicine, Division of Rheumatology, University of Michigan, Ann Arbor, Michigan, USA

SARAH R. ORMSETH
The Lundquist Institute, Harbor-UCLA Medical Center, Torrance, California, USA

DURGA PRASANNA MISRA, DM, MRCP(UK), FRCP(Edin)
Associate Professor, Department of Clinical Immunology and Rheumatology, Sanjay Gandhi Postgraduate Institute of Medical Sciences (SGPGIMS), Lucknow, India

ANJALI NIDHAAN, MD
Cleveland Clinic, Cleveland, Ohio, USA

MARCELLA PALUMBO, ScD
Department of Food and Drug, University of Parma, Parma, Italy

SOLBRITT RANTAPÄÄ-DAHLQVIST, MD, PhD
Department of Public Health and Clinical Medicine/Rheumatology, Umeå University, Umeå, Sweden

NICOLETTA RONDA, MD, PhD
Department of Food and Drug, University of Parma, Parma, Italy

ANNA SÖDERGREN, MD, PhD
Department of Public Health and Clinical Medicine/Rheumatology, Umeå University, Umeå, Sweden; Wallenberg Centre for Molecular Medicine (WCMM), Umeå University, Umeå, Sweden

AMAN SHARMA, MD, FRCP(London)
Professor, Clinical Immunology and Rheumatology Services, Department of Internal Medicine, Postgraduate Institute of Medical Education and Research (PGIMER), Chandigarh, India

W.H. WILSON TANG, MD
Cleveland Clinic Lerner College of Medicine at Case Western Reserve University, Kaufman Center for Heart Failure Treatment and Recovery, Heart Vascular and Thoracic Institute, Cleveland Clinic, Cleveland, Ohio, USA

BRITTANY WEBER, MD, PhD
Department of Medicine, Division of Cardiovascular Medicine, Cardiovascular Imaging Program, Department of Radiology, Brigham and Women's Hospital, Harvard Medical School, Boston, Massachusetts, USA

ALEXIA A. ZAGOURAS, MD, MA
Cleveland Clinic Lerner College of Medicine at Case Western Reserve University, Cleveland, Ohio, USA

FRANCESCA ZIMETTI, PhD
Department of Food and Drug, University of Parma, Parma, Italy

Contents

Cardiovascular diseases (CVDs) are the leading causes of death in the world, but declining trends for cardiovascular (CV) mortality and morbidity have been observed during the last decades. Reports on secular trends regarding the excess CV mortality and morbidity in rheumatoid arthritis show diverging results. Data support that also patients with inflammatory arthritis have benefited from improved treatment and prevention for CVD, which can be observed, for example, in decreased case fatality after CV event. However, several recent studies indicate a remaining excess CV risk in patients with inflammatory arthritis.

Cardiovascular disease (CVD) risk is increased in most inflammatory rheumatic diseases (IRDs), reiterating the role of inflammation in the initiation and progression of atherosclerosis. An inverse association of CVD risk with body weight and lipid levels has been described in IRDs. Coronary artery calcium scores, plaque burden and characteristics, and carotid plaques on ultrasound optimize CVD risk estimate in IRDs. Biomarkers of cardiac injury, autoantibodies, lipid biomarkers, and cytokines also improve risk assessment in IRDs. Machine learning and deep learning algorithms for phenotype and image analysis hold promise to improve CVD risk stratification in IRDs.

Systemic autoimmune rheumatic diseases (SARDs) are defined by the potential to affect multiple organ systems, and cardiac involvement is a prevalent but often overlooked sequela. Myocardial involvement in SARDs is medicated by macrovascular disease, microvascular dysfunction, and myocarditis. Systemic lupus erythematosus, rheumatoid arthritis, systemic sclerosis, eosinophilic granulomatosis with polyangiitis, and sarcoidosis are associated with the greatest risk of myocardial damage and heart failure, though myocardial involvement is also seen in other SARDs or their treatments. Management of myocardial involvement should be disease-specific. Further research is required to elucidate targetable mechanisms of myocardial involvement in SARDs.

There is a significant increase in risk of heart failure in several rheumatic diseases. Common cardiovascular risk factors and inflammatory processes, present in both rheumatic diseases and heart failure, are contributing to this increase. The opportunities for using immune-based strategies to fight development of heart failure in rheumatic diseases are evolving. The diversity of inflammation calls for a tailored characterization of inflammation, enabling differentiation of inflammation and subsequent introduction of precision medicine using target-specific strategies and immunomodulatory therapy. As the field of rheuma-cardiology is still evolving, clear recommendations cannot be given yet.

Takayasu's arteritis (TAK) and giant cell arteritis (GCA) are the 2 common primary large vessel vasculitides (LVV). They share common vascular targets, clinical presentations, and histopathology, but target a strikingly different patient demographic. While GCA predominantly affects elderly people of northern European ancestry, TAK preferentially targets young women of Asian heritage. Cardiovascular diseases (CVD), including ischemic heart disease, cerebrovascular disease, aortic disease, and thromboses, are significantly increased in LVV. In this review, we will compare and contrast the issue of CVD in patients with TAK and GCA, with respect to prevalence, risk factors, and mechanisms of events to gain an understanding of the relative contributions of active vasculitis, vascular damage, and accelerated atherosclerosis. Controversies and possible mitigation strategies will be discussed.

Venous thromboembolism (VTE), which includes deep venous thrombosis and pulmonary embolism, is a cardiovascular event whose risk is increased in most inflammatory rheumatic diseases (IRDs). Mechanisms that increase VTE risk include antiphospholipid antibodies (APLs), particularly anticardiolipin antibodies, anti-beta2glycoprotein I antibodies and lupus anticoagulant present together, and inflammation-mediated endothelial injury. Patients with IRDs should receive long-term anticoagulation drugs when the risk of VTE recurrence is high. In the light of recent warnings from regulatory agencies regarding heightened VTE risk with Janus kinase inhibitors, these drugs should be initiated only after a careful assessment of VTE risk in those with IRDs.

Feiring Heart Biopsy Study enables searching for potential pathogenetic mechanisms, therapeutic targets, and biomarkers through the assessment of clinical data and multiple blood and tissue samples from patients with and without inflammatory rheumatic diseases (IRDs), undergoing coronary artery bypass grafting. Some of our findings, for example, more inflammation (including the presence of immune cells and expression of proinflammatory cytokines) in vessels and the heart, and the presence of certain bacteria and autoantigens in vessels, could contribute to the increased risk of ischemia, aneurysms, and/or cardiac dysfunction in IRDs. Furthermore, some of the detected factors could be involved in the pathomechanisms of these conditions in general.

Immune and inflammatory mediators in autoimmune rheumatic diseases induce modification in the activity of enzymes pivotal for lipid metabolism and promote a proatherogenic serum lipid profile. However, disturbances in low- and high-density lipoprotein composition and increased lipid oxidation also occur. Therefore, lipoprotein dysfunction causes intracellular cholesterol accumulation in macrophages, smooth muscle cells, and platelets. Overall, both plaque progression and acute cardiovascular events are promoted. Single rheumatic diseases may present a particular pattern of lipid disturbances so that standard methods to evaluate cardiovascular risk may not be accurate enough. In general, antirheumatic drugs positively affect lipid metabolism in these patients.

Systemic auto-immune inflammatory arthritides are associated with increased cardiovascular (CV) risk compared to those without these conditions, and is a leading cause of morbidity and mortality. Newer biologic drug modifying antirheumatoid drugs (bDMARD) and small molecules have transformed treatment paradigms enabling tighter control of disease activity and in some cases, remission. There is evidence to suggest that the majority of bDMARDs may also reduce cardiovascular risk, although prospective interventional data remain sparse. Additionally, recent results raise concern for treatments targeting specific pathways that may negatively affect cardiovascular risk. This review will cover key biologic pathways targeted in rheumatoid arthritis, psoriatic arthritis, and spondyloarthropathies.

Nonsteroidal anti-inflammatory drugs (NSAIDs) are among the most prescribed pharmacologic therapies worldwide due to their therapeutic analgesic efficacy and relative tolerability. In the past several decades, various cardiovascular (CV) adverse events have emerged regarding both traditional NSAIDs (tNSAIDs) and cyclo-oxygenase 2 (COX-2) selective (coxibs). This review will provide an updated report on the CV risk profile of NSAIDs, focusing on several of the larger clinical trials, meta-analyses, and registry studies. We aim to provide rheumatologists with a framework for NSAID use in the context of rheumatologic chronic pain management. Recent findings: In patients with and without CV diseases, the use of NSAIDs, both tNSAIDs and coxibs, is associated with an increased risk of adverse CV events, myocardial infarction, heart failure, and cerebrovascular events. These CV risks have increased within weeks of coxib use and higher doses of tNSAIDs. The risk of adverse CV events is heterogenous across NSAIDs; naproxen and low-dose ibuprofen appear to have lower increased CV risk among NSAIDs. A variation in CV risk is associated with multiple factors, including NSAID class, COX-2 selectivity, treatment dose and duration, and baseline patient risk. Summary: Many important questions remain regarding the safety of NSAIDs and whether the culmination of research performed could inform us whether specific patient subtypes or NSAID class may have a more favorable profile. tNSAIDs such as naproxen and low-dose ibuprofen may have a lower CV risk profile, while coxibs have a more favorable GI risk profile. In general, any NSAID can be optimized if used at the lowest effective dose for the shortest amount of time, especially among individuals with increased CV risk.

RHEUMATIC DISEASE CLINICS OF NORTH AMERICA

FORTHCOMING ISSUES

May 2023
Scleroderma: Best Approaches to Patient Care
Tracy Frech, *Editor*

August 2023
Vasculitis
Eli Miloslavsky and Anisha Dua, *Editors*

RECENT ISSUES

November 2022
Environmental Triggers for Rheumatic Diseases
Bryant R. England, *Editor*

August 2022
Guideline development and implementation in Rheumatic Diseases
Michael Ward, *Editor*

SERIES OF RELATED INTEREST

Medical Clinics of North America
https://www.medical.theclinics.com/
Neurologic Clinics
https://www.neurologic.theclinics.com/
Dermatologic Clinics
https://www.derm.theclinics.com/
Physical Medicine and Rehabilitation Clinics of North America
https://www.pmr.theclinics.com/

THE CLINICS ARE AVAILABLE ONLINE!
Access your subscription at:
www.theclinics.com

Foreword

Cardiovascular Comorbidities in Inflammatory Rheumatic Diseases

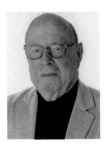

Michael H. Weisman, MD
Consulting Editor

Drs Karpouzas and Husni have assembled a series of articles that address one of the most important issues facing our management of systemic rheumatic disease patients in the modern era, the prevention and (hopefully) successful identification and avoidance of cardiovascular morbidity and mortality. In the 1960s and 1970s, patients with rheumatoid arthritis (RA) and systemic lupus erythematosus (SLE) actually died directly from the heart and vascular complications of their disease. This has been reversed. Today, modern management consists of early institution of aggressive combinations of disease-modifying agents, and the disease complications we saw 50 years ago are relegated to museum findings, and our Fellows in training may never see them, fortunately.

But what do we have in return? Patients die today not from the disease itself but from their experience of cardiovascular complications resulting from immune-mediated vascular responses to the underlying inflammatory nature of RA and SLE as well as from the drugs that are designed to control that inflammation. What is disconcerting and certainly becoming more evident is that drug development (recent example, JAK inhibition) may in fact add to the burden of cardiovascular morbidity and mortality in certain individuals at risk. What this issue is designed to do is to bring into focus the work that is being done to develop risk models and to identify mechanistic studies that can not only provide acceptable low disease activity but also avoid the effects of clinical and subclinical inflammatory burden of disease. We are grateful to George and

Rheum Dis Clin N Am 49 (2023) xiii–xiv
https://doi.org/10.1016/j.rdc.2022.09.002
0889-857X/23/© 2022 Published by Elsevier Inc.

Elaine, who have identified these clinical and research gaps and the attempts to bridge them.

Michael H. Weisman, MD
Division of Immunology and Rheumatology
Stanford University School of Medicine

E-mail address:
weisman@cshs.org

Preface

Cardiovascular Comorbidities in Inflammatory Rheumatic Diseases

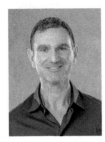 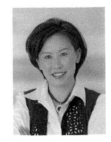

George A. Karpouzas, MD   M. Elaine Husni, MD, MPH
Editors

Patients with inflammatory rheumatic diseases experience higher cardiovascular morbidity and mortality compared with age- and gender-matched individuals in the general population. Those include atherosclerotic, ischemic complications as well as nonatherosclerotic events, such as venous thromboembolism, myocardial involvement, and heart failure. Disease flares and high cumulative inflammatory burden are characteristic of the systemic autoimmune diseases and constitute major, independent contributors to cardiovascular comorbidity. Moreover, chronic inflammation synergizes with traditional cardiac risk factors in promoting cardiovascular comorbidity, facilitates the development and appearance of some, like insulin resistance, diabetes mellitus, and hypertension, while altering the impact of others, such as lipids, lipoprotein levels, and obesity.

Disease-specific or -associated immune responses further contribute to atherosclerosis development by affecting lipoprotein composition and function, cholesterol loading to arterial wall macrophages, foam cell formation, plaque instability, and rupture. Several of them serve as predictive and prognostic biomarkers, optimizing risk estimates for atherosclerotic plaque presence, progression, and cardiovascular events above and beyond traditional risk factor models. The evaluation of subclinical atherosclerosis across various vascular territories and using different, noninvasive imaging modalities, additionally optimize cardiovascular risk estimates. Future risk prediction models combining traditional risk factors, disease-specific characteristics, information from disease-associated biomarkers, imaging, and synthesized with the help of machine- and deep-learning modalities of artificial intelligence may further optimize risk recognition and allow the development of more effective and comprehensive cardioprotective strategies.

The identification of disease-associated cellular and molecular processes and their specific targeting with biological or newer synthetic disease-modifying agents has

Rheum Dis Clin N Am 49 (2023) xv–xvi
https://doi.org/10.1016/j.rdc.2022.09.001
0889-857X/23/© 2022 Published by Elsevier Inc.

revolutionized our ability to achieve low-disease activity or remission and comprehensive inflammatory control. Above and beyond their potent anti-inflammatory effects, these agents may further optimize lipoprotein structure and function, cholesterol accumulation, and efflux from atherosclerotic plaques and influence body composition. Interestingly, most widely available analgesics, such as nonsteroidal anti-inflammatory drugs, used for short-term pain control can have long-term unintended cardiac risks. Overall, these treatment benefits should be judiciously weighed against the potential of harm in these patients. Beyond the development of highly efficient and disease-specific targeted therapies, the increasing and broader appreciation of accelerated risk, prompt and diligent clinical screening, and application of effective prevention campaigns have yielded significant improvements in inflammatory disease-associated and treatment-associated cardiovascular risk.

George A. Karpouzas, MD
David Geffen School of Medicine, UCLA
Division of Rheumatology
Harbor UCLA Medical Center
1124 West Carson Street, E4-R17A
Torrance, CA 90502, USA

M. Elaine Husni, MD, MPH
Department of Rheumatic and Immunologic Diseases
Arthritis and Musculoskeletal Center
Cleveland Clinic
9500 Euclid Avenue, Desk A50
Cleveland, OH 44195, USA

E-mail addresses:
gkarpouzas@lundquist.org (G.A. Karpouzas)
husnie@ccf.org (M.E. Husni)

Time Trends of Cardiovascular Disease in the General Population and Inflammatory Arthritis

Anna Södergren, MD, PhD[a,b,]*,
Solbritt Rantapää-Dahlqvist, MD, PhD[a], Lotta Ljung, MD, PhD[a,c]

KEYWORDS

- Time trends • Rheumatoid arthritis • Psoriatic arthritis • Spondarthritis
- Cardiovascular disease

KEY POINTS

- The cardiovascular (CV) mortality worldwide is decreasing, but due to the aging and growth of the world's population there is a rise of the absolute numbers of CV events.
- In patients with rheumatoid arthritis most studies have presented a decrease over time for the absolute risk of cardiovascular disease (CVD), but data are conflicting whether the relative risk compared with the general population is declining.
- There are limited data regarding secular time trends for other than atherosclerotic CVD manifestations in the general population as well as inflammatory arthritis.
- Data on CVD incidence and time trends for any CVD in patients with psoriatic arthritis or ankylosing spondylitis are limited.
- The trends for the exposure of risk factors diverge depending on the nature of the risk factor and between high- and low-income countries.

BACKGROUND

Cardiovascular diseases (CVDs) have long been recognized as the leading causes of death in the world. Most of these CV deaths are attributable to either ischemic heart disease (IHD) or cerebrovascular disease and are due to underlying atherosclerosis. CVD can also include heart failure (HF), peripheral arterial disease, arrhythmia, venous thrombosis and other vascular, and cardiac problems. In 2016, CVD was responsible

[a] Department of Public Health and Clinical Medicine/Rheumatology, Umeå University, 901 87 Umeå, Sweden; [b] Wallenberg Centre for Molecular Medicine (WCMM), Umeå University, Umeå, Sweden; [c] Center for Rheumatology, Academic Specialist Center, Stockholm Health Services, Box 6357, Stockholm 102 35, Sweden
* Corresponding author. Department of Public Health and Clinical Medicine/Rheumatology, Umeå University, 901 87 Umeå, Sweden.
E-mail address: anna.sodergren@umu.se
Twitter: @lotta_ljung (L.L.)

Rheum Dis Clin N Am 49 (2023) 1–17
https://doi.org/10.1016/j.rdc.2022.07.003
rheumatic.theclinics.com

for 45% of all deaths in Europe, making CVD the most frequently reported underlying cause of death.[1] In the past two decades, there has been a dramatic decline in CVD mortality rates worldwide, with the largest decline occurring between 2000 and 2005.[2] The same trends are obvious for the incidence of IHD and stroke, although the crude numbers of events have continued to rise due to larger, as well as aging, populations.[3] The improvement in CVD incidence between 1990 and 2013 has been similar among men and women; thus, CVD are still more common in the male population compared with females. Generally, there is an overall downward trend in CVD incidence and mortality rates worldwide, which become obvious after age-standardizing of the numbers (**Fig. 1**A and B).[4]

SECULAR TRENDS FOR THE CARDIOVASCULAR MORTALITY IN INFLAMMATORY ARTHRITIS

Most recent studies have presented a decrease of the all-cause mortality in rheumatoid arthritis (RA) comparable with the change in the general population,[5–10] but there are also studies presenting no improvement in the overall mortality over time or

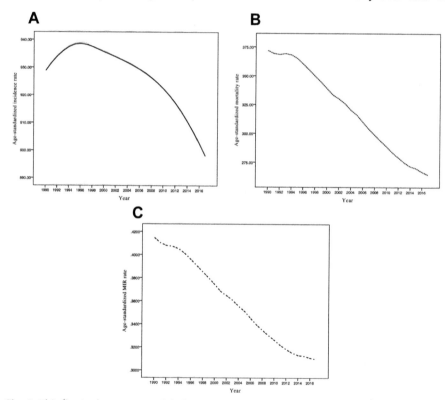

Fig. 1. This figure demonstrates (*A*) the age-standardized incidence rate, (*B*) mortality rate, and (*C*) MIR trends for the entire world from 1990 to 2017. As shown, the mean CVD mortality rate and MIR trend declined steeply over the study interval. CVD, cardiovascular disease; MIR, mortality-to-incidence ratio. (*From* Amini M, Zayeri F, Salehi M. Trend analysis of cardiovascular disease mortality, incidence, and mortality-to-incidence ratio: results from global burden of disease study 2017. BMC public health. 2021;21 (1):401. The figure is reprinted under is licensed under the Creative Commons Attribution 4.0 International License https://bmcpublichealth.biomedcentral.com/articles/10.1186/s12889-021-10429-0.)

compared with the mortality in the general population.[11–14] Furthermore, regarding excess risk of death from CVD and changes in CVD mortality over time in RA, the results are inconsistent.

During the second half of the previous century, the CV mortality was increased by 60% in RA, and there was no trend toward a decrease of the excess risk over time.[15] In one population, even an increase of the excess overall mortality was observed over the time span 1990 to 2006 in the seropositive RA population; an increase driven by CV and respiratory mortality.[16] A Swedish study presented a normalization of the 8-year all-cause mortality comparing patients with established RA in a cohort comprised in 1995 ($n = 161$) compared with a cohort from 1978 ($n = 161$), whereas the excess CV mortality remained.[17] However, in a North American cohort comprising patients with incident RA ($n = 3862$), a normalization of the acute myocardial infarction (AMI) standard mortality rate was observed already in patients with disease debut during the years 1980 to 1997.[18]

Several studies of the time period around and after the millennium indicate a faster decline of the CV mortality among patients with RA than in the general population.[5,8,9,18] The included studies on time trends for CV mortality are briefly presented in **Table 1**. In a large study including 24,914 patients with incident RA, Kaplan–Meier survival curves showed increased 5-year CV mortality in the 1996 to 2000 RA cohort, but not in the 2001 to 2006 RA cohort, compared with the CV mortality among population controls.[5] Similar findings were presented in a cohort study comprising 21,622 incident RA cases in which a statistically nonsignificant decline of the 5-year CV mortality associated with RA was observed, and no increased mortality associated with RA was observed for the years 2004 to 2006; adjusted hazard ratio (HR) 1.13 (95% CI 0.91, 1.40) and 2007 to 2009; adjusted HR 1.19 (95%CI 0.92, 1.54).[8] In a Norwegian study, the 10-year cardiovascular mortality rate among 1391 patients diagnosed with RA 1994 to 1998, 1999 to 2003, and 2004 to 2008 was 9.3%, 6.1%, and 2.9% for each of the time periods, respectively.[9] The patients diagnosed before 2004 had increased cardiovascular mortality; 1994 to 1998 cohort HR 1.55 (95% CI 1.11–2.17) and 1999 to 2003 cohort HR 1.80 (95% CI 1.20–2.70) for the risk of CV death among patients with RA compared with the general population, but in the 2004 to 2008 RA cohort no increase of the 10-year CV mortality was observed, HR 0.94 (95% CI 0.47–1.89).[9]

In the British Norfolk Arthritis Register similar 10-year mortality rates were observed in the cohort of patients with inflammatory arthritis included 2000 to 2004 compared with the cohort included 1990 to 1994 when the background risk in the general population was taken into account.[14] After full adjustments, the mortality rate ratio was 0.77 (95% CI 0.48, 1.24) comparing CV mortality in the later cohort compared with the earlier.[14] Furthermore, in the RA subgroup, no statistically significant improvement of the CV mortality rate was observed, which confirmed the results from an earlier study from the same register.[11] Another recent study presented a decline in the CV mortality parallel to the decline in the population.[19] In this cohort, comprising 813 patients diagnosed with RA 1989 to 2007, the presented unadjusted 10-year CV mortality decreased per decade of RA incidence; 13.6% (1980–1989), 7.1% (1990–1999), and 2.7% (2000–2007).[19] The mortality from coronary artery disease (CAD) in RA showed an even more marked decrease in recent years; 10-year CAD mortality 6.8% (1980–1989), 4.3% (1990–1999), and 1.1% (2000–2007). These mortality rates, although numerically higher for the years before 2000, did not significantly differ from the mortality rates among non-RA referents.[19]

Data for time trends for risks of CVD deaths in psoriatic arthritis (PsA) and ankylosing spondylitis (AS) are unfortunately lacking, but increasing evidence suggests that PsA and AS are associated with an excess CV mortality also during the last decades.[20,21]

Table 1
Overview of the studies on time trends for cardiovascular mortality in inflammatory arthritis included in the review

Author, Publishing Year	Study Area	Patient Identification	Number of Patients	Follow-Up	Study Period
Krishnan et al,[18] 2004	USA	Cohort, RA	3862	Up to 17 y	1980–97
Gonzalez et al,[16] 2008	Olmsted county, Minnesota, USA	Inception cohort, RA	603	Up to 30 y	1955–2006
Bergström et al,[17] 2009	Malmö, Sweden	Clinic-based cohort, RA	309	8 y	1978–85, 1995–2002
Humphreys et al,[11] 2014	Norfolk, UK	Inception cohort, RA	1419	7 y	1990–2011
Lacaille et al,[5] 2016	British Columbia, Canada	Incident RA, administrative database	24,914	5 y	1996–2010
Myasoedova et al,[19] 2017	Olmsted county, Minnesota, USA	Inception cohort, RA	813	10 y	1980–2014
Abhishek, et al,[8] 2018	UK	Incident RA, primary care database	21,622	5 y	1990–2009
Gwinnutt et al,[14] 2018	Norfolk, UK	Inception cohort, inflammatory arthritis (subgroup RA)	1653 (RA n = 961)	10 y	1990–2013
Provan et al,[9] 2020	Oslo, Norway	Inception cohort, RA	1391	5, 10, and 20 y	1994–2015

Abbreviation: CV, cardiovascular.

INFLAMMATORY ARTHRITIS AND TIME TRENDS FOR RISKS OF ATHEROSCLEROTIC CARDIOVASCULAR EVENTS

Despite the decline in mortality of CVD, the aging and growth of the world's population have led to rising numbers of the total numbers of CV events.[4] Still, a worldwide decline of age-standardized incidence of CV events in recent years is evident from large, global studies (see **Fig. 1A**).[4] In repeated cross-sectional samples of 50-year old men, almost 50% decline in AMI from 1975–79 to 2000–04 was observed.[22]

Secular trends in the incidence of atherosclerotic CV events in inflammatory arthritis (mainly RA), other than CV death exclusively, have been evaluated in some recent studies with diverging results.[17,23–29] The studies on secular trends of cardiovascular morbidity that are included in the review are summarized in **Table 2**.

Similar excess risks (>50%) of atherosclerotic CV events (CAD, stroke, and peripheral artery disease) were observed comparing patients with established RA 1978 and 1995.[17] A recently published study based on self-reported data from the National Health and Nutrition Examination Survey (NHANES) reported a doubled relative risk for CVD associated with RA in the three evaluated survey cycles: 1999 to 2006 odds ratio (OR) 2.32, 2007 to 2012 OR 2.19, and 2013 to 2018 OR 1.97, with a numerical, but not statistically significant, decreasing trend.[28] Another study evaluating CV events (AMI and stroke) found an excess risk for CV event (>50%) among patients with RA (n = 905) diagnosed in the 1980s and 1990s, but a risk comparable with the risk in the general population for patients diagnosed in the 2000s.[25] Evaluating the specific events the risk of AMI had decreased significantly in the latest cohort compared with the previous, but the risk of stroke was unchanged.[25] This indicated that the observed attenuation of the excess risk of CV events was mainly driven by a decreased risk of CAD. Similar findings, but for IHD and AMI, were presented in a study with patients diagnosed with RA (n = 1821) during the years 1972 to 2013, whereas the risk increase for IHD/AMI was attenuated for patients diagnosed after 1998.[29]

In contrast, in patients with incident RA (n = 23,237), the absolute risk of AMI was observed to describe a similar decline in patients with RA as in the general population, resulting in the excess 10-year risk of AMI of 21%, independent of year of RA debut (**Fig. 2**).[26] An evaluation of the risk of stroke in RA using the same methods in 23,545 patients with RA onset 1997 to 2004, showed a greater decline in patients with RA debut in 1999 or later than in the general population.[27]

In a more recent study comprising patients with incident RA 1997 to 2014 (n = 15,744), the time trends of risks of acute coronary syndrome (ACS; unstable angina or AMI) were evaluated.[23] The incidence of ACS in both patients and comparators decreased over time resulting in a remaining 40% to 60% excess risk of ACS in RA also in patients with a more recent RA diagnosis.[23] Similar results were presented in a study analyzing the risks of IHD and HF in patients with RA (n = 51,589).[24] In comparison with the general population, similar risks of IHD were observed among patients diagnosed with RA during the earlier part of the study period, 1995 to 2000; adjusted HR 1.37 (95% CI 1.26, 1.49), and during the later part 2001 to 2016; adjusted HR 1.34 (95% CI 1.26, 1.43).[24] Another study presented increasing absolute numbers of CVD diagnoses (AMI, HF, and atrial fibrillation) in hospital admissions with coexisting RA diagnosis during 2005 to 2014. However, the lack of population controls and the study design as such render interpretation of the results difficult.[30]

Reports on time trends for CV events in other inflammatory arthritis besides RA are scarce or lacking. The incidence of major CV events in PsA was not associated with decade of inclusion in the cohort, but in that study no comparison with the background

Table 2
Overview of the studies on time trends for atherosclerotic cardiovascular morbidity in inflammatory arthritis that is included in the review

Author, Publishing Year	Study Area	Patient Identification	Number of Arthritis Patients	Follow-Up	Study Period	Outcome
Bergström et al,[17] 2009	Malmö, Sweden	Clinic-based cohort, RA	309	8 y	1978–85, 1995–2002	CAD, stroke, PAD
Eder, et al,[31] 2016	Ontario, Canada	Clinic-based cohort, PsA	1091	Mean 9.8 y	1978–2013	CV event (AMI, ischaemic stroke, revascularization, CV death)
Holmqvist et al,[23] 2017	Sweden	Incident RA, register-based cohort	15,744	Up to 17 y	1997–2014	ACS (AMI, unstable angina)
Logstrup et al,[24] 2018	Denmark	Incident RA, administrative database	51,859	Up to 10 y	1995–2016	CAD (AMI and revascularization) and HF
Skielta et al,[36] 2020	Sweden	Incident AMI in RA, register-based cohort	4268	1 year after AMI	1998–2014	Prognosis after AMI
Myasoedova et al,[25] 2021	Olmsted county, Minnesota, USA	Inception cohort, RA	905	Up to 15 y as presented	1980–2016	CV events (AMI, stroke), prognosis after CV event
Yazdani et al,[26] 2021	British Columbia, Canada	Incident RA, administrative database	23,237	10 y	1997–2014	AMI
Yazdani et al,[27] 2021	British Columbia, Canada	Incident RA, administrative database	23,545	10 y	1997–2014	Ischaemic stroke
Jatwani, et al,[32] 2021	US	PsA, administrative database	4778 hospital admissions	—	2004–2014	AMI and in-patient mortality after MI
Bandyopadhyay et al,[30] 2021	US	RA, administrative database	774,808 hospital admissions	—	2005–2014	AMI, HF, AF
Hossain, et al,[28] 2022	US	RA, self-reported	2327	—	1999–2018	Self-reported CVD (HF, coronary heart disease, AMI, angina, stroke)
Alsing, et al,[29] 2022	Norway	RA, clinic-based cohort	1821	—	1972–2017	Ischaemic heart disease, AMI

Abbreviations: AF, atrial fibrillation; HF, heart failure; PAD, peripheral artery disease.

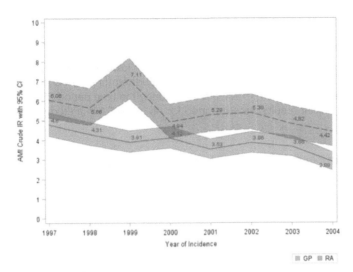

Fig. 2. Crude 10-year risk of AMI according to year of incidence (1997–2004) in RA and general population cohorts. (*From* Yazdani K, Xie H, Avina-Zubieta JA, Zheng Y, Abrahamowicz M, Lacaille D. Has the excess risk of acute myocardial infarction in rheumatoid arthritis relative to the general population declined? A population study of trends over time. Semin Arthritis Rheum. 2021 Apr;51(2):442–449.)

risk in the population was performed.[31] In a study of hospital admissions during the years 2004 to 2014, the total number of admissions for AMI varied over the years, but the number of admissions for AMI with PsA increased.[32] The properties of the database limited more precise analyses.[32]

TRENDS FOR THE PROGNOSIS AFTER ATHEROSCLEROTIC CARDIOVASCULAR EVENTS

As treatment for CV events improves, there has been an obvious decline in case fatality immediately after an event, evident in both sexes and in all race groups.[33,34] The case fatality during the first 28 days after a CV event was almost halved during the period 2000 to 2004 compared with the period 1975 to 1979.[22] The mortality-to-incidence ratio (MIR) can be used to evaluate the burden of disease by presenting mortality after accounting for incidence. In addition, it is a simple and common proxy for the 5-year relative survival of the patients. The overall trend of CVD MIR has continuously decreased, and the 26.8% reduction in mean global MIR imply a noticeable rise of the 5-year survival of CVD patients from 1990 to 2017 (**Fig. 1C**).[4] Furthermore, in Western Europe, the decline in incidence of CV event over three decades was slower than the decline in mortality of CV, again indicating improved treatment over the years.[35]

Evaluating patients ($n = 120$) with RA diagnosis in the 1980s, 1990s, or 2000s, the mortality after a CV event (follow-up median 3.3 years) was similar among patients with RA compared with the general population for all three cohorts.[25] In contrast, in a large register-based study, the 1-year mortality after a first AMI ($n = 245,377$) was analyzed.[36] A steady decrease was observed in the non-RA population during the years of 1998 to 2013, but not among patients with RA ($n = 4268$).[36] In-depth analyses suggested that this mainly was due to a negative trend regarding comorbidity (hypertension, atrial fibrillation, and HF) among RA patients, and RA was only independently associated with 1-year mortality after AMI in the youngest age group (≤62 years).[36]

Inpatient mortality after AMI in PsA was similar or lower than the inpatient mortality overall in a database of hospital admissions.[32] Furthermore, no trend in the inpatient mortality after admissions for AMI with PsA during the time period 2004 to 2014 was observed.[32] Similar results were reported for AMI with RA in a study using the same database.[30]

TRENDS IN RISK FACTORS FOR CARDIOVASCULAR DISEASE

The decline in CVD mortality can be attributed to more efficient treatment for CV events, but also better preventive strategies with treatment of CVD risk factors such as hypertension and hyperlipidemia.[22] The trend after 8-year follow-up concerning risk factors for CVD, for example, smoking, blood pressure, and blood lipids were evaluated in 259,753 patients showing improvement of these factors although only a smaller number of the patients researched adequate blood pressure.[37] Several population-based studies have described a decrease in blood pressure in high-income countries during the last decades.[38] Hence, the risk profile has changed in some countries, whereas metabolic risk factors, like obesity, are more common now compared with some decades ago.[39] Obviously, the prevalence of diabetes is increasing, being a more severe risk factor for CVD.[40] Physical activity, on the other hand, decreases the risk for CVD. However, studying physical activity in the population is complex.[41] Some attempts have still shown no or a slight increase in physical activity in the general population over recent years.[42,43] That is, today, the high burden of CVD can mostly be attributed to metabolic-related factors such as diabetes, obesity, lack of physical activity, hypertension, unhealthy diet, and excessive alcohol consumption.[4,44,45] Smoking, a strong risk factor for CVD has, however, decreased in high-income countries over the last years.[46] In low-income countries, the trend is the opposite, adding also air pollution as a significant risk factor.[46,47] Despite the overall decline in the past two decades, the adult smoking rate in the United States is still substantially higher than the national objective of Healthy People 2030 (i.e. 14.2% vs. 6.1%).[48] Suboptimal intake of fruits, vegetables, and nuts and increased intake of salt, meat, sweetened beverages, and trans-fat consumption are notably and an increasing risk factor, especially in high-income countries, making the United Nations General Assembly declaring years 2016 to 2025 as the Decade of Action on Nutrition.[15,46]

Although convincing evidence that the trend for CVD risk factors like diabetes, overweight, hypertension, and hyperlipidemia is changing in the general population, there is a lack of corresponding trend analyses of these CVD risk factors in patients with inflammatory arthritis.[49] Analyses of contextual factors, that is, socioeconomic vulnerability, depression, or anxiety identified in the general population have not been longitudinally analyzed in patients with inflammatory arthritides.[50]

In the general population, the risk for CVD declined substantially within the first 5 years after smoking cessation.[51] In a recent study including 3311 RA patients, from a number of different countries, former and never smokers had significantly lower CV event rates than current smokers.[52] Further, disease activity and the lipid profiles improved after smoking cessation. There are ongoing studies evaluating smoking cessation in patients with RA, although no results have yet been published.[53,54]

As in the general population, age increases the risk of CVD in patients with seropositive RA.[55] In an inception cohort of patients with RA followed until development of

CVD, the number of CV events exceeded what was expected, based on Framingham risk score calculation. The gap between observed and predicted CV events widened with increasing age in seropositive RA but not in seronegative.[55] A higher prevalence than expected in older patients was also noted in data from NHANES, where the absolute risk of CVD increased with age, even though the relative risks were higher in younger age groups.[28] In another study, the incidence rate increased sharply with age, although the age-specific incidence was not higher in older age groups due to a relative increase among controls.[56] Accelerated aging has been shown in RA patients with telomere deficiency and DNA instability resulting in an aging immune system.[57] In the population, telomere shortening has also been shown to precede the development of CVD.[58]

Increased risk for IHD was already detected within 1 to 4 years following RA diagnosis with similar risks after 5 to 12 years since diagnosis.[56] Other studies have reported similar findings.[24,59] Furthermore, prospective data from an early RA inception cohort (n = 855), where CVD was evaluated, did not show any differences between the groups after stratification for more or less than 10 years of disease duration.[60] However, in a cross-sectional study on patients with established RA, patients with CVD had significantly longer disease duration, yielding HR 1.57 (95% CI 1.09, 2.30) for longer duration at enrollment versus shorter.[61]

TRENDS IN ARRHYTHMIA, VALVULAR HEART DISEASE, HEART FAILURE, AND VENOUS THROMBOEMBOLISM

In the United States, a decline in incidence of atrial fibrillation, most evident in women has been reported.[62] Globally, the mortality associated with atrial fibrillation has increased 2-fold in women and 1.9-fold in men.[63] Still, recent data from a multicenter study in the United States suggest no change in the incidence rate but more frequent diagnostics of the atrial fibrillation.[64] Over the years, there has been a significant increase in pacemaker implantation as well as cardiac valve surgery due to technical and surgical progress.[65–69]

In patients with spondarthritis, and in patients with PsA with axial disease, conduction abnormalities and aortic insufficiency are suggested to be related to the rheumatic disease per se and possibly influenced by the disease activity of the rheumatic disease,[70,71] with a possible association of the conduction disorders to human leukocyte antigen B27 (HLAB27).[72] Studies on time trends of the prevalence of conduction disorders are sparse. An analysis of time trends on the risks of valvular heart disease and pacemaker placement in patients with AS greater than 65 years of age (n = 42,327) showed an increased incidence of aortic valve procedures over time in both patients with AS and controls, with resulting similar relative risks (ORs) over the time period 1999 to 2003, 2004 to 2008, and 2009 to 2013.[73] The incidence of pacemaker insertions in patients with AS, on the other hand, described a slightly decreasing trend with a corresponding slight reduction of the relative risk in AS in more recent years.[73] A trend toward an increasing prevalence of atrial fibrillation diagnoses in hospital admissions with concomitant RA diagnosis has been shown.[30]

Trends of HF are intricate to analyze; most data are on hospitalizations for HF with a decline during the last 20 to 30 years.[74,75] Data on development of HF are scarce; however, the improved diagnostics and treatment of HF over calendar years could contribute to the decrease in hospitalizations.[76]

An increased risk of HF has been reported in RA.[24,77,78] In a population-based inception cohort of RA patients, the risk of HF was particularly increased in seropositive patients and in this subgroup doubled compared with non-RA cases.[77] The cumulative incidence of HF increased more in RA patients and was independent of IHD.[77] A study comparing patients with both RA and HF ($n = 212$) with HF patients without RA observed a higher risk of hospitalization among patients with RA.[79] The risk of hospitalization among patients with HF declined after 2005, both in patients with RA and non-RA patients, and after 2010, the difference between the patient groups was decreasing. The risk of hospitalization associated with RA in the study was mainly due to non-CV diagnoses.[79] In a large cohort with patients with incident RA 1995 to 2016 ($n = 51,859$), the risk of HF was approximately 50% higher in patients with RA compared with the general population.[24] Similar excess risks of HF associated with RA was observed in patient diagnosed 1995 to 2000 (HR 1.61 [95% CI 1.49, 1.74]) as in RA patients diagnosed in the period 2001 to 2016 (HR 1.45 [95% CI 1.371.54]).[24] Corresponding analyses of trends in HF in patients with PsA or spondarthritis are currently lacking.

There is an increase in the global incidence of venous thromboembolic disease (VTE) which is especially pronounced in the elderly. The rates of hospitalization and mortality in VTE have changed dramatically after the introduction of warfarin and later of direct oral anticoagulants.[80] In Europe, there is a clear trend toward a decline in incidence as well as mortality in VTE during at least the last 20 years, most obvious for pulmonary embolism.[81,82]

A slight increase in the incidence of pulmonary embolism has been shown in patients with RA diagnosed in more recent years; however, the incidence of VTE was the same in patients diagnosed 1980-94 and 1995-2007.[83] Moreover, in one study, a decline in HR for VTE as well as pulmonary embolism was seen with disease duration in RA, with the highest risk of thrombotic disease the first year after diagnosis.[84] Data on secular time trends for incidence of VTE in the other inflammatory arthritides are lacking.

DISCUSSION

Despite the decreasing CV mortality worldwide, the aging and growth of the world's population have led to a rise of the absolute numbers of CVD-related deaths, a trend also obvious for the incidence of CV events following atherosclerotic disease. Consistently, among patients with RA, the absolute risk of death from CVD and risk of CV events have declined over time, and the excess mortality due to CVD in RA seem unchanged or attenuated over time in most populations. Regarding CV events, most studies from recent years still report an over-risk associated with RA. Results on time trends for risks of CVD deaths or incidence of CVD in other inflammatory arthritides are limited but indicate increased mortality also in recent years.

The decline in CV mortality in the population has been explained equally by improved control of risk factors and a wide range of advances from knowledge regarding preventive measures to pharmacological or technical inventions.[85] As the CV mortality associated with RA seem to decrease in parity with the CV mortality in the population, patients with RA are likely to have benefited from these advances to a similar extent or even more compared with the general population.

Life style factors might influence the development of inflammatory joint diseases as well as CVD.[86] Even so, the risk factors that are shared between RA and CVD seemingly do not increase the background risk for CVD significantly before RA onset, but do have an impact on the risk during the course of the RA disease.[87,88] Furthermore, the chronic systemic inflammation in inflammatory arthritides might contribute to the risk of CVD. Modern rheumatology with treat-to-target approaches and control of inflammation would minimize this contribution, but periods of inflammatory activity with the use of drugs with potential CV risks (ie, COX-inhibitors and glucocorticoids) and physical inactivity can be difficult to avoid before diagnosis and effective therapy and add to the CV risk even when optimal care is given. These, maybe inevitable, factors may partly explain the remaining gap of CV morbidity observed in several recent studies. Furthermore, disease duration was not associated with CV risk in RA, at least not during the first 10 or so years, indicating the influence of processes or alterations early and continuously during the disease course. Furthermore, for chronic diseases, generally a longer follow-up than 5 or 10 years would be preferable.[89]

Although smoking has become less common in the western world and primary prevention regarding blood pressure and blood lipids have been successful, a CVD risk factor profile with metabolic alterations, such as obesity and diabetes, is becoming more frequent in the general population. This change might contribute to the deceleration or inversion of the decreasing curve of CV mortality over time that has been observed in some populations.[85] It cannot be excluded that variability in the background mortality, such as an increase or slower decrease, could change the relative risk estimations for RA.

As acute treatment for CV event has improved, there has been a decline in case fatality immediately after an event; a trend also observed in patients with inflammatory arthritis. Comorbidity, cardiac or other, is likely to be more prevalent in RA, thus adjusting or matching for such factors might reduce the apparent impact of the inflammatory arthritic disease.[36,90] As no apparent differences in the prognosis after CV events between patients with RA and population referents is observed, it is likely that also patients with RA get the chance to benefit from the medical advances in recent years.

There is clearly a need for more data regarding CV morbidity and mortality in PsA, AS, and other spondarthritides. With a number of new treatment options, not only in RA but also specific drugs for PsA or AS, observational studies are needed to catch signals on how these might influence the CV risks. The recent studies on RA emphasize the importance of comparisons with general population, as the background risk needs to be acknowledged. Furthermore, observational studies should comprise a large number of individuals with a sufficient time of follow-up. There is also a need for more data on CVD risk factors and their interaction with rheumatic diseases as well as continuous research to identify specific disease related risk factors.

Studies of CV risks among patients with chronic diseases are affected by several time scales; the disease duration, the patients' own aging, and passing calendar time with progressive knowledge and technical advances in the society, but also potentially unfavorable changes in living conditions and habits. We have tried to give an overview of the present knowledge regarding these time scales for patients with inflammatory arthritis. Disease duration seem to be of minor importance, at least during the first decade of the disease course and in view of the effects of aging, which in turn may be even greater in inflammatory arthritis than in the population in general. It is tempting to speculate that the excess risk of CVD closely related to inflammation, such as atherosclerotic or thromboembolic disease, might be decreasing in patients with inflammatory arthritis. Most studies include patients with RA, no trends for spondarthritides could be reviewed, and data on trends for CV risk factors among patients with inflammatory arthritis are lacking. In short, we can summarize that more knowledge on optimal care is required to normalize the CVD risk for our patients in the future.

CLINICS CARE POINTS

- Time trends indicate that primary CVD prevention is at least as effective in patients with arthritis as in the general population.

- Ageing increase the absolute risk of most CVD and with a high absolute risk, also a limited increase in the relative risk due to arthritis requires clinical awareness.
- In recent years metabolic disorders such as obesity and diabetes have become common CVD risk factors in the general population, risk factors that may need specific considerations in patients with rheumatic disease.

FUNDING

This authors have financial support provided by Swedish Research Council ; King Gustaf V's 80-Year Fund; the Swedish Rheumatism Association; Knut and Alice Wallenberg association as well as through the regional agreement between Umeå University and Västerbotten County Council (ALF).

DISCLOSURE

The authors have nothing to disclose.

REFERENCES

1. Townsend N, Wilson L, Bhatnagar P, et al. Cardiovascular disease in Europe: epidemiological update 2016. Eur Heart J 2016;37(42):3232–45.
2. Roth GA, Huffman MD, Moran AE, et al. Global and regional patterns in cardiovascular mortality from 1990 to 2013. Circulation 2015;132(17):1667–78.
3. Morovatdar N, Avan A, Azarpazhooh MR, et al. Secular trends of ischaemic heart disease, stroke, and dementia in high-income countries from 1990 to 2017: the Global Burden of Disease Study 2017. Neurol Sci 2021. https://doi.org/10.1007/s10072-021-05259-2.
4. Amini M, Zayeri F, Salehi M. Trend analysis of cardiovascular disease mortality, incidence, and mortality-to-incidence ratio: results from global burden of disease study 2017. BMC Public Health 2021;21(1):401.
5. Lacaille D, Avina-Zubieta JA, Sayre EC, et al. Improvement in 5-year mortality in incident rheumatoid arthritis compared with the general population-closing the mortality gap. Ann Rheum Dis 2016. https://doi.org/10.1136/annrheumdis-2016-209562.
6. van den Hoek J, Boshuizen HC, Roorda LD, et al. Mortality in patients with rheumatoid arthritis: a 15-year prospective cohort study. Rheumatol Int 2017;37(4):487–93.
7. Zhang Y, Lu N, Peloquin C, et al. Improved survival in rheumatoid arthritis: a general population-based cohort study. Ann Rheum Dis 2017;76(2):408–13.
8. Abhishek A, Nakafero G, Kuo C-F, et al. Rheumatoid arthritis and excess mortality: down but not out. A primary care cohort study using data from Clinical Practice Research Datalink. Rheumatology (Oxford, England) 2018;57(6):977–81.
9. Provan SA, Lillegraven S, Sexton J, et al. Trends in all-cause and cardiovascular mortality in patients with incident rheumatoid arthritis: a 20-year follow-up matched case-cohort study. Rheumatology (Oxford, England) 2020;59(3):505–12.
10. Lee YK, Ahn GY, Lee J, et al. Excess mortality persists in patients with rheumatoid arthritis. Int J Rheum Dis 2021;24(3):364–72.
11. Humphreys JH, Warner A, Chipping J, et al. Mortality trends in patients with early rheumatoid arthritis over 20 years: results from the Norfolk Arthritis Register. Arthritis Care Res 2014;66(9):1296–301.

12. Jean S, Hudson M, Gamache P, et al. Temporal trends in prevalence, incidence, and mortality for rheumatoid arthritis in Quebec, Canada: a population-based study. Clin Rheumatol 2017;36(12):2667–71.

13. Holmqvist M, Ljung L, Askling J. Mortality following new-onset Rheumatoid Arthritis: has modern Rheumatology had an impact? Ann Rheum Dis 2017. https://doi.org/10.1136/annrheumdis-2017-212131.

14. Gwinnutt JM, Symmons DPM, MacGregor AJ, et al. Have the 10-year outcomes of patients with early inflammatory arthritis improved in the new millennium compared with the decade before? Results from the Norfolk Arthritis Register. Ann Rheum Dis 2018;77(6):848–54.

15. Meune C, Touze E, Trinquart L, et al. Trends in cardiovascular mortality in patients with rheumatoid arthritis over 50 years: a systematic review and meta-analysis of cohort studies. Rheumatology (Oxford, England) 2009;48(10):1309–13.

16. Gonzalez A, Icen M, Kremers HM, et al. Mortality trends in rheumatoid arthritis: the role of rheumatoid factor. J Rheumatol 2008;35(6):1009–14.

17. Bergstrom U, Jacobsson LT, Turesson C. Cardiovascular morbidity and mortality remain similar in two cohorts of patients with long-standing rheumatoid arthritis seen in 1978 and 1995 in Malmo, Sweden. Rheumatology (Oxford, England) 2009;48(12):1600–5.

18. Krishnan E, Lingala VB, Singh G. Declines in mortality from acute myocardial infarction in successive incidence and birth cohorts of patients with rheumatoid arthritis. Circulation 2004;110(13):1774–9.

19. Myasoedova E, Gabriel SE, Matteson EL, et al. Decreased Cardiovascular Mortality in Patients with Incident Rheumatoid Arthritis (RA) in Recent Years: Dawn of a New Era in Cardiovascular Disease in RA? J Rheumatol 2017. https://doi.org/10.3899/jrheum.161154.

20. Kerola AM, Kazemi A, Rollefstad S, et al. All-cause and cause-specific mortality in rheumatoid arthritis, psoriatic arthritis and axial spondyloarthritis: a nationwide registry study. Rheumatology (Oxford, England) 2022. https://doi.org/10.1093/rheumatology/keac210.

21. Chaudhary H, Bohra N, Syed K, et al. All-Cause and Cause-Specific Mortality in Psoriatic Arthritis and Ankylosing Spondylitis: A Systematic Review and Meta-Analysis. Arthritis Care Res 2021. https://doi.org/10.1002/acr.24820.

22. Wilhelmsen L, Welin L, Svärdsudd K, et al. Secular changes in cardiovascular risk factors and attack rate of myocardial infarction among men aged 50 in Gothenburg, Sweden. Accurate prediction using risk models. J Intern Med 2008;263(6):636–43.

23. Holmqvist M, Ljung L, Askling J. Acute coronary syndrome in new-onset rheumatoid arthritis: a population-based nationwide cohort study of time trends in risks and excess risks. Ann Rheum Dis 2017;76(10):1642–7.

24. Logstrup BB, Ellingsen T, Pedersen AB, et al. Development of heart failure in patients with rheumatoid arthritis: A Danish population-based study. Eur J Clin Invest 2018;48(5):e12915.

25. Myasoedova E, Davis JM 3rd, Roger VL, et al. Improved incidence of cardiovascular disease in patients with incident rheumatoid arthritis in the 2000s: a population-based cohort study. J Rheumatol 2021. https://doi.org/10.3899/jrheum.200842.

26. Yazdani K, Xie H, Avina-Zubieta JA, et al. Has the excess risk of acute myocardial infarction in rheumatoid arthritis relative to the general population declined? A population study of trends over time. Semin Arthritis Rheum 2021;51(2):442–9.

27. Yazdani K, Xie H, Avina-Zubieta JA, et al. Ten-year risk of cerebrovascular accidents in incident rheumatoid arthritis: a population-based study of trends over time. Rheumatology 2021;60(5):2267–76.
28. Hossain MB, Kopec JA, Atiquzzaman M, et al. The association between rheumatoid arthritis and cardiovascular disease among adults in the United States during 1999-2018, and age-related effect modification in relative and absolute scales. Ann Epidemiol 2022;71:23–30.
29. Alsing CL, Nystad TW, Igland J, et al. Trends in the occurrence of ischaemic heart disease over time in rheumatoid arthritis: 1821 patients from 1972 to 2017. Scand J Rheumatol 2022;1–10. https://doi.org/10.1080/03009742.2022.2040116.
30. Bandyopadhyay D, Banerjee U, Hajra A, et al. Trends of cardiac complications in patients with rheumatoid arthritis: analysis of the united states national inpatient sample; 2005-2014. Curr Probl Cardiol 2021;46(3):100455.
31. Eder L, Wu Y, Chandran V, et al. Incidence and predictors for cardiovascular events in patients with psoriatic arthritis. Ann Rheum Dis 2016;75(9):1680–6.
32. Jatwani S, Jatwani K, Tiwari P, et al. Trends in hospitalisations and inpatient mortality from acute myocardial infarction among patients with psoriatic arthritis: an analysis of nationwide inpatient sample 2004-2014. Clin Exp Rheumatol 2021;39(4):790–4.
33. Ergin A, Muntner P, Sherwin R, et al. Secular trends in cardiovascular disease mortality, incidence, and case fatality rates in adults in the United States. Am J Med 2004;117(4):219–27.
34. Vázquez-Troche JA, García-Fernández V, Hernández-Vásquez A, et al. Trends in mortality from ischemic heart disease in peru, 2005 to 2017. Int J Environ Res Public Health 2022;19(12). https://doi.org/10.3390/ijerph19127047.
35. Vancheri F, Tate AR, Henein M, et al. Time trends in ischaemic heart disease incidence and mortality over three decades (1990-2019) in 20 Western European countries: systematic analysis of the Global Burden of Disease Study 2019. Eur J Prev Cardiol 2022;29(2):396–403.
36. Skielta M, Söderström L, Rantapää-Dahlqvist S, et al. Trends in mortality, comorbidity and treatment after acute myocardial infarction in patients with rheumatoid arthritis 1998-2013. Eur Heart J Acute Cardiovasc Care 2020;9(8):931–8.
37. Bager JE, Mourtzinis G, Andersson T, et al. Trends in blood pressure, blood lipids, and smoking from 259 753 patients with hypertension in a Swedish primary care register: results from QregPV. Eur J Prev Cardiol 2021. https://doi.org/10.1093/eurjpc/zwab087.
38. Eliasson M, Eriksson M, Lundqvist R, et al. Comparison of trends in cardiovascular risk factors between two regions with and without a community and primary care prevention programme. Eur J Prev Cardiol 2018;25(16):1765–72.
39. Dai H, Much AA, Maor E, et al. Global, regional, and national burden of ischemic heart disease and its attributable risk factors, 1990-2017: results from the global Burden of Disease Study 2017. Eur Heart J Qual Care Clin Outcomes 2020. https://doi.org/10.1093/ehjqcco/qcaa076.
40. Fox CS. Cardiovascular disease risk factors, type 2 diabetes mellitus, and the Framingham Heart Study. Trends Cardiovasc Med 2010;20(3):90–5.
41. Ramírez Varela A, Cruz GIN, Hallal P, et al. Global, regional, and national trends and patterns in physical activity research since 1950: a systematic review. Int J Behav Nutr Phys Activity 2021;18(1):5.
42. Chau J, Chey T, Burks-Young S, et al. Trends in prevalence of leisure time physical activity and inactivity: results from Australian National Health Surveys 1989 to 2011. Aust N Z J Public Health 2017;41(6):617–24.

43. Sperlich S, Beller J, Epping J, et al. Trends in self-rated health among the elderly population in Germany from 1995 to 2015 - the influence of temporal change in leisure time physical activity. BMC Public Health 2020;20(1):113.

44. O'Hearn M, Lauren BN, Wong JB, et al. Trends and disparities in cardiometabolic health among U.S. adults, 1999-2018. J Am Coll Cardiol 2022;80(2):138–51.

45. Zhu Z, Bundy JD, Mills KT, et al. Secular trends in cardiovascular health in US adults (from NHANES 2007 to 2018). Am J Cardiol 2021;159:121–8.

46. Jagannathan R, Patel SA, Ali MK, et al. Global updates on cardiovascular disease mortality trends and attribution of traditional risk factors. Curr Diab Rep 2019; 19(7):44.

47. Wang T, Ma Y, Li R, et al. Trends of ischemic heart disease mortality attributable to household air pollution during 1990-2019 in China and India: an age-period-cohort analysis. Environ Sci Pollut Res Int 2022. https://doi.org/10.1007/s11356-022-21770-1.

48. ODPHP. Healthy People 2030. https://health.gov/healthypeople/objectives-and-data/browse-objectives/tobacco-use/reduce-current-cigarette-smoking-adults-tu-02. Accessed 31 August 2022.

49. Semb AG, Rollefstad S, Ikdahl E, et al. Diabetes mellitus and cardiovascular risk management in patients with rheumatoid arthritis: an international audit. RMD Open 2021;7(2). https://doi.org/10.1136/rmdopen-2021-001724.

50. Roest AM, Martens EJ, de Jonge P, et al. Anxiety and risk of incident coronary heart disease: a meta-analysis. J Am Coll Cardiol 2010;56(1):38–46.

51. Duncan MS, Freiberg MS, Greevy RA Jr, et al. Association of smoking cessation with subsequent risk of cardiovascular disease. JAMA 2019;322(7):642–50.

52. Roelsgaard IK, Ikdahl E, Rollefstad S, et al. Smoking cessation is associated with lower disease activity and predicts cardiovascular risk reduction in rheumatoid arthritis patients. Rheumatology (Oxford, England) 2020;59(8):1997–2004.

53. Aimer P, Treharne GJ, Stebbings S, et al. Efficacy of a rheumatoid arthritis-specific smoking cessation program: a randomized controlled pilot trial. Arthritis Care Res 2017;69(1):28–37.

54. Roelsgaard IK, Thomsen T, Østergaard M, et al. The effect of an intensive smoking cessation intervention on disease activity in patients with rheumatoid arthritis: study protocol for a randomised controlled trial. Trials 2017;18(1):570.

55. Crowson CS, Therneau TM, Davis JM 3rd, et al. Brief report: accelerated aging influences cardiovascular disease risk in rheumatoid arthritis. Arthritis Rheum 2013;65(10):2562–6.

56. Holmqvist ME, Wedrén S, Jacobsson LT, et al. Rapid increase in myocardial infarction risk following diagnosis of rheumatoid arthritis amongst patients diagnosed between 1995 and 2006. J Intern Med 2010;268(6):578–85.

57. Weyand CM, Fujii H, Shao L, et al. Rejuvenating the immune system in rheumatoid arthritis. Nat Rev Rheumatol 2009;5(10):583–8.

58. Samani NJ, van der Harst P. Biological ageing and cardiovascular disease. Heart (British Cardiac Society) 2008;94(5):537–9.

59. Baviera M, Cioffi G, Colacioppo P, et al. Temporal trends from 2005 to 2018 in deaths and cardiovascular events in subjects with newly diagnosed rheumatoid arthritis. Intern Emerg Med 2021. https://doi.org/10.1007/s11739-020-02581-z.

60. Arts EE, Fransen J, den Broeder AA, et al. The effect of disease duration and disease activity on the risk of cardiovascular disease in rheumatoid arthritis patients. Ann Rheum Dis 2015;74(6):998–1003.

61. Masuda H, Miyazaki T, Shimada K, et al. Disease duration and severity impacts on long-term cardiovascular events in Japanese patients with rheumatoid arthritis. J Cardiol 2014;64(5):366–70.

62. DeLago AJ, Essa M, Ghajar A, et al. Incidence and Mortality trends of atrial fibrillation/atrial flutter in the united states 1990 to 2017. Am J Cardiol 2021;148:78–83.

63. Chugh SS, Havmoeller R, Narayanan K, et al. Worldwide epidemiology of atrial fibrillation: a Global Burden of Disease 2010 Study. Circulation 2014;129(8):837–47.

64. Ghelani KP, Chen LY, Norby FL, et al. Thirty-year trends in the incidence of atrial fibrillation: the ARIC study. J Am Heart Assoc 2022;11(8):e023583.

65. Jiménez-García R, Perez-Farinos N, Miguel-Díez J, et al. National trends in utilization and in-hospital outcomes of surgical aortic valve replacements in spain, 2001-2015. Braz J Cardiovasc Surg 2020;35(1):65–74.

66. Paparella D, Fattouch K, Moscarelli M, et al. Current trends in mitral valve surgery: a multicenter national comparison between full-sternotomy and minimally-invasive approach. Int J Cardiol 2020;306:147–51.

67. Alkhouli M, Alqahtani F, Ziada KM, et al. Contemporary trends in the management of aortic stenosis in the USA. Eur Heart J 2020;41(8):921–8.

68. Kim K, Kim DY, Seo J, et al. Temporal trends in diagnosis, treatments, and outcomes in patients with bicuspid aortic valve. Front Cardiovasc Med 2021;8:766430.

69. Mauri V, Abdel-Wahab M, Bleiziffer S, et al. Temporal trends of TAVI treatment characteristics in high volume centers in Germany 2013-2020. Clin Res Cardiol 2021. https://doi.org/10.1007/s00392-021-01963-3.

70. Nurmohamed MT, van der Horst-Bruinsma I, Maksymowych WP. Cardiovascular and cerebrovascular diseases in ankylosing spondylitis: current insights. Curr Rheumatol Rep 2012;14(5):415–21.

71. Chiu HY, Chang WL, Huang WF, et al. Increased risk of arrhythmia in patients with psoriatic disease: A nationwide population-based matched cohort study. J Am Acad Dermatol 2015;73(3):429–38.

72. Bergfeldt L. HLA-B27-associated cardiac disease. Ann Intern Med 1997;127(8 Pt 1):621–9.

73. Ward MM. Lifetime risks of valvular heart disease and pacemaker use in patients with ankylosing spondylitis. J Am Heart Assoc 2018;7(20):e010016.

74. Schmidt M, Ulrichsen SP, Pedersen L, et al. Thirty-year trends in heart failure hospitalization and mortality rates and the prognostic impact of co-morbidity: a Danish nationwide cohort study. Eur J Heart Fail 2016;18(5):490–9.

75. Sulo G, Igland J, Øverland S, et al. Heart failure in Norway, 2000-2014: analysing incident, total and readmission rates using data from the Cardiovascular Disease in Norway (CVDNOR) Project. Eur J Heart Fail 2020;22(2):241–8.

76. Vinter N, Jensen M, Skjøth F, et al. Twenty-year time trends in use of evidence-based heart failure drug therapy in Denmark. Basic Clin Pharmacol Toxicol 2020;127(1):30–8.

77. Nicola PJ, Maradit-Kremers H, Roger VL, et al. The risk of congestive heart failure in rheumatoid arthritis: a population-based study over 46 years. Arthritis Rheum 2005;52(2):412–20.

78. Mantel Ä, Holmqvist M, Andersson DC, et al. Association between rheumatoid arthritis and risk of ischemic and nonischemic heart failure. J Am Coll Cardiol 2017;69(10):1275–85.

79. Myasoedova E, Davis JM 3rd, Matteson EL, et al. Increased hospitalization rates following heart failure diagnosis in rheumatoid arthritis as compared to the general population. Semin Arthritis Rheum 2020;50(1):25–9.

80. Merli GJ, Hollander JE, Lefebvre P, et al. Rates of hospitalization among patients with deep vein thrombosis before and after the introduction of rivaroxaban. Hosp Pract (1995) 2015;43(2):85–93.

81. Barco S, Mahmoudpour SH, Valerio L, et al. Trends in mortality related to pulmonary embolism in the European Region, 2000-15: analysis of vital registration data from the WHO Mortality Database. Lancet Respir Med 2020;8(3):277–87.

82. Valerio L, Fedeli U, Schievano E, et al. Decline in overall pulmonary embolism-related mortality and increasing prevalence of cancer-associated events in the Veneto region (Italy), 2008-2019. Thromb Haemost 2021. https://doi.org/10.1055/a-1548-4948.

83. Bacani AK, Gabriel SE, Crowson CS, et al. Noncardiac vascular disease in rheumatoid arthritis: increase in venous thromboembolic events? Arthritis Rheum 2012;64(1):53–61.

84. Li L, Lu N, Avina-Galindo AM, et al. The risk and trend of pulmonary embolism and deep vein thrombosis in rheumatoid arthritis: a general population-based study. Rheumatology (Oxford, England) 2021;60(1):188–95.

85. Mensah GA, Wei GS, Sorlie PD, et al. Decline in cardiovascular mortality: possible causes and implications. Circ Res 2017;120(2):366–80.

86. Kokkonen H, Stenlund H, Rantapaa-Dahlqvist S. Cardiovascular risk factors predate the onset of symptoms of rheumatoid arthritis: a nested case-control study. Arthritis Res Ther 2017;19(1):148.

87. Holmqvist ME, Wedren S, Jacobsson LT, et al. No increased occurrence of ischemic heart disease prior to the onset of rheumatoid arthritis: results from two Swedish population-based rheumatoid arthritis cohorts. Arthritis Rheum 2009;60(10):2861–9.

88. Innala L, Möller B, Ljung L, et al. Cardiovascular events in early RA are a result of inflammatory burden and traditional risk factors: a five year prospective study. Arthritis Res Ther 2011;13(4):R131.

89. Radovits BJ, Fransen J, Al Shamma S, et al. Excess mortality emerges after 10 years in an inception cohort of early rheumatoid arthritis. Arthritis Care Res 2010;62(3):362–70.

90. Mantel A, Holmqvist M, Jernberg T, et al. Rheumatoid arthritis is associated with a more severe presentation of acute coronary syndrome and worse short-term outcome. Eur Heart J 2015;36(48):3413–22.

Atherosclerotic Cardiovascular Risk Stratification in the Rheumatic Diseases:
An Integrative, Multiparametric Approach

Durga Prasanna Misra, DM, MRCP(UK), FRCP(Edin)[a],
Ellen M. Hauge, MD, PhD[b], Cynthia S. Crowson, PhD[c],
George D. Kitas, MD, PhD[d], Sarah R. Ormseth[e],
George A. Karpouzas, MD[e],*

KEYWORDS

- Cardiovascular risk factors • Cardiovascular risk score • Rheumatoid arthritis
- Systemic lupus erythematosus • Ankylosing spondylitis • Psoriatic arthritis

KEY POINTS

- Cardiovascular disease (CVD) risk is increased in most inflammatory rheumatic diseases (IRDs).
- Genetic, traditional, and disease-related risk factors drive increased CVD risk in IRDs.
- Efforts to develop a CVD risk score specific for IRDs are still underway.
- Imaging modalities including carotid ultrasound, cardiac computed tomography (CT), and PET-CT help characterize presence, burden, and composition of subclinical atherosclerotic plaque. However, concrete guidance regarding their optimal use and implementation in IRDs is still lacking.
- Traditional as well as disease-related biomarkers reflect CVD risk burden in IRDs.

[a] Department of Clinical Immunology and Rheumatology, Sanjay Gandhi Postgraduate Institute of Medical Sciences (SGPGIMS), Rae Bareli Road, Lucknow 226014, India; [b] Division of Rheumatology, Aarhus University Hospital, Palle Juul-Jensens Boulevard 99 DK-8200, Aarhus, Denmark; [c] Department of Quantitative Health Sciences and Division of Rheumatology, Mayo Clinic, 200 first St SW, Rochester, MN 55905, USA; [d] Dudley Group NHS Foundation Trust, United Kingdom; [e] The Lundquist Institute and Harbor-UCLA Medical Center, 1124 West Carson Street, Building E4-R17, Torrance, CA 90502, USA
* Corresponding author.
E-mail address: gkarpouzas@lundquist.org
Twitter: @AKarpouzas (G.A.K.)

Rheum Dis Clin N Am 49 (2023) 19–43
https://doi.org/10.1016/j.rdc.2022.07.004
0889-857X/23/© 2022 Elsevier Inc. All rights reserved.

INTRODUCTION

The rheumatic diseases are chronic systemic inflammatory syndromes affecting multiple tissues and organs. Cardiovascular involvement represents either a main clinical manifestation or an acquired comorbidity over time, linked to cumulative disease-related inflammation and/or its treatments.[1] Cardiovascular comorbidities are common, clinically and mechanistically diverse and have the greatest impact on mortality.[1,2] Yet, atherosclerosis is a shared feature and the main predictor of ischemic cardiovascular risk.[3] Therefore, accurate assessment of atherosclerotic cardiovascular disease (ASCVD) risk is instrumental to identify patients that might benefit from primary prevention strategies.[4] Although prompt detection and effective management of risk factors are pivotal, the mere presence of a rheumatic disease is not sufficient to justify the use of cardioprotective medications.[5]

In this review, the authors appraise the magnitude, secular trends, and rationale of heightened ASCVD risk in patients with rheumatic diseases. The authors discuss current practices and guidelines around risk evaluation, associated challenges, their shortcomings, and the role of imaging of subclinical atherosclerosis; serum biomarkers associated with plaque burden and clinical risk and the role of artificial intelligence (AI) in data synthesis and algorithm crafting to optimize risk prediction. Last, the authors address the exportability and clinical application of these advances in daily practice, enlist unanswered questions, areas of need, and propose a future research agenda.

SIZE OF THE PROBLEM AND SECULAR TRENDS

ASCVD pathogenesis in inflammatory rheumatic diseases (IRDs) is multifactorial, partly resulting from an interaction of chronic inflammation with traditional cardiac risk factors; disease-specific or related parameters, therapies, and metabolic perturbations further contribute to the enhanced risk. The increased risk of cardiovascular events is well recognized in rheumatoid arthritis (RA), systemic lupus erythematosus (SLE, particularly in association with antiphospholipid antibody syndrome) and the spondyloarthropathies (SpA, including psoriatic arthritis [PsA] and ankylosing spondylitis [AS]). Evidence is now accumulating for increased cardiovascular risk in systemic sclerosis (SSc), Sjogren's syndrome (SS), anti-neutrophil cytoplasmic antibody (ANCA)-associated vasculitis (AAV), large vessel vasculitides, gout, and osteoarthritis. Often, younger patients have greater ASCVD risk which is more prominent in the immediate years after disease onset. Although overall ASCVD risk and mortality have been declining worldwide, including in RA, the relative risk in RA compared with healthy controls still remains high. These findings are summarized in **Table 1**.

REASONS FOR DIFFERENTIAL RISK IN THE INFLAMMATORY RHEUMATIC DISEASES

All stages of the atherogenic process are accelerated and amplified in IRDs; this may reflect common genetic links between IRDs and atherosclerosis,[6–10] differential prevalence and contribution of traditional risk factors to cardiovascular risk,[11–18] qualitative and functional differences in lipoproteins in IRDs,[11] greater cumulative inflammation and interactions between inflammation and traditional risk factors on atherosclerotic plaque progression and composition, immune activation, and disease-specific[19–25] or related predictors. Lower body weight predicts greater cardiovascular disease (CVD) risk in RA.[13,14] Body composition changes occurring in RA, including sarcopenia, adipose tissue redistribution, and visceral fat expansion, are not captured by body mass index; instead, they are better reflected by waist circumference or waist-to-

Table 1
Burden of atherosclerotic cardiovascular disease in the inflammatory rheumatic diseases

Disease	Reference	Type of Study	Key Findings
Rheumatoid arthritis	Aviña-Zubieta et al,[74] 2008	SRMA	↑risk of CVD death (pooled SMR 1.50, 95%CI 1.39–1.61) ↑risk of death due to IHD (pooled SMR 1.59, 95%CI 1.46–1.73) ↑risk of death due to CVA (pooled SMR 1.52, 95%CI 1.40–1.67) Similar risk of death for both males and females
	Radovits et al,[75] 2010	Prospective cohort study	SMR for RA 1.40 (95%CI 1.09–1.77) after 20 y of follow-up. Excess mortality risk in RA becomes evident after about 10 y of disease.
	Aviña-Zubieta et al,[2] 2012	SRMA	↑risk of incident MI (pooled RR 1.68[95%CI 1.40–2.03]), stroke (pooled RR 1.41[95%CI 1.14–1.74]) and heart failure (RR 1.87 [95%CI 1.47–2.39]) in RA.
	Restivo et al,[3] 2022	SRMA	↑ risk of symptomatic CVE (pooled RR 1.55 [95%CI 1.18–2.02]) in RA vs controls, higher in >60 y (RR 1.98) vs < 60 y (RR 1.43).
	Nicola et al,[76] 2005	Retrospective cohort study	↑risk of heart failure in RA (HR 1.7 [95%CI 1.3–2.1]).
	Holmqvist et al,[77] 2010	Prospective cohort study	↑ CHD risk in RA becomes evident by the end of the first year after diagnosis.
	Myasoedova et al,[78] 2017	Prospective cohort study	Risk of CVD mortality, particularly CHD mortality, reduced gradually over time in RA diagnosed between 1980–89, 1990–99 and 2000–07.
	Kerola et al,[79] 2015	Retrospective cohort study	↓SMR for RA diagnosed between 2000–2007 (0.57[95%CI 0.52–0.62)
	Holmqvist et al,[19] 2017	Prospective cohort study	↓risk of ACS over time in RA as well as in the general population. HR for ACS remained higher by 19%–41% in RA than in the general population, although for the most recent observation period (2011–2014), was statistically similar in RA vs the general population (HR 1.19 [95%CI 0.85–1.67]). ACS risk was highest in those with active RA or those who were RF positive.

(continued on next page)

Table 1
(continued)

Disease	Reference	Type of Study	Key Findings
Systemic lupus erythematosus	Barbhaiya et al,[80] 2020	Retrospective cohort study	Risk of nonfatal CVD event ↑in SLE vs general population (HR 2.67 [95%CI 2.38–2.99]) and in SLE vs DM (IRR 1.27 [95%CI 1.23–1.30]). Highest risk in SLE was observed in younger patients between 18 and 39 y age (HR 7.79 [95%CI 5.77–10.50])
	Restivo et al,[3] 2022	SRMA	↑ risk of symptomatic CVE (pooled RR 1.98 [95%CI 1.18–3.31]) in SLE vs controls, higher in >46 y (RR 2.21) vs < 46 y (RR 1.89).
	Hermansen et al,[81] 2017	Retrospective cohort study	↑risk of MI (HR 8.5[95%CI 2.2–33] more for females and <55 y) but not for stroke (HR 1.9[95%CI 0.9–4.4)] comparing LN vs SLE without LN (both greater for females and for age <55 y). ↑risk of CVD mortality (HR 4.9 [95%CI 1.8–13.7]) in LN vs SLE without LN (greater for males and for age<55 y)
Psoriatic arthritis	Polachek et al,[82] 2017	SRMA	↑risk of CVE (RR 1.43 [95%CI 1.24–1.66]), MI (RR 1.68 [95%CI 1.31–2.15]), stroke (RR 1.22 [95%CI 1.05–1.41]) and heart failure (RR 1.32 [95%CI 1.11–1.57]) in PsA vs controls.
Ankylosing spondylitis	Mathieu et al,[83] 2019	SRMA	↑risk of MI (RR 1.44[95%CI 1.25–1.67]) and stroke (RR 1.37 [95% CI 1.08–1.73]) in AS vs controls.
Spondyloarthritis	Kim et al,[84] 2019	SRMA	↑risk of MI (RR 1.38[95%CI 1.18–1.61]) and stroke (RR 2.04[95%CI 1.11–3.78), however, no increase in risk of CVD death (RR 1.19 [95%CI 0.96–1.48]) with SpA vs controls.
Systemic sclerosis	Cen et al,[85] 2020	SRMA	↑risk of CVD (HR 2.36 [95%CI 1.97–2.81]), PVD (HR 5.27 [95%CI 4.27–6.51]), MI (HR 2.36 [95%CI 1.71–3.25]) & stroke (HR 1.52 [95%CI 1.18–1.96]) in SSc vs controls
Sjogren's syndrome	Yong et al,[86] 2018	SRMA	↑risk of overall cardiovascular or cerebrovascular disease (OR 1.28 [95%CI 1.11–1.46]) or cardiovascular disease alone (OR 1.30 [95%CI 1.09–1.55) but not for stroke alone (OR 1.31 [95%CI 0.96–1.79]) in SS vs controls.

(continued on next page)

Table 1
(continued)

Disease	Reference	Type of Study	Key Findings
ANCA-associated vasculitis	Houben et al,[87] 2018	SRMA	↑risk of all CVD events (RR 1.65 [95%CI 1.23–2.22]) & individually for IHD (RR 1.60 [95%CI 1.39–1.84]) but not for stroke (RR 1.20 [95%CI 0.98–1.40]) in AAV vs controls.
Giant cell arteritis	de Boysson et al,[88] 2022	Review	GCA ↑risk of cerebrovascular events (RR = 1.40 [95%CI 1.27–1.56]). Population-based studies, however, reported mixed result. GCA developing CVD display salient clinical phenotypes • predominantly male • vertebrobasilar territory involvement in 50%–100% of stroke cases vs 20% in the general population • LMCA involvement in the case of myocardial infarction Both vascular wall inflammation inherent to the disease patho-physiology and greater prevalence of traditional cardiac risk factors ↑CVD risk in GCA
Takayasu arteritis	Kim et al,[89] 2018	SRMA	Pooled prevalence of stroke or TIA 11.7 (9.2–14.1)% and of MI 3.4 (2.1–4.8)% in TAK
Gout	Scheier et al,[90] 2017	SRMA	Risk of incident MI ↑in gout [pooled age- and sex-adjusted RR 1.47 [95%CI 1.24–1.73])
Osteoarthritis	Scheier et al,[90] 2017	SRMA	Risk of incident MI ↑in OA [pooled age- and sex-adjusted RR 1.31 [95%CI 1.01–1.71])

Abbreviations: CI, confidence interval; AAV, ANCA-associated vasculitis; ANCA, anti-neutrophil cytoplasmic antibody; AS, ankylosing spondylitis; CHD, coronary heart disease; CS, acute coronary syndrome; CVA, cerebrovascular accident; CVD, cardiovascular disease; CVE, cardiovascular event; DM, diabetes mellitus; GCA, giant cell arteritis; HR, hazard ratio; IHD, ischemic heart disease; LMCA, left main coronary artery; LN, lupus nephritis; MI, myocardial infarction; OA, osteoarthritis; PsA, psoriatic arthritis; PVD, peripheral vascular disease; RA, rheumatoid arthritis; RR, risk ratio; SLE, systemic lupus erythematosus; SMR, standardized mortality ratio; SpA, spondyloarthritis; SRMA, systematic review and meta-analysis; SS, Sjogren's syndrome; SSc, systemic sclerosis; TIA, transient ischemic attack.

height ratio. Hyperhomocystinemia predisposes toward ASCVD in SLE.[12] Endothelial dysfunction might be driven by type I interferons[11,12] and by formation of neutrophil extracellular traps,[12] shared processes in the pathogenesis of ASCVD and SLE. CD4+CD28null cells are enriched in the rheumatoid synovium as well as in unstable atheromatous plaques.[26] **Fig. 1** summarizes processes involved in ASCVD risk in IRDs. **Box 1** delineates lipid abnormalities associated with CVD risk in RA.

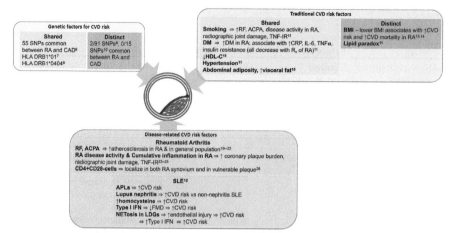

Fig. 1. Traditional, genetic, and disease-related cardiovascular risk factors in inflammatory rheumatic diseases. ACPA, anti-citrullinated peptide antibody; APLs, anti-phospholipid antibodies; BMI, body mass index; CAD, coronary artery disease; CRP, C-reactive protein; CVD, cardiovascular disease; DM, diabetes mellitus; FMD, flow-mediated dilation; HDL-C, high-density lipoprotein cholesterol; IFN, interferon; IL, interleukin; LDG, low-density granulocytes; NET, neutrophil extracellular traps; RA, rheumatoid arthritis; RF, rheumatoid factor; Rx, treatment; SLE, systemic lupus erythematosus; SNP, single nucleotide polymorphism; TNF-IR, inadequate response to TNF inhibitors; TNFα, tumor necrosis factor alpha.

CARDIOVASCULAR RISK CALCULATORS: PITFALLS AND CHALLENGES

Cardiovascular risk calculators used in the general population have demonstrated poor accuracy in patients with IRDs,[27,28] because traditional risk factors alone do not explain the increased CVD risk in those patients[29] and are also known to behave differently in patients with IRDs. Recent guidelines recommend the use of a multiplicative factor of 1.5 (except QRISK2, which includes RA as a risk factor) for all patients

---

Box 1
Lipid profile and cardiovascular disease risk in inflammatory rheumatic diseases

↓cholesterol and ↓LDL-C associate with ↑ myocardial infarction risk.[17]

RA patients with LDL <70 mg/dl display greater coronary atherosclerosis presence, burden, and high-risk plaque characteristics.[18]

Other studies have reported no relation with or increased CVD risk with LDL-C.[11]

Proatherogenic dyslipidemia—combination of low total cholesterol, LDL-C, HDL with high total cholesterol/HDL-C or ApoB/ApoAI ratio—is seen in 55%–65% of patients with RA.[11]

Classic dyslipidemia pattern in SLE—↑ VLDL-C, triglycerides and ↓ HDL—associates with disease activity.[12]

Lower cargo of ApoAI and paroxonase and higher serum alpha amyloid and oxidized fatty acids in the HDL particle attenuate its anti-inflammatory and antioxidant properties and its ability to perform cholesterol efflux from vessel wall macrophages.[11]

Abbreviations: CVD, cardiovascular disease; HDL-C, high-density lipoprotein cholesterol; LDL-C, low-density lipoprotein cholesterol; RA, rheumatoid arthritis; SLE, systemic lupus erythematosus; VLDL-C, very low-density lipoprotein cholesterol.

with RA.[5] However, the taskforce did not find sufficient evidence to recommend the use of a multiplier in other IRDs. Incorporation of measures of inflammation and disease-related factors is likely needed to improve the accuracy of CVD risk prediction. Unfortunately, efforts to develop a risk calculator that accurately predicts CVD in patients with RA have not demonstrated improvement over existing calculators.[30,31] Perhaps ongoing efforts to incorporate new biomarkers, carotid ultrasound, coronary artery calcium (CAC) score, or plaque burden and composition data into CVD risk assessment will demonstrate improved CVD risk prediction,[32–34] but more validation is needed before these approaches can be used clinically.

Imaging for Screening Atherosclerotic Cardiovascular Involvement in Inflammatory Rheumatic Diseases

Three main reasons justify the consideration of atherosclerosis imaging as part of primary prevention in patients with IRDs: (1) higher incidence rate, case fatality, and recurrence of cardiovascular events, (2) frequent atypical presentation, like silent myocardial infarction, or sudden cardiac death, and (3) poor performance and calibration of standard cardiovascular risk calculators in subjects with IRDs.[35]

Presence of Atherosclerosis on Carotid Ultrasound

Despite low agreement on the utility of carotid ultrasound for asymptomatic atherosclerotic plaque presence in RA and no imaging recommendation for other IRDs in EULAR guidelines, carotid ultrasound findings may reclassify RA patients into more appropriate risk groups.[35] Carotid plaques are more common, progress rapidly, and predict acute coronary syndromes in RA.[35,36] Carotid intima-media thickness (CIMT) has been extensively studied in general population cohorts and reported to be greater in both RA and PsA compared with controls.[35] However, CIMT may reflect either atherosclerosis or smooth muscle cell hypertrophy due to hypertension and its addition to the Framingham score did not improve risk prediction.[37] It is therefore no longer recommended in the cardiovascular risk evaluation in any population.[38]

Coronary Atherosclerosis Evaluation with Computed Tomography Angiography

Coronary atherosclerosis evaluation with computed tomography angiography (CCTA) is a reliable, noninvasive imaging modality evaluating the entire coronary arterial tree. CAC presence and score improves cardiovascular risk stratification beyond Framingham score in asymptomatic intermediate risk populations. The Multi-Ethnic Study of Atherosclerosis[39] and BioImage study[40] showed that CAC was superior to carotid plaque in predicting cardiovascular risk. Moreover, in inflammatory joint disease, carotid plaque presence and burden did not adequately reflect the presence and burden of coronary atherosclerosis.[41] Higher CAC scores have been reported in both long-term RA and SLE compared with early or no disease.[35] However, CAC is not sensitive for higher risk noncalcified or partially calcified plaques which are prevalent in IRDs. Coronary plaque burden and composition were shown to improve cardiovascular risk prediction beyond CAC.[11] RA patients displayed greater coronary plaque prevalence, burden, and vulnerability versus age and gender-matched controls and presence of at least moderate disease activity associated with higher risk plaques.[23] Importantly, coronary atherosclerosis burden predicted long-term cardiovascular events in RA independently of cardiac risk scores, RA characteristics, time-varying disease activity, prednisone, methotrexate, and bDMARD treatments.[25] Moreover, bDMARD therapy independently reduced long-term cardiovascular risk, attenuated new plaque formation and promoted stabilization and calcification of high-risk and noncalcified plaques respectively.[25] SLE duration associated with higher noncalcified plaque and immunosuppression attenuated noncalcified plaque progression.[42] Similarly, psoriasis patients displayed greater CAC scores, noncalcified plaque burden and high-risk features compared with matched controls, and biologic therapies reduced both total and noncalcified plaque burden compared with nonusers.[42] Of note, therapeutic adjustments based on coronary plaque presence on CCTA improved long-term cardiovascular outcomes and medication adherence in general patients with chest pain.[43] Although similar assessments in asymptomatic patients are lacking, coronary atherosclerosis on CCTA, as a risk-modifying tool, may impact adherence to preventive therapy.

International primary prevention guidelines recommend consideration of carotid plaques and CAC as additive risk prediction tools in individuals at borderline and intermediate risk.[44] Given the high likelihood of carotid plaque presence in RA, EULAR guidelines suggest screening ultrasound for carotid plaque evaluation in all patients with RA. Yet, despite at least equal prevalence of coronary plaque on CCTA, no clear recommendations are issued regarding its use.[5]

Coronary Vascular Inflammation and Injury

Coronary vascular inflammation evaluated as perivascular fat attenuation index (PFAI) on CCTA further improves cardiovascular risk prediction. Biologic therapies reduced PFAI in patients with psoriasis.[42] Arterial inflammation on fluoro-deoxy-glucose (FDG)-PET CT associated with coronary plaque presence, improved cardiovascular risk prediction beyond Framingham risk scores and displayed a dose-dependent reduction on statin treatment, suggesting attenuation of plaque inflammation.[42] Psoriasis patients showed greater FDG-PET uptake compared with controls. However, two recent randomized controlled trials—one with ustekinumab and another with adalimumab showed no difference in vascular inflammation despite reduction in systemic inflammatory markers.[42]

BIOMARKERS OF ATHEROSCLEROTIC CARDIOVASCULAR RISK IN INFLAMMATORY RHEUMATIC DISEASES

The immune activation, high inflammatory burden, oxidative stress, modifications in lipoprotein structure and function collectively inherent of several IRDs, and disease-specific mechanisms may underlie qualitative and quantitative differences in all stages of the atherogenic process. Distinct biomarkers may reflect various stages of this trajectory, from immune dysregulation (autoantibodies) to inflammation (c-reactive protein [CRP], cytokines), plaque vulnerability, thrombosis, myocardial stress (N-terminal pro-brain-type natriuretic peptide [NT-proBNP]) and myocardial necrosis (cardiac troponins).

Structural Cardiac Biomarkers Predicting Cardiovascular Risk

Blood levels of cardiac troponin I (cTnI) and T (cTnT) subunits increase during myocardial injury. Highly sensitive assays measure those in concentrations significantly lower than conventional assays. Hs-cTnI associated with coronary plaque presence, burden, vulnerability, and 5-year cardiovascular event risk in RA after adjusting for cardiac risk factors, obesity, and prednisone use. It further improved discrimination and optimized cardiovascular event prediction over cardiac risk scores alone. Likewise, hs-cTnI associated with carotid artery total area plaque in psoriasis and PsA. Detectable hs-cTnT yielded a 9-fold risk of carotid plaque presence in SLE. Hs-cTnT was further linked to noncalcified coronary plaque burden at baseline and 1-year follow-up in patients with psoriasis (**Table 2**).

Table 2
Biomarker association with atherosclerosis and cardiovascular events

Biomarker	Study (year)	Number	State	Outcome	Findings
Structural					
Hs-cTnl	Karpouzas et al,[91] 2018	150	RA	Coronary plaque 5-y CVD risk	Linked to presence, burden, extensive or obstructive disease and advanced plaque remodeling. Independently associates with 5-y CVD risk. If low, 82% lower CVD risk. Improves CVE prediction over clinical risk scores
	Hromádka et al,[92] 2016	44	RA	Coronary plaque	Independently associates with severe coronary stenosis (OR [95%CI] = 6.37[1.53, 26.48], P = .011)
	Bradhamet al,[93] 2012	164	RA	Coronary Calcium	Correlated in univariable but not multivariable analysis
	Colaco et al,[94] 2022	1000 (358)	PsO (PsA)	Carotid plaque	Associated with total carotid plaque area (b = 0.21 [0.0, 0.4]), but no improvement in predictive performance
Hs-cTnT	Zhou et al,[95] 2020	202	PsO	Coronary plaque	Burden of calcified plaque > median associated with positive hs-cTnT at baseline and at 1-y
	Divard et al,[96] 2017	63	SLE	Carotid plaque	Detectable cTnT (>3 ng/L) associates with plaque presence [OR for plaque 9.26 (95%CI 1.55–90.07)]
NT-proBNP	Mirjafari et al,[97] 2014	960	IP	All cause and CVD mortality	High NT-proBNP (>100pg/ml) associated with all cause as well as cardiovascular mortality, adjusted for age and sex
	Goldenberg et al,[98] 2012	124	SLE	Carotid plaque echo	No association with carotid plaque presence. Negative association with ejection fraction
	Colaco et al,[94] 2022	1000 (358)	PsO (PsA)	Carotid plaque	No association with total carotid plaque area (P = 0.21)
Autoantibody					
RF	Holmqvist et al,[19] 2017	15,744	RA	Acute coronary syndrome	50%–98% higher relative ACS risk in RF positive patients and 21%–59% higher relative ACS risk in those who have DAS28 > 3.2 at onset

(continued on next page)

Table 2
(continued)

Biomarker	Study (year)	Number	State	Outcome	Findings
ACPA	Lopez-Longo et al,[21] 2009	937	RA	Ischemic CVD / CVD mortality	Linked to greater risk of ischemic CVD (OR = 2.58, [1.17–5.65]) and CVD mortality (OR 1.72, [1.01–2.91]).
anti-PC	Anania et al,[99] 2010	114	SLE	Carotid plaque	Lowest tertile associated with higher plaque presence in patients without known CVD (OR = 2.92[95%CI 1.08–7.90])
Anti-oxLDL	Ahmed et al,[100] 2010	40	RA	Carotid IMT / Carotid plaque	Patients with plaques had higher anti-OxLDL vs those without. Anti-oxLDL linked to carotid plaque presence
	Cinoku et al, 2018[101]	79 / 121 / 63	RA / SLE pSS	Carotid plaque / Femoral plaque	Linked to lower presence of carotid or femoral plaques in pSS (OR = 0.14 [0.03–0.72]) but not in RA or SLE.
Anti-oxLDL IgG	Karpouzas et al,[18] 2022	150	RA	Coronary plaque	Associated with higher TNFa, presence and burden of lipid-rich noncalcified and high-risk plaque only in LDL <70 mg/dl
Anti-b2GPI IgA	Karpouzas et al,[102] 2021	150	RA	Coronary plaque / CVD risk	Linked to plaque, CAC progression, new mixed plaque formation and its persistence. Time-averaged CRP linked to CAC change and CVD risk in anti-β2GPI IgA positive patients but not in negative. Improved risk prediction for plaque progression over models with clinical score and inflammation.
Lipid					
HDL-CEC	Sánchez-Pérez et al,[103] 2020	195	SLE	Carotid IMT / Carotid plaque	CEC lower in SLE than controls. Inversely associated with presence of carotid plaques (OR = 0.87 [0.78, 0.97])
	Tejera-Segura et al,[104] 2017	178	RA	Carotid IMT / Carotid plaque	No association with IMT. Higher CEC linked to lower risk of carotid plaque presence (OR = 0.94 [0.89–0.98])

Biomarker	Study	N	Disease	Measure	Findings
HDL-H5%	Chang et al,[105] 2021	69	RA	Carotid IMT / Carotid plaque	H5 subfraction linked to SCA (AUC 71.1%). H5 amplified IL-1 and IL-8 elaboration from monocytes and macrophages and foam cell formation.
LDL-CLC	Karpouzas et al,[106,107] 2022	140	RA	Coronary plaque / CVD events	Associated with CVD risk independently of ASCVD and plaque burden. CLC associated with presence and burden of partially-calcified, LAP, obstructive plaques and CAC in bDMARD nonusers
LDL-L5%	Chang et al,[108] 2019	64	RA	Carotid IMT / Carotid plaque	Associated with SCA (adjusted OR = 4.94, $P < 0.05$) and predicted SCA with AUC 78.8%. Decreased at 6 mo after adalimumab/tocilizumab with methotrexate.
Lp(a)	Karpouzas et al,[14] 2022	150	RA	Coronary plaque	Associated with OxLDL and anti-OxLDL IgG levels. In LDL-C<70 mg/dL, anti-OxLDL linked to presence and burden of lipid-rich, high-risk and obstructive plaques.
	García-Gómez et al,[109] 2019	426 / 412	AS PsA	CVD events	Trend for association between Lp(a) and prior CVD events [adjusted OR = 2.47 (0.95–6.41), $P = 0.06$]
Apolipoproteins	Kiani et al,[110] 2015	58	SLE	Carotid IMT / Carotid plaque	Neither cardioprotective, nor proatherogenic apolipoproteins linked to either CAC or CIMT.
Proteins					
Proprotein convertase subtilisin/kexin type 9	Arida et al,[111] 2021	85	RA	AI / Carotid IMT / Carotid plaque	Serum PCSK9 levels (adjusted for age and sex) associated with CIMT, carotid plaques, and arterial stiffness (augmentation index).
	Fang et al,[112] 2018	90	SLE	Carotid IMT	Higher in SLE with subclinical atherosclerosis.
	Ferraz-Amaro et al,[113] 2020	73	SSc	Carotid IMT / Carotid plaque	Associated with CIMT but not with carotid plaques (adjusted for traditional CVD risk factors).
	de Armas-Rillo et al,[114] 2021	299	AxSpA	Carotid IMT / Carotid plaque	No association with CIMT or carotid plaques (adjusted for disease-related and traditional CVD risk factors).
	Ferraz-Amaro et al,[115] 2016	326	RA	Carotid IMT / Carotid plaque	Serum PCSK9 levels (adjusted for traditional CVD risk factors) did not associate with CIMT or carotid plaques.
	Liu et al,[116] 2020	109	SLE	Carotid IMT / Carotid plaque / CVD events	Serum PCSK9 levels did not associate with CIMT or carotid plaques or with CVD events (adjusted for age).

(continued on next page)

Table 2
(continued)

Biomarker	Study (year)	Number	State	Outcome	Findings
Inflammatory/Cytokines					
CRP	Goodson et al,[117] 2005	506	IP	CVD death	CRP independent predicts CVD death [HR = 3.3 (1.4–7.6)] after controlling for age, gender, smoking, HAQ, RF, swollen joint counts
	Karpouzas et al,[24,25] 2020	150	RA	Coronary plaque CVD events	Cumulative CRP independently predicted long-term coronary atherosclerosis progression and CVD events
ESR	Myasedoeva et al,[17] 2011	651	RA	CVD events	Increased risk of CVD events (HR = 1.2 [1.1–1.3] for per 10 mm/h increase in ESR). Trend for increased CVD event risk with higher CRP (P = 0.07)
	Innala et al,[118] 2011	442	RA	CVD events	Baseline ESR, cumulative DAS28 (AUC), DAS28 AUC at 6 mo all associated with greater CVD risk (all P < 0.01)
	Wallberg-Johnsson et al,[119] 1999	211	RA	CVD events	Increased last registered ESR before event and high disease activity at onset associate with high risk of CVD events
MBDA	Curtis et al,[34] 2020	30,751	RA	CVD events	Improved discrimination; reclassified 42% of patients when compared with a model comprising age and sex alone; reclassified 28% patients vs the model with clinical risk factors with best performance (age, se, diabetes, HTN, smoking, prior CVD, CRP).
IL-33	Shen et al,[120] 2015	98	RA	Carotid plaque	Predicted new carotid plaques over 1 y despite adjustment for classical CVD risk factors.
	López-Mejías et al,[121] 2015	576	RA	Carotid IMT	rs3939286 polymorphism in IL-33 gene associated with lower CIMT after adjusting for age and sex.
TNFa	Verma et al,[122] 2015	30	AS	Carotid IMT	Moderately associated with CIMT
IL-6	Garg et al,[123] 2016	18	PsA	Carotid IMT	Serum IL-6 and soluble ICAM-1 had a moderate positive correlation with CIMT

| sST2 | Shen et al, 2016[124] | 80 | PsA | Carotid plaque | Independent positive association with the presence of carotid plaques after adjustment for age, disease duration, statin use, and traditional CVD risk factors |

Abbreviations: ACPA, anti-citrullinated peptide antibody; ACS, acute coronary syndrome; AI, augmentation index; anti-PC, anti-phosphorylcholine; anti-β2GPI, anti-beta2 glycoprotein 1; AS, ankylosing spondylitis; ASCVD, atherosclerotic cardiovascular disease; AUC, area under the curve; bDMARD, biologic disease-modifying anti-rheumatic drugs; CI, confidence interval; CAC, coronary artery calcium score; CEC, cholesterol efflux capacity; CIMT, carotid intima medial thickness; CRP, C-reactive protein; CVD, cardiovascular disease; DAS28, disease activity score in RA using 28 joint count; ESR, erythrocyte sedimentation rate; HAQ, health assessment questionnaire disability index; HDL, high-density lipoprotein cholesterol; HR, hazard ratio; Hs-cTnI, high-sensitivity cardiac troponin I; Hs-cTnT, high-sensitivity cardiac troponin T; HTN, Hypertension; ICAM-1, intercellular adhesion molecule 1; IL, interleukin; IMT, intima-medial thickness; LAP, low attenuation plaques; LDL, low-density lipoprotein cholesterol; Lp(a), lipoprotein a; MBDA, multi-biomarker disease activity score; NT-proBNP, N-terminal pro-brain natriuretic peptide; OR, odds ratio; oxLDL, oxidized LDL; P, inflammatory polyarthritis; PC, phosphorylcholine; PsA, psoriatic arthritis; PsO, psoriasis; pSS, primary Sjogren's syndrome; RA, rheumatoid arthritis; RF, rheumatoid factor; SCA, subclinical atherosclerosis; SCA, subclinical atherosclerosis; SLE, systemic lupus erythematosus; sST2, soluble ST2; Th17, T-helper 17 lymphocytes; TNF-α, tumor necrosis factor alpha; Treg, regulatory T lymphocytes.

NT-proBNP is released from ventricular cardiomyocytes in response to strain or ischemia. High NT-proBNP (>100 pg/ml) associated with all cause and cardiovascular mortality independently of cardiac risk factors in patients with early inflammatory polyarthritis. NT-proBNP associated with left ventricular ejection fraction but not carotid plaque presence in SLE. Finally, NT-proBNP did not associate with carotid artery total area plaque in psoriasis and PsA (see **Table 2**).

Autoantibodies as Biomarkers of Cardiovascular Risk

Rheumatoid factor (RF) positive patients incur higher CVD risk[19]; likewise, anti-citrullinated peptide antibody (ACPA)-positive patients—especially those with high titers—experience higher likelihood of ischemic heart disease and cardiovascular death.[21]

Low-density lipoprotein (LDL) oxidation and macrophage uptake is pivotal in foam cell formation, atherosclerosis initiation, and progression. Oxidized LDL (oxLDL) was linked to coronary plaque and predicted atherosclerotic events in general patients with or without known CVD.[45] Higher oxLDL levels have been reported in IRDs. Moreover, high-titer antibodies against oxLDL (anti-oxLDL) were reported in patients with rapidly progressive carotid atherosclerosis, angiographic evidence of coronary artery disease, and myocardial infarction.[46] OxLDL can bind b2-glycoprotein-1 (b2GPI) in the plaque and anti-b2GPI antibodies against the complex can promote oxLDL uptake by macrophages. oxLDL/b2GPI complexes are higher in patients with antiphospholipid syndrome, SLE, and SScl compared with controls.[47] Antibodies against oxLDL, oxidized phospholipids, or oxLDL/b2GPI complexes associate with atherosclerosis presence and burden in IRDs.[48] In SLE, lower anti-oxLDL immunoglobulin M (IgM) titers and higher anti-oxLDL IgG associated with CVD and carotid plaque[49-51] (see **Table 2**). In RA, higher anti-oxLDL immunoglobulin G (IgG) associated with carotid plaque, as well as presence and burden of lipid-rich and high-risk coronary plaque specifically in patients with LDL-C less than 70 mg/dl.[18,52] High prevalence of anti-b2GPI immunoglobulin A (IgA) was seen in RA; they associated with development and progression of coronary atherosclerosis, formation and persistence of high-risk plaques and improved prediction accuracy for plaque progression over models based on cardiac risk factors and inflammation (see **Table 2**).

Lipoprotein Levels, Structure, and Function as Biomarkers of Cardiovascular Risk

High-grade chronic inflammation impacts on levels and composition of circulating lipoproteins and on cell cholesterol homeostasis through the regulation of cholesterol transporters. High-density lipoprotein (HDL) levels are lower due to accelerated clearance or reduced synthesis of HDL particles. Modifications of HDL composition including increased inflammatory molecules (serum alpha amyloid [SAA], oxidized fatty acids), displacement of apoA-I, reduction in antioxidant proteins (paroxonase) and rearrangement of the HDL proteome impair its ability to perform cholesterol efflux from arterial wall macrophages.[53] Cholesterol efflux capacity (CEC) is impaired in RA, SLE, PsA, and AS compared with controls and inversely correlated with disease activity. In contrast, DMARD therapies associated with improvement in CEC.[53,54] CEC inversely associated with atherosclerosis and events in general patients, independently of HDL levels. Likewise, CEC inversely correlated with carotid atherosclerosis in SLE and RA (see **Table 2**).

Cholesterol loading capacity (CLC) is the ability of serum to deliver cholesterol to cells and is related to foam cell formation. RA serum increased cholesterol content in macrophages and promoted foam cell formation significantly more than control serum.[55] CLC was linked to long-term cardiovascular event risk in RA overall and associated with high-risk low-attenuation and obstructive coronary plaque presence and burden in biologic disease modifying anti-rheumatic drugs (bDMARD) nonusers. Of note, oxLDL influenced CLC directly in dual seropositive patients regardless of CRP levels. Two additional and independent pathways—via anti-oxLDL IgG and PCSK9—mediated the effects of oxidized LDL on CLC depending on CRP and seropositivity status. Lipoprotein(a)-cholesterol [LP(a)-C] content was linked to both oxidized LDL and anti-oxLDL IgG levels in RA serum. Lp(a)-C content was higher in RA patients with LDL-C less than 70 mg/dl versus those with higher LDL-C and anti-oxLDL IgG associated with presence and burden of lipid-rich and high-risk coronary plaque specifically in those patients,[18] providing anatomic and mechanistic plausibility to the lipid paradox theory. Studies addressing the association between serum lipoproteins and clinical or subclinical atherosclerosis in IRDs are summarized in **Table 2**.

Proprotein Convertase Subtilisin/Kexin Type 9

Clearance of LDL-C is a protective mechanism against atherosclerosis. Proprotein convertase subtilisin/kexin type 9 (PCSK9) is the main inhibitor of hepatic LDL-receptor expression; high PCSK9 leads to high LDL-C. An association between serum PCSK9 and subclinical atherosclerosis was reported in RA, SLE, and SSc but not in SpA (see **Table 2**). Higher PCSK9 was seen in RA patients with LDL-C less than 70 mg/dl after adjustment for Framingham CVD risk score, statin use and HDL-C, and associated with LDL oxidation, suggesting that non-LDL-receptor-mediated clearance of LDL accounts for low-LDL-C in that group.[18]

Cytokines and Other Circulating Proteins as Biomarkers of Atherosclerosis

The role of inflammation in atherogenesis both in general patients and those with IRDs is well recognized. Serum CRP independently predicted CVD death in an inception cohort of inflammatory polyarthritis over 10 years. Cumulative CRP independently predicted long-term coronary atherosclerosis progression and cardiovascular events in RA.[24,25] Each 10 mm/h increment in erythrocyte sedimentation rate (ESR) associated with 20% greater CVD risk in a population-based study of RA patients.[17] Baseline ESR and the last ESR registered prior a CVD event associated with increased CVD risk in two long-term Swedish RA studies (see **Table 2**).

A multibiomarker disease activity (MBDA) test for RA that measures 12 protein serum biomarkers and provides a score on a scale from 0 to 100 was validated against DAS28-CRP. It showed good accuracy in predicting 3-year CVD risk in RA outperforming clinical models with or without CRP.[34] Proinflammatory cytokines including tumor necrosis factor alpha (TNF-α), interleukin (IL)-1β, IL-6, and IL-17 associated with atherosclerosis as well as CVD events.[56–59] Some reports associated IL-33 and polymorphisms in IL-33 gene with carotid plaques in RA and PsA. Studies exploring the relationship between soluble mediators and CVD events or subclinical atherosclerosis are summarized in **Table 2**.

ROLE OF ARTIFICIAL INTELLIGENCE IN DATA SYNTHESIS AND ALGORITHM CRAFTING

AI is an emerging tool to make sense out of very large volumes of data collected from different settings.[60] AI uses machine learning (ML) to make sense out of such enormous volumes of data. The concepts of data analysis via ML, involving analysis of data points in relation to predefined outcomes (supervised ML, further subcategorized into classification techniques for discrete outcomes, or regression techniques for continuous outcomes) or leaves the identification of outcomes to the artificial neural network while providing the raw information (unsupervised ML, using either clustering or dimensionality reduction).[61] Deep learning (DL) relates particularly to the analysis of images (such as carotid ultrasound scans) from different angles and layers of imaging using convoluted neural networks.[62]

AI has already been successfully used to facilitate detection and management of cardiovascular risk in diabetes mellitus.[63] However, the use of ML techniques for CVD risk stratification in IRDs is in its infancy. Available studies use relatively small cohorts that were not set-up for this purpose and with little external validation. In an RA cohort from Greece followed over 3 years, the risk prediction accuracy using traditional calculators (SCORE, ASCVD, and framingham risk score [FRS]) was compared with ML algorithms using information from 46 different CVD risk factors (clinical, laboratory, and imaging—carotid and femoral ultrasound). The ML approaches used were linear discriminant analysis (LDA), random forest (RF), and support vector machine (SVM) modeling. At baseline, whereas traditional CVD risk scores had an area under curve (AUC) from 72% to 79%, the AUC for LDA (90%–99%), RF, and SVM (both 100%) was superior. At 3 years, AUC for CVD risk scores was 73% to 80%, LDA 92% to 98%, SVM and RF were both 100%. For the overall cohort, traditional risk scores had an AUC of 76% for CVD risk prediction, whereas a combination of ML algorithms had an AUC of 100%.[64] Another study in PsA compared CVD risk predicted by FRS versus ML approaches using the same clinical and laboratory variables included in the FRS. The AUC was better with the ML models (85% using SVM, 83% using RF and 80% using K nearest neighbor technique) than the FRS alone (76%).[65] The association between CVD events and clinical features was also evaluated in pSS patients using ML techniques of automated hierarchical clustering (AHC) and auto contracting maps (Auto-CM). Although AHC failed to identify associations, Auto-CM identified two groups (non-ischemic heart failure [associated with glandular features], and ischemic CVD [associated with disease duration and extraglandular features]).[66] ML approaches also predicted arrhythmic events from cardiac MRI images of cardiac sarcoidosis[67] and deep learning techniques identified cardiac sarcoidosis from routine echocardiographic images.[68] The use of AI to predict or stratify CVD risk with greater accuracy, using data from large, longitudinal cohorts of IRDs is an important research agenda item in the near future.

CLINICAL APPLICATION AND EXPORTABILITY

The EULAR recommendations for cardiovascular risk management in patients with IRDs[5] including SLE and antiphospholipid syndrome (APLS)[69] stresses that cardiovascular risk factor assessments are performed regularly in all individuals in rheumatology clinic, that inflammation is reduced, that defined treatment targets are reached, and that CVD risk management should follow national guidelines. Cardiovascular treatments may vary by location but include antihypertensive, antiplatelet, diabetes management, lipid-lowering, and anticoagulant therapies.[4]

Age, sex, smoking status, diabetes, hypertension, hypercholesterolaemia, and kidney disease are included in the risk prediction models for primary prevention.[44,70] SCORE in its updated versions SCORE2 and SCORE2-OP for older persons are recommended to predict 10-year risk of first-onset CVD in the general European population[71,72] and the ASCVD 10-year risk estimator based on the pooled cohort equation in the United States.[73]

The burden of ASCVD in IRDs is best described for RA (**Table 1**), but inflammatory conditions may be included as effect modifiers in the conventional risk prediction models to identify patients who might benefit from primary prevention strategies.[70]

Thus, the EULAR recommendations for CVD risk management in patients with RA suggest that conventional CVD risk prediction models should use a 1.5 multiplication factor if not already included in the algorithm.[5] This approach lowers the threshold for assessment of total CVD risk based on the presence of a chronic inflammatory condition; however, it is also suggested that the threshold be lowered based on the level of disease activity but no recommendation concerning the indication or type of anti-inflammatory treatment is given.[5,70]

In patients classified at borderline or intermediate risk CAC score may be added to improve CVD risk stratification and reclassify patients as eligible for treatment.[44,70] CAC scoring was proven to be a superior imaging modality to modify CVD risk stratification by reclassification, but ultrasound for carotid plaque detection may be used, when CAC measurements are unavailable or not feasible.[44,70] High-sensitivity CRP, lipoprotein(a), other biomarkers, genetic risk scores or other potential modifiers are not yet sufficiently studied to be recommended for routine use in ASCVD risk stratification.[70]

UNANSWERED QUESTIONS/FUTURE RESEARCH ADDENDA

Despite significant improvements in cardiovascular outcomes in RA over time as a result of successful prevention campaigns, more streamlined risk stratification algorithms and guidelines, and a higher relative CVD risk versus controls still remains. Several questions linger and present a series of actionable research agenda items. The generation of accurate, disease-specific cardiovascular risk calculator(s) is still a fruitful endeavor. Enrichment with disease-restricted features, metrics of cumulative inflammation, disease-process or stage-related biomarkers, structural cardiac or plaque-vulnerability indices, atherosclerosis burden, and composition characteristics may optimize risk prediction estimates. In the era of precision medicine, advanced analytical methods including machine or deep learning techniques may integrate high volumes of such information, manage and consider significant population heterogeneities and assist in the generation of testable algorithms, calculators, and ultimately guidelines for accurate cardiovascular risk assessment and prevention.

Large scale validation of the impact of cumulative inflammation, cytokine, lipid, and structural biomarkers on atherosclerotic plaque formation, burden, progression, and hard events is still lacking. Also lacking is comprehensive, prospective evaluation of the impact of atherosclerotic plaque burden and characteristics on hard cardiovascular outcomes across various IRDs, presently limiting their concrete endorsement in available international society guidelines. Moreover, it is currently unknown whether traditional cardiac risk factor management using targets similar to the general population is equally effective in patients with IRDs, nor whether such targets should be adapted or revised for patients with IRDs, commensurate to their heightened risk.

Design of adequately powered large-scale, long-term prospective clinical trials with comprehensive data collections encompassing the aforementioned modalities in isolation or combination and prespecified hard event outcomes in various IRDs may foster optimization of cardiovascular risk estimates and prevention.

CLINICS CARE POINTS

- Cardiovascular disease (CVD) risk factors should be carefully sought and addressed in every individual with an inflammatory rheumatic disease (IRD).
- Smoking cessation, timely diagnosis and adequate control of diabetes mellitus and hypertension, regular physical exercise, and lipid-lowering therapy as per existing recommendations are essential CVD risk mitigation strategies.

- Cardiovascular risk algorithms approved for use according to local recommendation, and practice should be used for cardiovascular risk stratification in the respective populations.
- If the cardiovascular risk algorithm does not account for the presence of IRD as a CVD risk factor, then the risk estimate should be multiplied by 1.5.
- Screening for carotid plaques or coronary atherosclerosis using computerized tomography might be useful helpful to further delineate CVD risk in IRDs.

DISCLOSURE

The authors have nothing to disclose.

FUNDING

None of the authors have any funding to declare in relation to the current manuscript.

REFERENCES

1. Nurmohamed MT, Heslinga M, Kitas GD. Cardiovascular comorbidity in rheumatic diseases. Nat Rev Rheumatol 2015;11(12):693–704.
2. Avina-Zubieta JA, Thomas J, Sadatsafavi M, et al. Risk of incident cardiovascular events in patients with rheumatoid arthritis: a meta-analysis of observational studies. Ann Rheum Dis 2012;71(9):1524–9.
3. Restivo V, Candiloro S, Daidone M, et al. Systematic review and meta-analysis of cardiovascular risk in rheumatological disease: Symptomatic and non-symptomatic events in rheumatoid arthritis and systemic lupus erythematosus. Autoimmun Rev 2022;21(1):102925.
4. Semb AG, Ikdahl E, Wibetoe G, et al. Atherosclerotic cardiovascular disease prevention in rheumatoid arthritis. Nat Rev Rheumatol 2020;16(7):361–79.
5. Agca R, Heslinga SC, Rollefstad S, et al. EULAR recommendations for cardiovascular disease risk management in patients with rheumatoid arthritis and other forms of inflammatory joint disorders: 2015/2016 update. Ann Rheum Dis 2017;76(1):17–28.
6. Karczewski KJ, Dudley JT, Kukurba KR, et al. Systematic functional regulatory assessment of disease-associated variants. Proc Natl Acad Sci U S A 2013;110(23):9607–12.
7. Paakkanen R, Lokki ML, Seppänen M, et al. Proinflammatory HLA-DRB1*01-haplotype predisposes to ST-elevation myocardial infarction. Atherosclerosis 2012;221(2):461–6.
8. Gonzalez-Gay MA, Gonzalez-Juanatey C, Lopez-Diaz MJ, et al. HLA-DRB1 and persistent chronic inflammation contribute to cardiovascular events and cardiovascular mortality in patients with rheumatoid arthritis. Arthritis Rheum 2007;57(1):125–32.
9. Ferraz-Amaro I, Winchester R, Gregersen PK, et al. Coronary Artery Calcification and Rheumatoid Arthritis: Lack of Relationship to Risk Alleles for Coronary Artery Disease in the General Population. Arthritis Rheumatol 2017;69(3):529–41.
10. López-Mejías R, Corrales A, Vicente E, et al. Influence of coronary artery disease and subclinical atherosclerosis related polymorphisms on the risk of atherosclerosis in rheumatoid arthritis. Sci Rep 2017;7:40303.

11. Karpouzas GA, Bui VL, Ronda N, et al. Biologics and atherosclerotic cardiovascular risk in rheumatoid arthritis: a review of evidence and mechanistic insights. Expert Rev Clin Immunol 2021;17(4):355–74.
12. Giannelou M, Mavragani CP. Cardiovascular disease in systemic lupus erythematosus: A comprehensive update. J Autoimmun 2017;82:1–12.
13. Escalante A, Haas RW, del Rincón I. Paradoxical effect of body mass index on survival in rheumatoid arthritis: role of comorbidity and systemic inflammation. Arch Intern Med 2005;165(14):1624–9.
14. Kremers HM, Nicola PJ, Crowson CS, et al. Prognostic importance of low body mass index in relation to cardiovascular mortality in rheumatoid arthritis. Arthritis Rheum 2004;50(11):3450–7.
15. Giles JT, Allison M, Blumenthal RS, et al. Abdominal adiposity in rheumatoid arthritis: association with cardiometabolic risk factors and disease characteristics. Arthritis Rheum 2010;62(11):3173–82.
16. Gonzalez A, Maradit Kremers H, Crowson CS, et al. Do cardiovascular risk factors confer the same risk for cardiovascular outcomes in rheumatoid arthritis patients as in non-rheumatoid arthritis patients? Ann Rheum Dis 2008;67(1):64–9.
17. Myasoedova E, Crowson CS, Kremers HM, et al. Lipid paradox in rheumatoid arthritis: the impact of serum lipid measures and systemic inflammation on the risk of cardiovascular disease. Ann Rheum Dis 2011;70(3):482–7.
18. Karpouzas GA, Ormseth SR, Ronda N, et al. Lipoprotein oxidation may underlie the paradoxical association of low cholesterol with coronary atherosclerotic risk in rheumatoid arthritis. J Autoimmun 2022;129:102815.
19. Holmqvist M, Ljung L, Askling J. Acute coronary syndrome in new-onset rheumatoid arthritis: a population-based nationwide cohort study of time trends in risks and excess risks. Ann Rheum Dis 2017;76(10):1642–7.
20. Edwards CJ, Syddall H, Goswami R, et al. The autoantibody rheumatoid factor may be an independent risk factor for ischaemic heart disease in men. Heart 2007;93(10):1263–7.
21. López-Longo FJ, Oliver-Miñarro D, de la Torre I, et al. Association between anti-cyclic citrullinated peptide antibodies and ischemic heart disease in patients with rheumatoid arthritis. Arthritis Rheum 2009;61(4):419–24.
22. Cambridge G, Acharya J, Cooper JA, et al. Antibodies to citrullinated peptides and risk of coronary heart disease. Atherosclerosis 2013;228(1):243–6.
23. Karpouzas GA, Malpeso J, Choi TY, et al. Prevalence, extent and composition of coronary plaque in patients with rheumatoid arthritis without symptoms or prior diagnosis of coronary artery disease. Ann Rheum Dis 2014;73(10):1797–804.
24. Karpouzas GA, Ormseth SR, Hernandez E, et al. Impact of Cumulative Inflammation, Cardiac Risk Factors, and Medication Exposure on Coronary Atherosclerosis Progression in Rheumatoid Arthritis. Arthritis Rheumatol 2020;72(3):400–8.
25. Karpouzas GA, Ormseth SR, Hernandez E, et al. Biologics May Prevent Cardiovascular Events in Rheumatoid Arthritis by Inhibiting Coronary Plaque Formation and Stabilizing High-Risk Lesions. Arthritis Rheumatol 2020;72(9):1467–75.
26. Liuzzo G, Goronzy JJ, Yang H, et al. Monoclonal T-cell proliferation and plaque instability in acute coronary syndromes. Circulation 2000;101(25):2883–8.
27. Crowson CS, Matteson EL, Roger VL, et al. Usefulness of risk scores to estimate the risk of cardiovascular disease in patients with rheumatoid arthritis. Am J Cardiol 2012;110(3):420–4.

28. Arts EE, Popa C, Den Broeder AA, et al. Performance of four current risk algorithms in predicting cardiovascular events in patients with early rheumatoid arthritis. Ann Rheum Dis 2015;74(4):668–74.
29. Esdaile JM, Abrahamowicz M, Grodzicky T, et al. Traditional Framingham risk factors fail to fully account for accelerated atherosclerosis in systemic lupus erythematosus. Arthritis Rheum 2001;44(10):2331–7.
30. Crowson CS, Gabriel SE, Semb AG, et al. Rheumatoid arthritis-specific cardiovascular risk scores are not superior to general risk scores: a validation analysis of patients from seven countries. Rheumatology (Oxford) 2017;56(7):1102–10.
31. Crowson CS, Rollefstad S, Kitas GD, et al. Challenges of developing a cardiovascular risk calculator for patients with rheumatoid arthritis. PLoS One 2017; 12(3):e0174656.
32. Corrales A, González-Juanatey C, Peiró ME, et al. Carotid ultrasound is useful for the cardiovascular risk stratification of patients with rheumatoid arthritis: results of a population-based study. Ann Rheum Dis 2014;73(4):722–7.
33. Skaggs BJ, Grossman J, Sahakian L, et al. A Panel of Biomarkers Associates With Increased Risk for Cardiovascular Events in Women With Systemic Lupus Erythematosus. ACR open Rheumatol 2021;3(4):209–20.
34. Curtis JR, Xie F, Crowson CS, et al. Derivation and internal validation of a multi-biomarker-based cardiovascular disease risk prediction score for rheumatoid arthritis patients. Arthritis Res Ther 2020;22(1):282.
35. Sade LE, Akdogan A. Imaging for screening cardiovascular involvement in patients with systemic rheumatologic diseases: more questions than answers. Eur Heart J Cardiovasc Imaging 2019;20(9):967–78.
36. Evans MR, Escalante A, Battafarano DF, et al. Carotid atherosclerosis predicts incident acute coronary syndromes in rheumatoid arthritis. Arthritis Rheum 2011;63(5):1211–20.
37. Den Ruijter HM, Peters SA, Anderson TJ, et al. Common carotid intima-media thickness measurements in cardiovascular risk prediction: a meta-analysis. JAMA 2012;308(8):796–803.
38. Mach F, Baigent C, Catapano AL, et al. 2019 ESC/EAS Guidelines for the management of dyslipidaemias: lipid modification to reduce cardiovascular risk. Eur Heart J 2020;41(1):111–88.
39. Gepner AD, Young R, Delaney JA, et al. Comparison of Carotid Plaque Score and Coronary Artery Calcium Score for Predicting Cardiovascular Disease Events: The Multi-Ethnic Study of Atherosclerosis. J Am Heart Assoc 2017;6(2).
40. Mortensen MB, Fuster V, Muntendam P, et al. A Simple Disease-Guided Approach to Personalize ACC/AHA-Recommended Statin Allocation in Elderly People: The BioImage Study. J Am Coll Cardiol 2016;68(9):881–91.
41. Svanteson M, Rollefstad S, Kløw NE, et al. Associations between coronary and carotid artery atherosclerosis in patients with inflammatory joint diseases. RMD Open 2017;3(2):e000544.
42. Choi H, Uceda DE, Dey AK, et al. Application of Non-invasive Imaging in Inflammatory Disease Conditions to Evaluate Subclinical Coronary Artery Disease. Curr Rheumatol Rep 2019;22(1):1.
43. Newby DE, Adamson PD, Berry C, et al. Coronary CT Angiography and 5-Year Risk of Myocardial Infarction. N Engl J Med 2018;379(10):924–33.
44. Arnett DK, Blumenthal RS, Albert MA, et al. 2019 ACC/AHA Guideline on the Primary Prevention of Cardiovascular Disease: A Report of the American College of Cardiology/American Heart Association Task Force on Clinical Practice Guidelines. Circulation 2019;140(11):e596–646.

45. Byun YS, Yang X, Bao W, et al. Oxidized Phospholipids on Apolipoprotein B-100 and Recurrent Ischemic Events Following Stroke or Transient Ischemic Attack. J Am Coll Cardiol 2017;69(2):147–58.
46. Salonen JT, Ylä-Herttuala S, Yamamoto R, et al. Autoantibody against oxidised LDL and progression of carotid atherosclerosis. Lancet 1992;339(8798):883–7.
47. Lopez LR, Simpson DF, Hurley BL, et al. OxLDL/beta2GPI complexes and auto-antibodies in patients with systemic lupus erythematosus, systemic sclerosis, and antiphospholipid syndrome: pathogenic implications for vascular involve-ment. Ann N Y Acad Sci 2005;1051:313–22.
48. Suciu CF, Prete M, Ruscitti P, et al. Oxidized low density lipoproteins: The bridge between atherosclerosis and autoimmunity. Possible implications in accelerated atherosclerosis and for immune intervention in autoimmune rheumatic disorders. Autoimmun Rev 2018;17(4):366–75.
49. Svenungsson E, Jensen-Urstad K, Heimbürger M, et al. Risk factors for cardio-vascular disease in systemic lupus erythematosus. Circulation 2001;104(16): 1887–93.
50. Grönwall C, Reynolds H, Kim JK, et al. Relation of carotid plaque with natural IgM antibodies in patients with systemic lupus erythematosus. Clin Immunol 2014;153(1):1–7.
51. Fesmire J, Wolfson-Reichlin M, Reichlin M. Effects of autoimmune antibodies anti-lipoprotein lipase, anti-low density lipoprotein, and anti-oxidized low density lipoprotein on lipid metabolism and atherosclerosis in systemic lupus erythema-tosus. Rev Bras Reumatol 2010;50(5):539–51.
52. Nowak B, Madej M, Łuczak A, et al. Disease Activity, Oxidized-LDL Fraction and Anti-Oxidized LDL Antibodies Influence Cardiovascular Risk in Rheumatoid Arthritis. Adv Clin Exp Med 2016;25(1):43–50.
53. Adorni MP, Ronda N, Bernini F, et al. High Density Lipoprotein Cholesterol Efflux Capacity and Atherosclerosis in Cardiovascular Disease: Pathophysiological Aspects and Pharmacological Perspectives. Cells 2021;10(3).
54. Soria-Florido MT, Schröder H, Grau M, et al. High density lipoprotein function-ality and cardiovascular events and mortality: A systematic review and meta-analysis. Atherosclerosis 2020;302:36–42.
55. Voloshyna I, Modayil S, Littlefield MJ, et al. Plasma from rheumatoid arthritis pa-tients promotes pro-atherogenic cholesterol transport gene expression in THP-1 human macrophages. Exp Biol Med (Maywood) 2013;238(10):1192–7.
56. Arida A, Protogerou AD, Kitas GD, et al. Systemic Inflammatory Response and Atherosclerosis: The Paradigm of Chronic Inflammatory Rheumatic Diseases. Int J Mol Sci 2018;19(7).
57. Skeoch S, Bruce IN. Atherosclerosis in rheumatoid arthritis: is it all about inflam-mation? Nat Rev Rheumatol 2015;11(7):390–400.
58. López P, Rodríguez-Carrio J, Martínez-Zapico A, et al. IgM anti-phosphorylcholine antibodies associate with senescent and IL-17+ T cells in SLE patients with a pro-inflammatory lipid profile. Rheumatology (Oxford) 2020;59(2):407–17.
59. Xing H, Pang H, Du T, et al. Establishing a Risk Prediction Model for Atheroscle-rosis in Systemic Lupus Erythematosus. Front Immunol 2021;12:622216.
60. Rajkomar A, Dean J, Kohane I. Machine Learning in Medicine. N Engl J Med 2019;380(14):1347–58.
61. Badillo S, Banfai B, Birzele F, et al. An Introduction to Machine Learning. Clin Pharmacol Ther 2020;107(4):871–85.

62. Khanna NN, Jamthikar AD, Gupta D, et al. Rheumatoid Arthritis: Atherosclerosis Imaging and Cardiovascular Risk Assessment Using Machine and Deep Learning-Based Tissue Characterization. Curr Atheroscler Rep 2019;21(2):7.

63. Triantafyllidis A, Kondylakis H, Katehakis D, et al. Deep Learning in mHealth for Cardiovascular Disease, Diabetes, and Cancer: Systematic Review. JMIR Mhealth Uhealth 2022;10(4):e32344.

64. Konstantonis G, Singh KV, Sfikakis PP, et al. Cardiovascular disease detection using machine learning and carotid/femoral arterial imaging frameworks in rheumatoid arthritis patients. Rheumatol Int 2022;42(2):215–39.

65. Navarini L, Sperti M, Currado D, et al. A machine-learning approach to cardiovascular risk prediction in psoriatic arthritis. Rheumatology (Oxford) 2020;59(7):1767–9.

66. Bartoloni E, Baldini C, Ferro F, et al. Application of artificial neural network analysis in the evaluation of cardiovascular risk in primary Sjögren's syndrome: a novel pathogenetic scenario? Clin Exp Rheumatol 2019;37:133–9. Suppl 118(3).

67. Okada DR, Xie E, Assis F, et al. Regional abnormalities on cardiac magnetic resonance imaging and arrhythmic events in patients with cardiac sarcoidosis. J Cardiovasc Electrophysiol 2019;30(10):1967–76.

68. Katsushika S, Kodera S, Nakamoto M, et al. Deep Learning Algorithm to Detect Cardiac Sarcoidosis From Echocardiographic Movies. Circ J 2021;86(1):87–95.

69. Drosos GC, Vedder D, Houben E, et al. EULAR recommendations for cardiovascular risk management in rheumatic and musculoskeletal diseases, including systemic lupus erythematosus and antiphospholipid syndrome. Ann Rheum Dis 2022;81(6):768–79.

70. Visseren FLJ, Mach F, Smulders YM, et al. ESC Guidelines on cardiovascular disease prevention in clinical practice. Eur Heart J 2021;42(34):3227–337.

71. SCORE2 risk prediction algorithms: new models to estimate 10-year risk of cardiovascular disease in Europe. Eur Heart J 2021;42(25):2439–54.

72. SCORE2-OP risk prediction algorithms: estimating incident cardiovascular event risk in older persons in four geographical risk regions. Eur Heart J 2021;42(25):2455–67.

73. Goff DC Jr, Lloyd-Jones DM, Bennett G, et al. ACC/AHA guideline on the assessment of cardiovascular risk: a report of the American College of Cardiology/American Heart Association Task Force on Practice Guidelines. J Am Coll Cardiol 2014;63(25 Pt B):2935–59.

74. Aviña-Zubieta JA, Choi HK, Sadatsafavi M, et al. Risk of cardiovascular mortality in patients with rheumatoid arthritis: a meta-analysis of observational studies. Arthritis Rheum 2008;59(12):1690–7.

75. Radovits BJ, Fransen J, Al Shamma S, et al. Excess mortality emerges after 10 years in an inception cohort of early rheumatoid arthritis. Arthritis Care Res (Hoboken) 2010;62(3):362–70.

76. Nicola PJ, Maradit-Kremers H, Roger VL, et al. The risk of congestive heart failure in rheumatoid arthritis: a population-based study over 46 years. Arthritis Rheum 2005;52(2):412–20.

77. Holmqvist ME, Wedrén S, Jacobsson LT, et al. Rapid increase in myocardial infarction risk following diagnosis of rheumatoid arthritis amongst patients diagnosed between 1995 and 2006. J Intern Med 2010;268(6):578–85.

78. Myasoedova E, Gabriel SE, Matteson EL, et al. Decreased Cardiovascular Mortality in Patients with Incident Rheumatoid Arthritis (RA) in Recent Years: Dawn of a New Era in Cardiovascular Disease in RA? J Rheumatol 2017;44(6):732–9.

79. Kerola AM, Nieminen TV, Virta LJ, et al. No increased cardiovascular mortality among early rheumatoid arthritis patients: a nationwide register study in 2000-2008. Clin Exp Rheumatol 2015;33(3):391–8.

80. Barbhaiya M, Feldman CH, Chen SK, et al. Comparative Risks of Cardiovascular Disease in Patients With Systemic Lupus Erythematosus, Diabetes Mellitus, and in General Medicaid Recipients. Arthritis Care Res (Hoboken) 2020;72(10): 1431–9.

81. Hermansen ML, Lindhardsen J, Torp-Pedersen C, et al. The risk of cardiovascular morbidity and cardiovascular mortality in systemic lupus erythematosus and lupus nephritis: a Danish nationwide population-based cohort study. Rheumatology (Oxford) 2017;56(5):709–15.

82. Polachek A, Touma Z, Anderson M, et al. Risk of Cardiovascular Morbidity in Patients With Psoriatic Arthritis: A Meta-Analysis of Observational Studies. Arthritis Care Res (Hoboken) 2017;69(1):67–74.

83. Mathieu S, Soubrier M. Cardiovascular events in ankylosing spondylitis: a 2018 meta-analysis. Ann Rheum Dis 2019;78(6):e57.

84. Kim J, Choi IA. SAT0321 cardiovascular events in spondyloarthritis : a meta-analysis. Ann Rheum Dis 2019;78(Suppl 2):1239.

85. Cen X, Feng S, Wei S, et al. Systemic sclerosis and risk of cardiovascular disease: A PRISMA-compliant systemic review and meta-analysis of cohort studies. Medicine (Baltimore) 2020;99(47):e23009.

86. Yong WC, Sanguankeo A, Upala S. Association between primary Sjögren's syndrome, cardiovascular and cerebrovascular disease: a systematic review and meta-analysis. Clin Exp Rheumatol 2018;36:190–7. Suppl 112(3).

87. Houben E, Penne EL, Voskuyl AE, et al. Cardiovascular events in anti-neutrophil cytoplasmic antibody-associated vasculitis: a meta-analysis of observational studies. Rheumatology (Oxford) 2018;57(3):555–62.

88. de Boysson H, Aouba A. An Updated Review of Cardiovascular Events in Giant Cell Arteritis. J Clin Med 2022;11(4).

89. Kim H, Barra L. Ischemic complications in Takayasu's arteritis: A meta-analysis. Semin Arthritis Rheum 2018;47(6):900–6.

90. Schieir O, Tosevski C, Glazier RH, et al. Incident myocardial infarction associated with major types of arthritis in the general population: a systematic review and meta-analysis. Ann Rheum Dis 2017;76(8):1396–404.

91. Karpouzas GA, Estis J, Rezaeian P, et al. High-sensitivity cardiac troponin I is a biomarker for occult coronary plaque burden and cardiovascular events in patients with rheumatoid arthritis. Rheumatology (Oxford) 2018;57(6):1080–8.

92. Hromádka M, Seidlerová J, Baxa J, et al. Relationship between hsTnI and coronary stenosis in asymptomatic women with rheumatoid arthritis. BMC Cardiovasc Disord 2016;16(1):184.

93. Bradham WS, Bian A, Oeser A, et al. High-sensitivity cardiac troponin-I is elevated in patients with rheumatoid arthritis, independent of cardiovascular risk factors and inflammation. PloS one 2012;7(6):e38930.

94. Colaco K, Lee KA, Akhtari S, et al. Association of Cardiac Biomarkers With Cardiovascular Outcomes in Patients With Psoriatic Arthritis and Psoriasis: A Longitudinal Cohort Study. Arthritis Rheumatol 2022;74(7):1184–92.

95. Zhou W, Abdelrahman KM, Dey AK, et al. Association Among Noncalcified Coronary Burden, Fractional Flow Reserve, and Myocardial Injury in Psoriasis. J Am Heart Assoc 2020;9(22):e017417.

96. Divard G, Abbas R, Chenevier-Gobeaux C, et al. High-sensitivity cardiac troponin T is a biomarker for atherosclerosis in systemic lupus erythematous patients: a cross-sectional controlled study. Arthritis Res Ther 2017;19(1):132.

97. Mirjafari H, Welsh P, Verstappen SM, et al. N-terminal pro-brain-type natriuretic peptide (NT-pro-BNP) and mortality risk in early inflammatory polyarthritis: results from the Norfolk Arthritis Registry (NOAR). Ann Rheum Dis 2014;73(4):684–90.

98. Goldenberg D, Miller E, Perna M, et al. Association of N-terminal pro-brain natriuretic peptide with cardiac disease, but not with vascular disease, in systemic lupus erythematosus. Arthritis Rheum 2012;64(1):316–7.

99. Anania C, Gustafsson T, Hua X, et al. Increased prevalence of vulnerable atherosclerotic plaques and low levels of natural IgM antibodies against phosphorylcholine in patients with systemic lupus erythematosus. Arthritis Res Ther 2010;12(6):R214.

100. Ahmed HM, Youssef M, Mosaad YM. Antibodies against oxidized low-density lipoprotein are associated with subclinical atherosclerosis in recent-onset rheumatoid arthritis. Clin Rheumatol 2010;29(11):1237–43.

101. Cinoku I, Mavragani CP, Tellis CC, et al. Autoantibodies to ox-LDL in Sjögren's syndrome: are they atheroprotective? Clin Exp Rheumatol 2018;36:61–7. Suppl 112(3).

102. Karpouzas GA, Ormseth SR, Hernandez E, et al. Beta-2-glycoprotein-I IgA antibodies predict coronary plaque progression in rheumatoid arthritis. Semin Arthritis Rheum 2021;51(1):20–7.

103. Sánchez-Pérez H, Quevedo-Abeledo JC, de Armas-Rillo L, et al. Impaired HDL cholesterol efflux capacity in systemic lupus erythematosus patients is related to subclinical carotid atherosclerosis. Rheumatology (Oxford) 2020;59(10):2847–56.

104. Tejera-Segura B, Macía-Díaz M, Machado JD, et al. HDL cholesterol efflux capacity in rheumatoid arthritis patients: contributing factors and relationship with subclinical atherosclerosis. Arthritis Res Ther 2017;19(1):113.

105. Chang CK, Cheng WC, Ma WL, et al. The Potential Role of Electronegative High-Density Lipoprotein H5 Subfraction in RA-Related Atherosclerosis. Int J Mol Sci 2021;22(21).

106. Karpouzas G, Papotti B, Ormseth S, et al. OP0136 SERUM CHOLESTEROL LOADING CAPACITY ON MACROPHAGES AND INTERACTIONS WITH TREATMENTS ON CORONARY ATHEROSCLEROSIS BURDEN AND EVENT RISK IN RHEUMATOID ARTHRITIS. Ann Rheum Dis 2022;81(Suppl 1):87.

107. Karpouzas G, Papotti B, Ormseth S, et al. POS0596 serum cholesterol loading capacity on macrophages is linked to oxidized low-density lipoprotein and regulated by seropositivity and c-reactive protein in patients with rheumatoid arthritis. Ann Rheum Dis 2022;81(Suppl 1):565.

108. Chang CY, Chen CH, Chen YM, et al. Association between Negatively Charged Low-Density Lipoprotein L5 and Subclinical Atherosclerosis in Rheumatoid Arthritis Patients. J Clin Med 2019;8(2).

109. García-Gómez C, Martín-Martínez MA, Fernández-Carballido C, et al. Hyperlipoproteinaemia(a) in patients with spondyloarthritis: results of the Cardiovascular in Rheumatology (CARMA) project. Clin Exp Rheumatol 2019;37(5):774–82.

110. Kiani AN, Fang H, Akhter E, et al. Apolipoprotein-containing lipoprotein subclasses and subclinical atherosclerosis in systemic lupus erythematosus. Arthritis Care Res (Hoboken) 2015;67(3):442–6.

111. Arida A, Legaki AI, Kravvariti E, et al. PCSK9/LDLR System and Rheumatoid Arthritis-Related Atherosclerosis. Front Cardiovasc Med 2021;8:738764.
112. Fang C, Luo T, Lin L. Elevation of serum proprotein convertase subtilisin/kexin type 9 (PCSK9) concentrations and its possible atherogenic role in patients with systemic lupus erythematosus. Ann Transl Med 2018;6(23):452.
113. Ferraz-Amaro I, Delgado-Frías E, Hernández-Hernández V, et al. Proprotein convertase subtilisin/kexin type 9 in patients with systemic sclerosis. Clin Exp Rheumatol 2020;38:18–24. Suppl 125(3).
114. de Armas-Rillo L, Quevedo-Abeledo JC, de Vera-González A, et al. Proprotein convertase subtilisin/kexin type 9 in the dyslipidaemia of patients with axial spondyloarthritis is related to disease activity. Rheumatology (Oxford) 2021; 60(5):2296–306.
115. Ferraz-Amaro I, López-Mejías R, Ubilla B, et al. Proprotein convertase subtilisin/kexin type 9 in rheumatoid arthritis. Clin Exp Rheumatol 2016;34(6):1013–9.
116. Liu A, Rahman M, Hafström I, et al. Proprotein convertase subtilisin kexin 9 is associated with disease activity and is implicated in immune activation in systemic lupus erythematosus. Lupus 2020;29(8):825–35.
117. Goodson NJ, Symmons DP, Scott DG, et al. Baseline levels of C-reactive protein and prediction of death from cardiovascular disease in patients with inflammatory polyarthritis: a ten-year followup study of a primary care-based inception cohort. Arthritis Rheum 2005;52(8):2293–9.
118. Innala L, Möller B, Ljung L, et al. Cardiovascular events in early RA are a result of inflammatory burden and traditional risk factors: a five year prospective study. Arthritis Res Ther 2011;13(4):R131.
119. Wållberg-Jonsson S, Johansson H, Ohman ML, et al. Extent of inflammation predicts cardiovascular disease and overall mortality in seropositive rheumatoid arthritis. A retrospective cohort study from disease onset. J Rheumatol 1999; 26(12):2562–71.
120. Shen J, Shang Q, Wong CK, et al. IL-33 and soluble ST2 levels as novel predictors for remission and progression of carotid plaque in early rheumatoid arthritis: A prospective study. Semin Arthritis Rheum 2015;45(1):18–27.
121. López-Mejías R, Genre F, Remuzgo-Martínez S, et al. Protective Role of the Interleukin 33 rs3939286 Gene Polymorphism in the Development of Subclinical Atherosclerosis in Rheumatoid Arthritis Patients. PLoS One 2015;10(11): e0143153.
122. Verma I, Krishan P, Syngle A. Predictors of Atherosclerosis in Ankylosing Spondylitis. Rheumatol Ther 2015;2(2):173–82.
123. Garg N, Krishan P, Syngle A. Atherosclerosis in Psoriatic Arthritis: A Multiparametric Analysis Using Imaging Technique and Laboratory Markers of Inflammation and Vascular Function. Int J Angiol 2016;25(4):222–8.
124. Shen J, Shang Q, Wong CK, et al. Carotid plaque and bone density and microarchitecture in psoriatic arthritis: the correlation with soluble ST2. Sci Rep 2016; 6:32116.

Myocardial Involvement in Systemic Autoimmune Rheumatic Diseases

Alexia A. Zagouras, MD, MA[a], W.H. Wilson Tang, MD[a,b],*

KEYWORDS

- Systemic autoimmune rheumatic diseases • Cardiomyopathy • Myocarditis
- Coronary microvascular dysfunction

KEY POINTS

- Cardiac disease contributes significantly to morbidity and mortality in patients with systemic autoimmune rheumatic diseases (SARDs).
- Myocardial involvement in SARDs can arise from multiple pathophysiological mechanisms, including coronary artery disease, coronary microvascular dysfunction, and myocarditis.
- Systemic lupus erythematosus, rheumatoid arthritis, systemic sclerosis, eosinophilic granulomatosis with polyangiitis, and sarcoidosis are particularly associated with myocardial involvement and heart failure (HF).
- Acute myocarditis is associated with significant morbidity and mortality, especially in sarcoidosis where it can cause sudden cardiac death.
- Further research is required to elucidate targetable mechanisms of myocardial involvement in SARDs.

INTRODUCTION

Systemic autoimmune rheumatic diseases (SARDs) are defined by a pathological disruption in self-tolerance that results in cellular- and/or antibody-mediated immune responses affecting at least two organ systems. Cardiac involvement in SARDs is a relatively common but underappreciated phenomenon that has significant implications for morbidity and mortality. A recent study of mortality in a group of Dutch patients with SARDs from 2013 to 2017 found that diseases of the circulatory system accounted for 55.5% of listed causes of death, with 35.7% of mortalities attributable to nonischemic heart disease and 10.1% attributable to ischemic heart disease.[1]

a Cleveland Clinic Lerner College of Medicine at Case Western Reserve University, , EC-10 Cleveland Clinic, 9501 Euclid Avenue, Cleveland, OH 44195, USA; b Kaufman Center for Heart Failure Treatment and Recovery, Heart Vascular and Thoracic Institute, Cleveland Clinic, Cleveland, OH, USA
* Corresponding author. 9500 Euclid Avenue, Desk J3-4, Cleveland, OH 44195.
E-mail address: tangw@ccf.org

Rheum Dis Clin N Am 49 (2023) 45–66
https://doi.org/10.1016/j.rdc.2022.08.002   rheumatic.theclinics.com
0889-857X/23/© 2022 Elsevier Inc. All rights reserved.

Inflammation in SARDs can affect many heart tissues, including the myocardium, pericardium, valves, and coronary vasculature.[2] Myocardial involvement in SARDs is often overlooked, but with greater access to advanced cardiac imaging modalities detection and more aggressive immunosuppressive therapies, the natural history of SARDs has been favorably impacted. In this review, the authors focus specifically on myocardial involvement in SARDs, including effects of vascular pathology on heart muscle. Potential mechanisms of myocardial damage in SARDs include coronary artery disease (CAD), microvascular dysfunction, and myocarditis. The authors detail current evidence regarding myocardial involvement in systemic lupus erythematosus (SLE), rheumatoid arthritis (RA), systemic sclerosis (SSc), eosinophilic granulomatosis with polyangiitis (EGPA), granulomatosis with polyangiitis (GPA), primary Sjogren's syndrome (pSS), sarcoidosis, spondyloarthropathies, and inflammatory myopathies. Potential myocardial toxicities of immunomodulatory medications used in these conditions are also discussed. Finally, the authors review current recommendations for the evaluation and treatment of myocardial disease in patients with SARDs.

MECHANISMS OF MYOCARDIAL INVOLVEMENT IN SYSTEMIC AUTOIMMUNE RHEUMATIC DISEASES

Myocardial involvement in SARDs falls into three general categories of pathophysiology: macrovascular disease, microvascular dysfunction, and myocarditis.[3,4] Significant overlap exists among these three pathophysiological mechanisms, though each may predominate in different SARDs or under different conditions. All three may contribute to clinically apparent cardiomyopathy (CM), conduction abnormalities, and/or heart failure (HF), or to subclinical cardiac damage. Although subclinical myocardial involvement may not contribute to disease morbidity in terms of symptomatology, both clinical and subclinical CM are associated with increased mortality in several SARDs (**Fig. 1**). The authors discuss these three general mechanisms contributing to clinical and subclinical myocardial damage in SARDs before diving into disease-specific implications.

Coronary Artery Disease

Macrovascular disease in SARDs refers to the increased development of atherosclerosis leading to CAD. Although not intrinsic to the myocardium, ischemia secondary to CAD causes myocardial injury and aberrant remodeling, which may in turn lead to ischemic CM and HF. Several SARDs are associated with accelerated atherosclerosis and increased prevalence of CAD, with most studies focusing on RA and SLE.[5–7] The relationship between chronic systemic inflammation and atherosclerosis is thought to

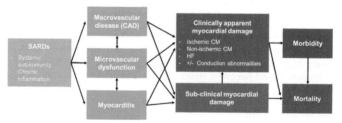

Fig. 1. Mechanisms and manifestations of myocardial involvement in systemic autoimmune rheumatic disease (SARDs). CAD, coronary artery disease; CM, cardiomyopathy; HF, heart failure.

stem from shared inflammatory mechanisms that drive both processes, such as the release of the pro-inflammatory cytokines tumor necrosis factor (TNF)-α and interleukin (IL)-6.[8] TNF-α and IL-6 activate the nuclear factor κ-B pathway, contributing to downstream vascular endothelial cell dysfunction, promoting leukocyte infiltration of the subendothelial space, and thereby perpetuating local inflammation and promoting atherosclerosis.[8,9] Vascular cell adhesion protein 1 expression on endothelial cells further contributes to this pathological leukocyte migration and has also been associated with accelerated atherosclerosis in SARDs.[10] Meanwhile, dyslipidemia is also common in patients with SARDs and likely contributes to increased atherosclerotic burden with various proinflammatory pathophysiologic processes.

Coronary Microvascular Dysfunction

Coronary microvascular dysfunction (CMD) also contributes to myocardial disease in chronic inflammatory diseases. Although macrovascular dysfunction refers to atherosclerosis at the level of the epicardial coronary arteries (diameter range of ~500 μm to ~5 mm), mechanisms of microvascular dysfunction affect the pre-arterioles (~100–500 μm) and arterioles (<100 μm).[11] CMD is characterized by failure of the coronary microcirculation to adequately match the myocardial oxygen supply with demand.[12] CMD can arise in the setting of CAD but can also manifest independently from CAD via other pathogenic mechanisms that promote microvascular remodeling, endothelial cell dysfunction, and/or smooth muscle dysfunction.[12] Of note, CMD has been implicated in the pathogenesis of HF with preserved ejection fraction (HFpEF), where is it also associated with myocardial oxidative stress, myocardial fibrosis, cardiac hypertrophy, and resulting diastolic dysfunction.[13,14] Unlike CAD, which can be observed directly via angiography, CMD is often difficult to diagnose and cannot be visualized in vivo without physiologic perturbations. Rather, CMD is assessed by measuring the coronary flow reserve (CFR), the ratio of blood flow in response to vasoactive stimuli to baseline blood flow.[12,15] CFR may be measured invasively during coronary angiography using an intracoronary pressure wire, or estimated from echocardiography, computed tomography, or positron emission tomography (PET) imaging.[12,15] CMD may also be assessed using cardiac magnetic resonance (CMR) imaging with gadolinium contrast under vasoactive stress, as gadolinium uptake in the myocardium correlates with microvascular function.[12] Abnormal myocardial blood flow estimated by PET or CMR imaging may also be suggestive.

Although the mechanisms of microvascular damage are not as well understood, the proinflammatory mechanisms that contribute to CAD in SARDs likely also contribute to CMD.[12] Several studies have demonstrated a close relationship between CMD and chronic inflammation. One such study of 268 asymptomatic male twins demonstrated an association between lower CFR (measured via PET) and higher white blood cell count, as well as C-reactive protein (CRP), IL-6, and intercellular adhesion molecule-1 levels.[16] The relationship between CMD and inflammatory mechanisms has also been shown in patients with SARDs. Yilmaz and colleagues[17] demonstrated an association between increased oxidative stress markers and decreased CFR a measured via Doppler echocardiography. The inflammatory marker soluble urokinase-type plasminogen activator receptor, which has been implicated in several mechanisms of RA and SLE pathogenesis, is also associated with CMD in patients without obstructive CAD.[18–20] CMD is an especially important contributor to cardiac pathology in SSc and appears to be mediated by similar pathogenic mechanisms that contribute to the characteristic systemic vasculopathy and fibrosis in these patients.[21] As demonstrated by studies of the murine Fos-related antigen-2 overexpression model of SSc, endothelial cell dysfunction and apoptosis cause microvascular dysfunction, leading to leukocyte infiltration of perivascular myocardial tissue and subsequent fibroblast activation.[22–24]

Finally, there is evidence to suggest that in addition to coronary microvascular dysfunction, lymphatic microvascular dysfunction may also play a role in the pathogenesis of myocardial damage in SARDs. A recent study by Rossitto and colleagues[25] demonstrated rarefaction of small peripheral blood and lymphatic vessels in patients with HFpEF compared with controls, associated with impaired lymphatic drainage in the HFpEF cohort. The investigators conclude that reduced lymphatic reserve secondary to peripheral blood and lymphatic microvascular dysfunction may contribute to the pathophysiology of HFpEF. Studies in SARD patients, particularly in SSc and RA, have also demonstrated the role of autoimmune-mediated lymphatic microvascular damage in the perpetuation of organ damage in these patients.[26–28] It is possible that in addition to the direct effects of coronary microvascular dysfunction on the myocardium, peripheral lymphatic microvascular dysfunction in SARDs also contributes to myocardial strain and damage by altering systemic fluid homeostasis. However, as there are limited imaging modalities to visualize lymphatic dysfunction or reserve, the true prevalence and clinical significance of lymphatic microvascular dysfunction in patients with SARDs is not well understood.

Myocarditis

A third major mechanism of myocardial damage in SARDs is myocarditis. The term myocarditis can be used to describe both a chronic pathophysiological phenomenon of inflammation directly affecting the myocardium, which can contribute either clinically or subclinically to cardiac pathology in SARDs, and the clinical syndrome arising from fulminant myocardial inflammation, which can lead to dilated CM and/or HF. Myocarditis in SARDs can be both cell- and antibody-mediated. The classic histopathological findings of myocarditis on endomyocardial biopsy (EMB) include patchy T cell, macrophage ("giant cell"), and/or eosinophil infiltration, which may be followed by fibrosis and scarring.[29] Although not visible on histology, pathogenic cardiac autoimmunization also seems to play a role in the development and perpetuation of myocarditis. Autoantibodies to the beta-1 and beta-2 adrenergic receptors (ARs), myosin, troponin T, and other cardiac proteins have been studied in myocarditis and dilated CM.[30–32] The antigenic role of myosin in myocarditis has been particularly well studied. Murine models of myocarditis have been generated by immunization with cardiac myosin, and anti-myosin antibodies have been detected in human myocarditis.[33,34] Interestingly, human cardiac myosin also seems to function as an endogenous toll-like receptor ligand, directly stimulating CD14+ monocytes, leading to an exaggerated proinflammatory cytokine response promoting myocardial inflammation, fibrosis, and eventual CM.[35] In addition, beta-1 AR autoantibodies have been linked to a potential autoimmune mechanism of dilated CM and HF, with antibody binding to the beta-1 receptor on cardiomyocytes perpetuating a sustained pro-adrenergic response, and leading to cardiomyocyte apoptosis and eventual fibrosis.[36] Recent studies, however, have also described a potential cardioprotective role of the immunoglobulin G3 subclass of beta-1 AR autoantibodies, indicating that anticardiac autoantibodies may serve other pathophysiological roles besides perpetuating myocardial damage.[37] Although studies of anticardiac antibodies have mostly focused on patients with acute myocarditis, dilated CM, or HF, some have examined their role in patients with SARDs. Activating antibodies again the endothelin-1 type A receptor and the angiotensin II type 1 receptor have been associated with profibrotic mechanisms in SSc.[38] Autoantibodies against ion channels as well as contractile or intercalated proteins have also been implicated in arrhythmic syndromes including atrial or ventricular tachyarrhythmia or heart blocks.[30] Further research is required to establish the role of anticardiac antibodies in autoimmune myocarditis and to identify targetable mechanisms of cellular and humoral autoimmunity affecting the myocardium in patients with SARDs.

DISEASE-SPECIFIC IMPLICATIONS FOR MYOCARDIAL INVOLVEMENT
Systemic Lupus Erythematosus

SLE is a heterogenous autoimmune condition characterized by autoreactive antinuclear antibodies and immune complex and complement deposition resulting in inflammation and damage to multiple organs.[39,40] Cardiac involvement occurs in over 50% of SLE patients, with pericarditis being the most common manifestation. Although up to 25% of patients with SLE develop pericarditis, clinically apparent myocarditis and CM are less common.[4,41] Patients who do develop clinically apparent SLE myocarditis can present with symptoms of HF, chest pain, fever, or pericarditis. A retrospective multicenter French study of lupus myocarditis patients from 2000 to 2014 found that in 58%, myocarditis was the presenting sign of SLE.[42] The rate of subclinical SLE myocarditis discovered on autopsy seems to have decreased with improved corticosteroid treatment; however, more recent imaging studies have revealed a significant rate of subclinical myocarditis.[43,44] Of note, Mavrogeni and colleagues[44] found that CMR was a reliable and noninvasive method for detecting subclinical myocarditis in SLE patients, with signs of myocarditis on CMR (specifically, increased T2 ratio and early gadolinium enhancement) present in 16/20 active SLE patients. Interestingly, they found CMR to be a more reliable method of diagnosis than EMB, likely due to the patchy nature of myocardial involvement in SLE.[44,45]

SLE diagnosis is associated with an increased risk of HF independent of cardiovascular (CV) risk factors and chronic kidney disease (CKD).[46] Left ventricular (LV) systolic and diastolic function are decreased in SLE patients compared with controls in a 2016 meta-analysis of case-control studies.[47] Imaging studies have also identified a significant rate of subclinical LV diastolic dysfunction in SLE patients, with increased SLE disease severity associated with the development of diastolic dysfunction.[48–50] In a study of 82 pairs of SLE patients and controls, Shang and colleagues[51] found a significant relationship between the long-term inflammatory burden of SLE as measured by the Systemic Lupus International Collaborating Clinics/American College of Rheumatology (SLICC/ACR) damage index and the development of diastolic dysfunction. In addition, in a recent study by Chorin and colleagues,[52] serum levels of the SLE disease activity markers ST2 and CXCL-10 were significantly correlated with diastolic dysfunction parameters on echocardiography. Taken together, these findings indicate a likely connection between chronic subclinical myocarditis in SLE and the development of LV diastolic dysfunction and possible HF; however, additional research is required to elucidate the mechanisms driving this myocardial pathology. Among the SARD population, SLE patients are more likely to present in the form of HF with reduced ejection fraction (HFrEF).[53] Fortunately, many SLE patients demonstrate some improvement in their impaired systolic function with intensification of immunosuppressive therapy and guideline-directed HF therapies, such as neurohormonal antagonists.

Another component to the spectrum of SLE myocardial disease is congenital heart block in neonatal lupus.[41,54] Several studies have suggested that maternal anti-Ro/SSA autoantibodies that cross the placenta during gestation are associated with the development of fetal myocarditis and heart block characteristic of neonatal lupus in 60% to 90% of cases.[55,56] It is unclear why the same association between anti-Ro/SSA autoantibodies and heart block has not been seen in adults, but it is thought that an unknown circulating fetal factor may play a role. Children affected with neonatal lupus and congenital heart block may also develop dilated CM, endomyocardial fibroelastosis and mitral insufficiency, and ultimately HF requiring cardiac transplantation.[57] A recent study by Izmirly and colleagues[58] of 54 anti-SSA positive mothers who had a previous pregnancy complicated by congenital heart block, demonstrated a greater than 50% reduction in recurrence of congenital heart block among women who took hydroxychloroquine during pregnancy. Further research is required to understand the pathophysiology and treatment of congenital heart block in children of mothers with SLE and other rheumatological conditions.

Rheumatoid Arthritis

RA is among the most prevalent SARDs and is characterized by synovial inflammation, adjacent bone and cartilage destruction, autoantibody production, and multiorgan involvement.[59] The primary cardiac burden in RA is CAD and ischemic heart disease, with multiple large cohort studies identifying increased risk of CV disease and myocardial infarction in this population.[60–62] There is also an established link between inflammation in RA and increased atherosclerosis risk.[6,7,9] Incident HF risk is also increased in RA. This is attributable in part to ischemic CM, but the association between HF and RA also persists independent of traditional CV risk factors. A population-based retrospective study over 46 years in Rochester, Minnesota, found that RA diagnosis was associated with an 87% increased risk of incident HF after adjusting for demographics, ischemic heart disease, and other CV risk factors.[63] Interestingly, in this study, RA patients who were rheumatoid factor positive had a higher risk of incident HF compared with those that were negative, indicating a correlation between increased disease severity and risk of HF.[63] Prasada and colleagues[46] reported a similar finding, with RA diagnosis associated with an approximate 40% increased risk of HF in their cohort, after adjusting for CV risk factors and CKD (**Fig. 2**). They also found that higher CRP levels were associated with increased risk of incident HF, with RA patients with peak CRP level greater than 3 having a 2.6-fold increased risk of HF compared with controls.[46] These results indicate that an underlying inflammatory mechanism affecting the myocardium contributes to HF risk in RA patients. In fact, 3% to 30% of cases of CM in RA are associated with focal lymphocytic, diffuse

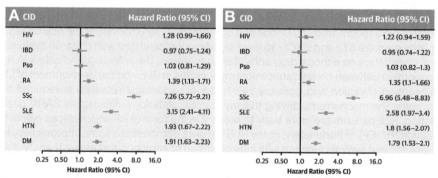

Fig. 2. Heart failure risks according to subtypes of chronic inflammatory diseases. Model adjusted for (*A*) age, sex, race, insurance status, baseline diabetes (DM), and hypertension (HTN); (*B*) all variables in (*A*) plus chronic kidney disease. HIV, human immunodeficiency syndrome; IBD, inflammatory bowel disease; Pso, psoriatic arthritis; RA, rheumatoid arthritis; SSc, systemic sclerosis; SLE, systemic lupus erythematosus. (*Reproduced from Ref.*[46]; *with permission*.)

necrotizing, or granulomatous myocarditis.[4,64,65] Histologically, cardiac granulomas detected in RA patients at autopsy are identical to rheumatoid nodules. Recent CMR studies have revealed cardiac involvement in asymptomatic RA patients as well, including signs of inflammation and fibrosis, indicating that subclinical myocardial involvement may be more common than previously thought.[66,67]

Systemic Sclerosis

SSc is a rare SARD characterized by systemic vascular dysfunction and multiorgan fibrosis, most notably of the skin. Patients with SSc can be subcategorized into three distinct categories based on extent of skin tightness: in limited cutaneous SSc (lcSSc) skin tightness is confined distally to the elbows and knees; in diffuse cutaneous SSc (dcSSc) skin tightness affects the proximal extremities, chest, and/or abdomen; and in SSc sine scleroderma skin tightness is not present but internal organs are involved.[68] SSc has the highest mortality rate of all SARDs and is associated with a high rate of clinical and subclinical cardiac involvement, with the prevalence of SSc-CM ranging from 7% to 39% per comprehensive review.[69]

SSc patients are often closely monitored with echocardiography to assess for pulmonary hypertension (PH), which is common in this population and can arise from primary pulmonary arterial hypertension (PAH) or secondary to intrinsic lung disease (most commonly pulmonary fibrosis) or intrinsic left heart disease.[70,71] Although PAH has historically been thought to account for the majority of PH burden in SSc, recent studies have suggested that the LV dysfunction is relatively common in these patients as well, especially in the form of HF with mildly reduced or preserved ejection fraction. In fact, a recent retrospective study of 53 SSc patients with PH found that 55% had PAH and 45% had evidence of left heart disease on routine right or left heart catheterization.[72] Prasada and colleagues[46] report that SSc is associated with a 7-fold increased incident HF risk when controlling for CV risk factors and CKD (see **Fig. 2**). There is also evidence that mortality is increased in SSc when there is concomitant left heart dysfunction. Bourji and colleagues[73] studied 117 patients with SSc and PH and found that those patients with PH secondary to HFpEF experienced twice the mortality risk of those with PAH, after adjusting for hemodynamic prognostic factors. Subclinical diastolic dysfunction is also common, with up to a third of SSc patients demonstrating evidence of diastolic dysfunction on routine echocardiography.[74,75] In addition, diastolic dysfunction in the absence of HF is associated with mortality in SSc, with one study reporting a 57% mortality rate for patients with diastolic dysfunction versus 13% without, after a median 3.4 year follow-up.[76]

Advanced cardiac imaging has also revealed evidence of myocardial involvement in SSc. CFR measured by echocardiographic pulsed-wave Doppler analysis is reduced in SSc patients, even without clinical signs of cardiac dysfunction.[77–79] Studies of SSc patients using speckle tracking echocardiography have demonstrated heterogenous patterns of regional heart strain, including decreased global longitudinal and circumferential strain, suggestive of occult myocardial disease.[80,81] CMR studies in SSc have also demonstrated a significant prevalence of silent myocarditis and subclinical fibrosis that is correlated with disease severity (increased fibrosis in SSc versus lcSSc).[82,83]

Myocardial damage in SSc is thought to be mediated largely by CMD, low-grade chronic myocarditis, cardiomyocyte apoptosis, and replacement fibrosis.[84] This fibrosis mirrors fibrosis occurring in other organs, such as the skin and the lungs, and results in increased myocardial stiffness, decreased ventricular compliance, resulting in diastolic dysfunction.[85,86] A recent histological study by De Luca and colleagues[87] showed increased fibrosis in SSc-myocarditis EMB tissue compared with non-SSc virus-negative samples. In addition, there was a close correlation between SSc-myocarditis on histology and HF diagnosis, but the degree of fibrosis was not significantly different between those SSc patients with and without HF, indicating that myocardial fibrosis may be an early sign of subclinical SSc-CM. There is evidence that autoantibodies play a role in SSc myocarditis and CM. Seropositivity for anti-Ku, anti-RNA polymerase III, or anti-U3-ribonculeoprotein (RNP) antibodies is associated with increased risk of SSc-CM.[88] Although these characteristic SSc autoantibodies are directed against nuclear antigens, antibodies directed against certain intrinsic vascular and cardiac proteins, such as titin, the endothelin-1 type A receptor, and the angiotensin II type 1 receptor, have been detected in SSc as well.[38,89,90] As mentioned previously, lymphatic microvascular dysfunction may also play a role in abnormal fluid homeostasis contributing to HF in SSc, as lymphatic microangiopathy has been observed in SSc.[25,91]

Eosinophilic Granulomatosis with Polyangiitis

Formerly called Churg-Strauss syndrome, this relatively rare but serious multisystemic disease is an eosinophil-rich, antineutrophilic cytoplasmic antibody (ANCA)-associated vasculitis that predominantly affects small to medium vessels. EGPA is often associated with asthma and eosinophilia that often do not respond to immunosuppressive treatment, with common findings of nasal polyps and necrotizing granulomatous and non-granulomatous extravascular inflammation.[92] Cardiac involvement in EGPA is estimated to occur in 15% to 60% of patients, and CM affects up to 30%.[93] CM is more prevalent in ANCA-negative cases of EGPA and is associated with higher eosinophil counts.[94,95] There is an association of ANCA positivity (~40% of cases) with more kidney and peripheral nervous system involvement and constitutional symptoms.

Cardiac involvement shows mixture of eosinophilic infiltration in myocardium and endocardium causing myocarditis and endocarditis and small vessel vasculitis.[4,96] The presence of CM in EGPA is associated with worse prognosis and should always be evaluated when diagnosis of EGPA is confirmed. Specifically, about half of the deaths in EGPA are related to cardiac disease and occur within the first few months after diagnosis.[95,97] Cardiac involvement in EGPA can also be subclinical, with 60% of patients in apparent clinical remission demonstrating abnormalities on echocardiography (ECG), or CMR in one study.[98] Therefore, patients with EGPA, even in asymptomatic cases, should be routinely assessed for cardiac involvement by CMR imaging to detect a wide range of presentations from pericarditis, pericardial effusion, acute HF, acute myocardial infarction, valvular heart disease, to myocarditis.[95,99] Cardiac involvement usually warrants more aggressive immunosuppressive therapy such as high-dose corticosteroids, cyclophosphamide (CP), or considerations for mepolizumab (an IL-5 inhibitor).[100,101]

Granulomatosis with Polyangiitis

GPA, formally called Wegener's granulomatosis, is another rare ANCA-associated vasculitis that may present with myocardial involvement, though less frequently than EGPA.[93] GPA is a small and medium vessel vasculitis that mostly affects the upper and lower respiratory tract, kidneys, and central nervous system.[102] Cardiac involvement has been observed in 3% to 13% of patients with GPA, and of those with cardiac involvement, CM accounts for 30%.[4,103,104] In some studies, cardiac involvement in GPA is associated with negative prognosis including symptomatic vasculitis relapse.[104,105] Cases of acute myocarditis have been reported in GPA as well.[106,107] Immunosuppressive treatment is necessary to avoid fatality in GPA, and because cardiac involvement has been associated with worse prognosis, escalation of immunomodulatory treatment may be warranted in such cases.[4,108] There is also evidence of subclinical myocardial involvement in GPA. One retrospective study of 85 patients identified echocardiographic abnormalities attributable to GPA in 36%, with a significantly increased mortality rate among this group of patients with subclinical myocardial involvement.[109]

Primary Sjögren's Syndrome

Sjögren's syndrome can occur secondary to another autoimmune condition or, less commonly, as a primary autoimmune disease. SS mainly affects exocrine glands, but more than a third of patients with pSS also have extraglandular involvement.[110] There is conflicting evidence regarding increased risk of MI and cerebrovascular events in pSS and that question remains unclear.[111,112] Several echocardiographic studies have demonstrated the increased rates of subclinical LV diastolic dysfunction and/or PH in primary pSS.[113–115] Myocarditis is relatively uncommon in pSS, though a few isolated cases have been reported.[4,116,117] As seen in SLE, the presence of maternal SSA or SSB antibodies in pSS have been associated with congenital heart block, which can lead to pediatric HF.[118] Of note, infant CHB can be a presenting symptom of pSS in yet asymptomatic mothers carrying the SSA/SSB antibodies who may develop clinically apparent pSS in the future.[118] Therefore, mothers of infants with CHB should be tested for the presence of SSA/SSB antibodies and followed up long term.[119]

Sarcoidosis

Sarcoidosis is unique among SARDs, in that it is characterized by systemic granuloma formation, most commonly affecting the hilar lymph nodes, lungs, skin, and heart.[119,120] The environmental antigen that triggers granuloma formation in individuals genetically susceptible to sarcoid is unknown, but the resulting T cell and inflammatory cytokine immune response leads to the formation of granulomas with a core of mononuclear cells surrounded by majority CD4+ T cells with some CD8+ T cells and B cells.[120] Cardiac granuloma characteristics of cardiac sarcoidosis have been reported in up to 25% of sarcoidosis patients at autopsy, though in keeping with the pattern seen in other SARDs, more than half of these cases are likely subclinical.[120–122] The prevalence of clinically apparent cardiac sarcoidosis is debated and may vary due to the lack of standardized diagnostic criteria.[120] The ACCESS study found that only 2.3% of sarcoidosis patients ($n = 736$) were diagnosed with cardiac sarcoid based on their defined criteria.[123] Interestingly, cardiac sarcoidosis seems to be more prevalent in the Japanese population compared with the United States population, with 68% prevalence of cardiac sarcoidosis on autopsy in Japan versus 16% in the United States.[124]

  Cardiac involvement of sarcoidosis is perhaps most familiar to the cardiology consultants because of its primary CV manifestations. The morbidity and mortality burden of cardiac sarcoidosis is high due to the potential of significant cardiac tissue disruption caused by granulomas. Although granulomatous inflammation in cardiac sarcoidosis can present anywhere, the most commonly affected locations are the LV free wall, posterior interventricular septum, papillary muscles, right ventricle, and atria.[4,125] Patients with symptomatic cardiac sarcoidosis can present with palpitations, syncope, or HF, and the presence of these symptoms in a patient with known sarcoidosis should raise concern for cardiac involvement.[120] Cardiac involvement in sarcoidosis can also present as sudden onset ventricular tachycardia and nonischemic CM, even in the absence of initial systemic symptoms, and up to 25% of patients present with sudden cardiac death.[120,126,127] Other possible presentations of cardiac sarcoid include atrioventricular block, brady-tachyarrhythmias, HF signs or symptoms, LV diastolic or systolic dysfunction on echocardiography or CMR imaging, or abnormal tissue uptake patterns on CMR or PET.[4,120] These clinical symptoms or findings can be linked directly to granulomatous infiltration and adjacent scar tissue development causing disruption of electrical conduction and/or myocardial function.[120] Although corticosteroids and other immunomodulatory drugs can be used to treat cardiac sarcoidosis, often patients will require pacemaker or internal cardioverter defibrillator (ICD) implantation, or even cardiac transplant.[120,125] Further study is required to establish methods to prevent cardiac sarcoidosis and associated potentially lethal complications in these patients.

Spondyloarthropathies

Spondyloarthropathies are characterized by axial joint involvement and include psoriatic arthritis (PsA), ankylosing spondylitis (AS), and arthritis associated with inflammatory bowel disease (IBD). CV disease is the leading cause of death in PsA, attributable to 20% to 56% of mortality.[128,129] There is conflicting data regarding the burden of CV mortality in PsA compared with the general population, with some studies demonstrating increased CV mortality, with a standardized mortality ratio of 1.4 to 1.6, and others demonstrating no change.[129–131] Similar heterogeneity of data exists for AS, though several studies have an increased risk of CV death among AS patients compared with the general population.[131,132] Interestingly, there is an increased prevalence of risk factors for CVD and HF, including hypertension, obesity, hyperlipemia, type 2 diabetes mellitus, and past CV events, in patients with PsA compared with those with psoriasis limited to the skin.[133,134] This indicates that the systemic inflammation present in PsA and absent in psoriasis may contribute to increased CV risk. In their 2020 study, Prasada and colleagues[46] found that PsA and IBD were not associated with increased risk of incident HF when controlling for traditional HF risk factors. This indicates that CV and HF risk in PsA is likely primarily mediated by increased metabolic risk factors rather than an autoimmune mechanism directly affecting the myocardium.

Inflammatory Myopathy

The category of inflammatory myopathy (IM) includes dermatomyositis, polymyositis, necrotizing autoimmune myositis, inclusion body myositis, and overlap myositis. All of these conditions are characterized by inflammation affecting skeletal muscles. CV mortality in IM is between 5% and 17%, and the most frequent causes are myocardial infarction, HF, and myocarditis.[4,135] A systematic review of literature regarding cardiac involvement in adult polymyositis or dermatomyositis found that HF is the most common clinical manifestation of cardiac involvement, with clinically apparent HF documented in 32% to 77% of patients studied.[135] The investigators additionally found a wide range of rates of subclinical cardiac involvement in these patients of 13% to 72%, with 42% of patients exhibiting LV diastolic dysfunction on echocardiography in one study ($n = 32$).[135,136] Myocarditis can occur in IM patients with imflammatory myopathies, including biopsy-proven lymphocytic and giant cell myocarditis.[135,137,138] However, most myocarditis in IM seems to be subclinical, with histological myocarditis present in up to 30% of autopsied patients.[139] In a longitudinal study of 162 cases of IM, cardiac involvement was a significant independent prognostic factor for death.[140]

Disease-Modifying Antirheumatic Drug Cardiotoxicity

Several disease-modifying antirheumatic drugs (DMARDs) used to treat SARDs are associated with adverse CV effects, including myocardial damage. Hydroxychloroquine (HCQ) is an antimalarial drug used widely in SARDs, particularly in SLE, RA, and SS. Its rheumatological mechanism of action is not completely elucidated but likely involves disruption of lysosomal activity, autophagy, and signaling pathways, including toll-like receptor signaling on antigen-presenting immune cells.[141] HCQ is has been associated with QT-segment prolongation, and rare cases of HCQ-induced CM have been reported.[141-143] However, evidence that HCQ therapy increases risk of CM or HF on a population level is lacking.

TNF-α antagonists represent a large class of biologic DMARDs used primarily in the treatment of RA, spondyloarthropathies, psoriasis, and other autoimmune conditions.[144] TNF-α inhibitors have also been associated with adverse cardiac outcomes in patients with HF. Although TNF-α-mediated inflammation is thought to play a role in HF, clinical trials of TNF-α inhibitors in HF have demonstrated no effect at low doses and adverse effect on clinical condition in patients with moderate-to-severe HFrEF at high doses.[145-147] As a result, this class of drugs is contraindicated in patients with existing HF, although there is no evidence that TNF-α inhibitor therapy increases risk of incident HF.

Cyclophosphamide is an anticancer drug that is also used in the treatment of certain SARDs, including RA and SLE.[148] CP is an alkylating agent that is metabolized by cytochrome P450 and other enzymes into toxic metabolites that act on DNA, causing tumor death or immunosuppression, and can also damage endothelial cells and cardiomyocytes.[148,149] Cardiotoxic effects of CP are dose-related and manifest as an acute CM over days to weeks following treatment.[150] Although the incidence is higher among patients with cancer receiving high doses in chemotherapy regimens, CP cardiotoxicity has been reported in a wide range of doses and therefore should always be considered when using CP in SARDs.[150]

Clinical Recommendations

Because myocardial involvement in SARDs presents in a disease-specific manner, there is no one diagnostic algorithm to encompass assessment or management of all SARDs. However, some guiding principles can be useful in the approach to myocardial disease in this population. In any SARD patient (or yet undiagnosed SARD patient), acute myocarditis should be suspected with the presence of certain concerning symptoms, such as unexplained dyspnea, chest pain, syncope, new arrythmia, acute or chronic HF, sudden cardiac death or aborted lethal arrythmia, or cardiogenic shock.[119,151] In addition to autoimmune etiology of myocarditis in a SARD patient presenting with such symptoms, it is also important to consider the possibility of infectious myocarditis, especially in the setting of therapeutic chronic immunosuppression.[119] Owing to the increased risk of CAD and CMD in many SARDs, ischemic etiology of new or worsening cardiac symptoms should also be ruled out. Biomarkers such as troponin or natriuretic peptides, such as N-terminal-pro hormone BNP (NT-proBNP), may be used to assess cardiac function in such a case, though it is important to note that myocarditis can present with or without elevation of either.[119] Doppler echocardiography is recommended for all SARD patients with concern for myocardial involvement and is additionally useful for evaluation of possible pericardial or valvular involvement as well. Annual echocardiography is recommended for SSc patients due to the high rate of PH and should also be used to evaluate for LV systolic or diastolic function.[152] As advanced imaging modalities are becoming more widely available, CMR and PET imaging provide greater sensitivity in detecting cardiac involvement and has the benefit of providing better resolution and tissue characterization for diagnosis and risk stratification for SARD patients. CMR can be used to differentiate ischemic versus inflammatory myocardial damage, when echocardiography is inconclusive, and PET imaging can be useful in visualizing inflammation in sarcoidosis specifically.[119] EMB is the gold standard for the diagnosis of myocarditis and histopathological analysis can distinguish between different etiologies.[119]

Treatment guidelines for myocarditis in SARDs include optimizing immunosuppressive therapy with disease-specific indications. Despite risks of immunosuppression, diagnosis of acute myocarditis with evidence of impaired LV function often indicates escalation to aggressive immunosuppression with corticosteroids to prevent irreversible organ damage and improve survival.[4,119,120] The approach to cardiac sarcoidosis management is similar, as consensus guidelines are lacking. A modified Delphi study among sarcoid experts in the United states in 2021 revealed low to moderate agreement overall, although there was agreement in the use of steroids ($\leq$40 mg prednisone daily) for treatment of cardiac sarcoid with evidence of myocardial or conduction system damage on imaging or electrocardiogram.[120,153] DMARDs, such as TNF-α inhibitors, may also be used in the treatment of cardiac sarcoidosis. A recent retrospective study of 77 cardiac sarcoidosis patients by Baker and colleagues[154] found that those that were treated with TNF-α inhibitors ($n = 20$) did not experience worsening HF, and in fact saw clinical benefit as assessed by changes in advanced imaging, echocardiography, and steroid use. In the case of refractory and potentially lethal tachy- or brady-arrythmias, pacemaker or ICD implantation may be indicated, and in the case of refractory HF, cardiac transplantation may be necessary in these patients.[120,125]

HF in SARDs, especially when presented with impaired LV ejection fraction or cardiac remodeling, should be aggressively treated according to current goal-directed standards of management with beta-blockers, angiotensin receptor neprilysin inhibitors, mineralocorticoid-receptor antagonists, and sodium-glucose transporter 2 inhibitors, in addition to optimization of disease-modifying immunosuppression and management of comorbidities that also contribute to HF risk, such as hypertension, diabetes, dyslipidemia, and thyroid dysfunction. SARD patients with HF should be routinely monitored with echocardiography, ECG, and cardiac biomarkers. Although routine CFR measurement to assess for microvascular dysfunction is not current practice, this may change in the future with more advanced cardiac imaging and a greater appreciation for the role of microvascular coronary dysfunction in SARDs.[15] Because most myocardial involvement in SARDs is subclinical, routine cardiac and risk factor screening is very important in this population to ensure that overt myocardial involvement is not missed. Finally, multidisciplinary and collaborative management of myocardial disease in SARDs patients is of great importance, as many of these patients will require close follow-up by both rheumatology and cardiology.

SUMMARY

Systemic autoimmune diseases are defined by their potential to affect multiple organ systems, and when treating patients with SARDs it is important to consider the possibility of myocardial involvement to avoid missing life-threatening complications. Myocardial involvement in SARDs is mediated by macrovascular disease (CAD), microvascular dysfunction, and myocarditis. These three mechanisms manifest differently by SARD diagnosis. SLE, RA, SSc, EGPA, and sarcoidosis are associated with the greatest risks of clinical and subclinical myocardial damage and HF, though myocardial involvement can be seen in other SARDs, such as pSS, spondyloarthropathies, and IM as well. Certain DMARDs are associated with cardiotoxicity and may also contribute to myocardial damage in SARD patients. Management of myocardial involvement must be disease-specific, but general guidelines include treating acute myocarditis with increased corticosteroids and optimization of the immunosuppressive medication regimen. Myocardial disease is associated with increased morbidity and mortality in patients with SARDs. Further research is needed to reveal the mechanisms or genetic predispositions underlying myocardial autoinflammation to identify biological targets to prevent or improve management of cardiac damage in these patients.

CLINICS CARE POINTS

- Myocardial involvement in systemic autoimmune rheumatic diseases (SARDs) is prevalent and can be subclinical, making regular cardiac screening imperative in this population.

- Systemic lupus erythematosus, rheumatoid arthritis, systemic sclerosis, eosinophilic granulomatosis with polyangiitis, and sarcoidosis are particularly associated with myocardial involvement and heart failure.

- Cyclophosphamide is associated with significant cardiotoxicity and should be used with caution in SARD patients.

- Cardiac imaging modalities, such as echocardiography, cardiac magnetic resonance, and PET, are essential in diagnosing myocarditis and in monitoring long-term myocardial function in SARDs.

- Myocarditis is associated with significant morbidity and mortality, especially in sarcoidosis where it can cause sudden cardiac death.

- Acute myocarditis should be treated with corticosteroids or other appropriate immunomodulatory agents and optimization of chronic immunosuppression regimen according to disease-specific guidelines.

- Further research is required to elucidate targetable mechanisms of myocardial involvement in SARDs.

DISCLOSURE

Dr. A.A. Zagouras has no relationships to disclose. Dr. W.H.W. Tang is partially supported by grants from the National Institutes of Health (R01HL126827, R01HL146754), and has served as a consultant for Sequana Medical A.G., Owkin Inc, Relypsa Inc, preCARDIA Inc, Cardiol Therapeutics Inc, Genomics plc, and has received honorarium from Springer Nature for authorship/editorship and American Board of Internal Medicine for exam writing committee participation–all unrelated to the subject and contents of this article.

REFERENCES

1. Mitratza M, Klijs B, Hak AE, et al. Systemic autoimmune disease as a cause of death: mortality burden and comorbidities. Rheumatology 2021;60(3):1321-30.
2. Lee KS, Kronbichler A, Eisenhut M, et al. Cardiovascular involvement in systemic rheumatic diseases: an integrated view for the treating physicians. Autoimmun Rev 2018;17(3):201-14.

3. De Lorenzis E, Gremese E, Bosello S, et al. Microvascular heart involvement in systemic autoimmune diseases: The purinergic pathway and therapeutic insights from the biology of the diseases. Autoimmun Rev 2019;18(4):317–24.

4. Caforio ALP, Marcolongo R, Baritussio A, et al. Myocarditis in systemic immune-mediated diseases. In: Caforio ALP, editor. Myocarditis: pathogenesis, diagnosis and treatment. Springer International Publishing; 2020. p. 195–221. https://doi.org/10.1007/978-3-030-35276-9_11.

5. Bartoloni E, Shoenfeld Y, Gerli R. Inflammatory and autoimmune mechanisms in the induction of atherosclerotic damage in systemic rheumatic diseases: two faces of the same coin. Arthritis Care Res (Hoboken) 2011;63(2):178–83.

6. Full LE, Ruisanchez C, Monaco C. The inextricable link between atherosclerosis and prototypical inflammatory diseases rheumatoid arthritis and systemic lupus erythematosus. Arthritis Res Ther 2009;11(2):217.

7. Ku IA, Imboden JB, Hsue PY, et al. Rheumatoid arthritis: model of systemic inflammation driving atherosclerosis. Circ J 2009;73(6):977–85.

8. Prasad M, Hermann J, Gabriel SE, et al. Cardiorheumatology: cardiac involvement in systemic rheumatic disease. Nat Rev Cardiol 2015;12(3):168–76.

9. Montecucco F, Mach F. Common inflammatory mediators orchestrate pathophysiological processes in rheumatoid arthritis and atherosclerosis. Rheumatology (Oxford) 2009;48(1):11–22.

10. Breland UM, Hollan I, Saatvedt K, et al. Inflammatory markers in patients with coronary artery disease with and without inflammatory rheumatic disease. Rheumatology (Oxford) 2010;49(6):1118–27.

11. Faccini A, Kaski JC, Camici PG. Coronary microvascular dysfunction in chronic inflammatory rheumatoid diseases. Eur Heart J 2016;37(23):1799–806.

12. Camici PG, d'Amati G, Rimoldi O. Coronary microvascular dysfunction: mechanisms and functional assessment. Nat Rev Cardiol 2015;12(1):48–62.

13. Mohammed SF, Hussain S, Mirzoyev SA, et al. Coronary microvascular rarefaction and myocardial fibrosis in heart failure with preserved ejection fraction. Circulation 2015;131(6):550–9.

14. Sorop O, Heinonen I, van Kranenburg M, et al. Multiple common comorbidities produce left ventricular diastolic dysfunction associated with coronary microvascular dysfunction, oxidative stress, and myocardial stiffening. Cardiovasc Res 2018;114(7):954–64.

15. Zanatta E, Colombo C, D'Amico G, et al. Inflammation and coronary microvascular dysfunction in autoimmune rheumatic diseases. Int J Mol Sci 2019;20(22): 5563.

16. Vaccarino V, Khan D, Votaw J, et al. Inflammation is related to coronary flow reserve detected by positron emission tomography in asymptomatic male twins. J Am Coll Cardiol 2011;57(11):1271–9.

17. Yılmaz S, Caliskan M, Kulaksızoglu S, et al. Association between serum total antioxidant status and coronary microvascular functions in patients with SLE. Echocardiography 2012;29(10):1218–23.

18. Dinesh P, Rasool M. uPA/uPAR signaling in rheumatoid arthritis: Shedding light on its mechanism of action. Pharmacol Res 2018;134:31–9.

19. Toldi G, Szalay B, Bekő G, et al. Plasma soluble urokinase plasminogen activator receptor (suPAR) levels in systemic lupus erythematosus. Biomarkers 2012;17(8):758–63.

20. Mekonnen G, Corban MT, Hung OY, et al. Plasma soluble urokinase-type plasminogen activator receptor level is independently associated with coronary

microvascular function in patients with non-obstructive coronary artery disease. Atherosclerosis 2015;239(1):55–60.

21. Cutolo M, Soldano S, Smith V. Pathophysiology of systemic sclerosis: current understanding and new insights. Expert Rev Clin Immunol 2019;15(7):753–64.

22. Maurer B, Distler JHW, Distler O. The Fra-2 transgenic mouse model of systemic sclerosis. Vasc Pharmacol 2013;58(3):194–201.

23. Venalis P, Kumánovics G, Schulze-Koops H, et al. Cardiomyopathy in murine models of systemic sclerosis. Arthritis Rheumatol 2015;67(2):508–16.

24. Maurer B, Busch N, Jüngel A, et al. Transcription factor fos-related antigen-2 induces progressive peripheral vasculopathy in mice closely resembling human systemic sclerosis. Circulation 2009;120(23):2367–76.

25. Giacomo R, Sheon M, Christine M, et al. Reduced lymphatic reserve in heart failure with preserved ejection fraction. J Am Coll Cardiol 2020;76(24):2817–29.

26. Schwartz N, Chalasani MLS, Li TM, et al. Lymphatic function in autoimmune diseases. Front Immunol 2019;10:519.

27. Rossi A, Sozio F, Sestini P, et al. Lymphatic and blood vessels in scleroderma skin, a morphometric analysis. Hum Pathol 2010;41(3):366–74.

28. Bouta EM, Bell RD, Rahimi H, et al. Targeting lymphatic function as a novel therapeutic intervention for rheumatoid arthritis. Nat Rev Rheumatol 2018;14(2): 94–106.

29. Bracamonte-Baran W, Čiháková D. Cardiac autoimmunity: myocarditis. Adv Exp Med Biol 2017;1003:187–221.

30. Ryabkova VA, Shubik YV, Erman MV, et al. Lethal immunoglobulins: autoantibodies and sudden cardiac death. Autoimmun Rev 2019;18(4):415–25.

31. Myers JM, Fairweather D, Huber SA, et al. Autoimmune myocarditis, valvulitis, and cardiomyopathy. Curr Protoc Immunol 2013;1–51. Chapter 15:Unit 15.14.

32. Nagatomo Y, Tang WHW. Autoantibodies and cardiovascular dysfunction: cause or consequence? Curr Heart Fail Rep 2014;11(4):500–8.

33. Li Y, Heuser JS, Kosanke SD, et al. Cryptic epitope identified in rat and human cardiac myosin S2 region induces myocarditis in the Lewis rat. J Immunol 2004; 172(5):3225–34.

34. Mascaro-Blanco A, Alvarez K, Yu X, et al. Consequences of unlocking the cardiac myosin molecule in human myocarditis and cardiomyopathies. Autoimmunity 2008;41(6):442–53.

35. Myers JM, Cooper LT, Kem DC, et al. Cardiac myosin-Th17 responses promote heart failure in human myocarditis. JCI Insight 2016;1(9):85851.

36. Düngen H-D, Dordevic A, Felix SB, et al. β1-adrenoreceptor autoantibodies in heart failure: physiology and therapeutic implications. Circ Heart Fail 2020; 13(1):e006155.

37. Nagatomo Y, Li D, Kirsop J, et al. Autoantibodies specifically against β1 adrenergic receptors and adverse clinical outcome in patients with chronic systolic heart failure in the β-blocker era: the importance of immunoglobulin G3 subclass. J Card Fail 2016;22(6):417–22.

38. Kill A, Tabeling C, Undeutsch R, et al. Autoantibodies to angiotensin and endothelin receptors in systemic sclerosis induce cellular and systemic events associated with disease pathogenesis. Arthritis Res Ther 2014;16(1):R29.

39. Kiriakidou M, Ching CL. Systemic lupus erythematosus. Ann Intern Med 2020; 172(11):ITC81–96.

40. Durcan L, O'Dwyer T, Petri M. Management strategies and future directions for systemic lupus erythematosus in adults. Lancet 2019;393(10188):2332–43.

41. Miner JJ, Kim AHJ. Cardiac manifestations of systemic lupus erythematosus. Rheum Dis Clin North Am 2014;40(1):51–60.
42. Thomas G, Cohen Aubart F, Chiche L, et al. Lupus Myocarditis: Initial Presentation and Longterm Outcomes in a Multicentric Series of 29 Patients. J Rheumatol 2017;44(1):24–32.
43. Bulkley BH, Roberts WC. The heart in systemic lupus erythematosus and the changes induced in it by corticosteroid therapy. A study of 36 necropsy patients. Am J Med 1975;58(2):243–64.
44. Mavrogeni S, Bratis K, Markussis V, et al. The diagnostic role of cardiac magnetic resonance imaging in detecting myocardial inflammation in systemic lupus erythematosus. Differentiation from viral myocarditis. Lupus 2013;22(1):34–43.
45. Jain D, Halushka MK. Cardiac pathology of systemic lupus erythematosus. J Clin Pathol 2009;62(7):584–92.
46. Prasada S, Rivera A, Nishtala A, et al. Differential associations of chronic inflammatory diseases with incident heart failure. JACC: Heart Fail 2020;8(6):489–98.
47. Chen J, Tang Y, Zhu M, et al. Heart involvement in systemic lupus erythematosus: a systemic review and meta-analysis. Clin Rheumatol 2016;35(10): 2437–48.
48. Leone P, Cicco S, Prete M, et al. Early echocardiographic detection of left ventricular diastolic dysfunction in patients with systemic lupus erythematosus asymptomatic for cardiovascular disease. Clin Exp Med 2020;20(1):11–9.
49. Roldan CA, Alomari IB, Awad K, et al. Aortic stiffness is associated with left ventricular diastolic dysfunction in systemic lupus erythematosus: a controlled transesophageal echocardiographic study. Clin Cardiol 2014;37(2):83–90.
50. Seneviratne MG, Grieve SM, Figtree GA, et al. Prevalence, distribution and clinical correlates of myocardial fibrosis in systemic lupus erythematosus: a cardiac magnetic resonance study. Lupus 2016;25(6):573–81.
51. Shang Q, Yip GWK, Tam LS, et al. SLICC/ACR damage index independently associated with left ventricular diastolic dysfunction in patients with systemic lupus erythematosus. Lupus 2012;21(10):1057–62.
52. Chorin E, Hochstadt A, Arad U, et al. Soluble ST2 and CXCL-10 may serve as biomarkers of subclinical diastolic dysfunction in SLE and correlate with disease activity and damage. Lupus 2020;29(11):1430–7.
53. Dhakal BP, Kim CH, Al-Kindi SG, et al. Heart failure in systemic lupus erythematosus. Trends Cardiovasc Med 2018;28(3):187–97.
54. Wainwright B, Bhan R, Trad C, et al. Autoimmune-mediated congenital heart block. Best Pract Res Clin Obstet Gynaecol 2020;64:41–51.
55. Scott JS, Maddison PJ, Taylor PV, et al. Connective-tissue disease, antibodies to ribonucleoprotein, and congenital heart block. N Engl J Med 1983;309(4): 209–12.
56. Jayaprasad N, Johnson F, Venugopal K. Congenital complete heart block and maternal connective tissue disease. Int J Cardiol 2006;112(2):153–8.
57. Moak JP, Barron KS, Hougen TJ, et al. Congenital heart block: development of late-onset cardiomyopathy, a previously underappreciated sequela. J Am Coll Cardiol 2001;37(1):238–42.
58. Izmirly P, Kim M, Friedman DM, et al. Hydroxychloroquine to prevent recurrent congenital heart block in fetuses of Anti-SSA/Ro-positive mothers. J Am Coll Cardiol 2020;76(3):292–302.
59. McInnes IB, Schett G. The pathogenesis of rheumatoid arthritis. N Engl J Med 2011;365(23):2205–19.

60. Solomon DH, Karlson EW, Rimm EB, et al. Cardiovascular morbidity and mortality in women diagnosed with rheumatoid arthritis. Circulation 2003;107(9): 1303–7.

61. Gabriel SE. Cardiovascular morbidity and mortality in rheumatoid arthritis. Am J Med 2008;121(10 Suppl 1):S9–14.

62. Elbadawi A, Ahmed HMA, Elgendy IY, et al. Outcomes of acute myocardial infarction in patients with rheumatoid arthritis. Am J Med 2020;133(10): 1168–79.e4.

63. Nicola PJ, Maradit-Kremers H, Roger VL, et al. The risk of congestive heart failure in rheumatoid arthritis: a population-based study over 46 years. Arthritis Rheum 2005;52(2):412–20.

64. Lebowitz WB. The heart in rheumatoid arthritis (rheumatoid disease). A clinical and pathological study of sixty-two cases. Ann Intern Med 1963;58:102–23.

65. Pappas DA, Taube JM, Bathon JM, et al. A 73-year-old woman with rheumatoid arthritis and shortness of breath. Arthritis Rheum 2008;59(6):892–9.

66. Ntusi NAB, Piechnik SK, Francis JM, et al. Diffuse myocardial fibrosis and inflammation in rheumatoid arthritis: insights from CMR T1 mapping. JACC Cardiovasc Imaging 2015;8(5):526–36.

67. Greulich S, Mayr A, Kitterer D, et al. Advanced myocardial tissue characterisation by a multi-component CMR protocol in patients with rheumatoid arthritis. Eur Radiol 2017;27(11):4639–49.

68. Denton CP, Khanna D. Systemic sclerosis. The Lancet 2017;390(10103): 1685–99.

69. Bissell L-A, Md Yusof MY, Buch MH. Primary myocardial disease in scleroderma-a comprehensive review of the literature to inform the UK Systemic Sclerosis Study Group cardiac working group. Rheumatology (Oxford) 2017; 56(6):882–95.

70. Chatterjee S. Pulmonary hypertension in systemic sclerosis. Semin Arthritis Rheum 2011;41(1):19–37.

71. Launay D, Sobanski V, Hachulla E, et al. Pulmonary hypertension in systemic sclerosis: different phenotypes. Eur Respir Rev 2017;26(145). https://doi.org/ 10.1183/16000617.0056-2017.

72. Fox BD, Shimony A, Langleben D, et al. High prevalence of occult left heart disease in scleroderma-pulmonary hypertension. Eur Respir J 2013;42(4):1083–91.

73. Bourji KI, Kelemen BW, Mathai SC, et al. Poor survival in patients with scleroderma and pulmonary hypertension due to heart failure with preserved ejection fraction. Pulm Circ 2017;7(2):409–20.

74. Rubio-Rivas M, Corbella X, Guillén-Del-Castillo A, et al. Spanish scleroderma risk score (RESCLESCORE) to predict 15-year all-cause mortality in scleroderma patients at the time of diagnosis based on the RESCLE cohort: derivation and internal validation. Autoimmun Rev 2020;19(5):102507.

75. Ciurzyński M, Bienias P, Lichodziejewska B, et al. Assessment of left and right ventricular diastolic function in patients with systemic sclerosis. Kardiol Pol 2008;66(3):269–76 [discussion: 277-278].

76. Tennøe AH, Murbræch K, Andreassen JC, et al. Left ventricular diastolic dysfunction predicts mortality in patients with systemic sclerosis. J Am Coll Cardiol 2018;72(15):1804–13.

77. Sulli A, Ghio M, Bezante GP, et al. Blunted coronary flow reserve in systemic sclerosis. Rheumatology (Oxford) 2004;43(4):505–9.

78. Valentini G, Vitale DF, Giunta A, et al. Diastolic abnormalities in systemic sclerosis: evidence for associated defective cardiac functional reserve. Ann Rheum Dis 1996;55(7):455–60.
79. Zanatta E, Famoso G, Boscain F, et al. Nailfold avascular score and coronary microvascular dysfunction in systemic sclerosis: a newsworthy association. Autoimmun Rev 2019;18(2):177–83.
80. Mukherjee M, Chung S-E, Ton VK, et al. Unique Abnormalities in right ventricular longitudinal strain in systemic sclerosis patients. Circ Cardiovasc Imaging 2016; 9(6). https://doi.org/10.1161/CIRCIMAGING.115.003792.
81. Yiu KH, Schouffoer AA, Marsan NA, et al. Left ventricular dysfunction assessed by speckle-tracking strain analysis in patients with systemic sclerosis: relationship to functional capacity and ventricular arrhythmias. Arthritis Rheum 2011; 63(12):3969–78.
82. Rodríguez-Reyna TS, Morelos-Guzman M, Hernández-Reyes P, et al. Assessment of myocardial fibrosis and microvascular damage in systemic sclerosis by magnetic resonance imaging and coronary angiotomography. Rheumatology (Oxford) 2015;54(4):647–54.
83. Mavrogeni S, Koutsogeorgopoulou L, Karabela G, et al. Silent myocarditis in systemic sclerosis detected by cardiovascular magnetic resonance using Lake Louise criteria. BMC Cardiovasc Disord 2017;17(1):187.
84. Mohameden M, Vashisht P, Sharman T. Scleroderma and primary myocardial disease. In: StatPearls. StatPearls Publishing; 2020. Available at: http://www.ncbi.nlm.nih.gov/books/NBK557686/. Accessed July 22, 2020.
85. Allanore Y, Meune C. Primary myocardial involvement in systemic sclerosis: evidence for a microvascular origin. Clin Exp Rheumatol 2010;28(5 Suppl 62): S48–53.
86. West SG, Killian PJ, Lawless OJ. Association of myositis and myocarditis in progressive systemic sclerosis. Arthritis Rheum 1981;24(5):662–8.
87. De Luca G, Campochiaro C, De Santis M, et al. Systemic sclerosis myocarditis has unique clinical, histological and prognostic features: a comparative histological analysis. Rheumatology (Oxford) 2020. https://doi.org/10.1093/rheumatology/kez658.
88. Hesselstrand R, Scheja A, Shen GQ, et al. The association of antinuclear antibodies with organ involvement and survival in systemic sclerosis. Rheumatology (Oxford) 2003;42(4):534–40.
89. Machado C, Sunkel CE, Andrew DJ. Human autoantibodies reveal titin as a chromosomal protein. J Cell Biol 1998;141(2):321–33.
90. Riemekasten G, Philippe A, Näther M, et al. Involvement of functional autoantibodies against vascular receptors in systemic sclerosis. Ann Rheum Dis 2011; 70(3):530–6.
91. Manetti M, Milia AF, Guiducci S, et al. Progressive loss of lymphatic vessels in skin of patients with systemic sclerosis. J Rheumatol 2011;38(2):297–301.
92. Furuta S, Iwamoto T, Nakajima H. Update on eosinophilic granulomatosis with polyangiitis. Allergol Int 2019;68(4):430–6.
93. Miloslavsky E, Unizony S. The heart in vasculitis. Rheum Dis Clin North Am 2014; 40(1):11–26.
94. Chang H-C, Chou P-C, Lai C-Y, et al. Antineutrophil cytoplasmic antibodies and organ-specific manifestations in eosinophilic granulomatosis with polyangiitis: a systematic review and meta-analysis. J Allergy Clin Immunol Pract 2021;9(1): 445–52.e6.

95. Dalia T, Parashar S, Patel NV, et al. Eosinophilic myocarditis demonstrated using cardiac magnetic resonance imaging in a patient with eosinophilic granulomatosis with polyangiitis (churg-strauss disease). Cureus 2018;10(6):e2792.

96. Comarmond C, Pagnoux C, Khellaf M, et al. Eosinophilic granulomatosis with polyangiitis (Churg-Strauss): clinical characteristics and long-term followup of the 383 patients enrolled in the French Vasculitis Study Group cohort. Arthritis Rheum 2013;65(1):270–81.

97. Szczeklik W, Miszalski-Jamka T. Cardiac involvement in eosinophilic granulomatosis with polyangitis (Churg Strauss) (RCD code: I-3A.7a). J Rare Cardiovasc Dis 2014;1(3):91–5.

98. Dennert RM, van Paassen P, Schalla S, et al. Cardiac involvement in Churg-Strauss syndrome. Arthritis Rheum 2010;62(2):627–34.

99. Brucato A, Maestroni S, Masciocco G, et al. [Cardiac involvement in Churg-Strauss syndrome]. G Ital Cardiol (Rome) 2015;16(9):493–500.

100. Moosig F, Bremer JP, Hellmich B, et al. A vasculitis centre based management strategy leads to improved outcome in eosinophilic granulomatosis and polyangiitis (Churg-Strauss, EGPA): monocentric experiences in 150 patients. Ann Rheum Dis 2013;72(6):1011–7.

101. Steinfeld J, Bradford ES, Brown J, et al. Evaluation of clinical benefit from treatment with mepolizumab for patients with eosinophilic granulomatosis with polyangiitis. J Allergy Clin Immunol 2019;143(6):2170–7.

102. Jennette JC, Falk RJ, Bacon PA, et al. 2012 Revised international chapel hill consensus conference nomenclature of vasculitides. Arthritis Rheum 2013; 65(1):1–11.

103. McGeoch L, Carette S, Cuthbertson D, et al. Cardiac involvement in granulomatosis with polyangiitis. J Rheumatol 2015;42(7):1209–12.

104. Guillevin L, Pagnoux C, Seror R, et al. The Five-Factor Score revisited: assessment of prognoses of systemic necrotizing vasculitides based on the French Vasculitis Study Group (FVSG) cohort. Medicine (Baltimore) 2011;90(1):19–27.

105. Walsh M, Flossmann O, Berden A, et al. Risk factors for relapse of antineutrophil cytoplasmic antibody-associated vasculitis. Arthritis Rheum 2012;64(2):542–8.

106. Hanna RM, Lopez E, Wilson J. Granulomatosis with polyangiitis with myocarditis and ventricular tachycardia. Case Rep Med 2017;2017:6501738.

107. Munch A, Sundbøll J, Høyer S, et al. Acute myocarditis in a patient with newly diagnosed granulomatosis with polyangiitis. Case Rep Cardiol 2015;2015: 134529.

108. Guillevin L, Pagnoux C, Karras A, et al. Rituximab versus azathioprine for maintenance in ANCA-associated vasculitis. N Engl J Med 2014;371(19):1771–80.

109. Oliveira GHM, Seward JB, Tsang TSM, et al. Echocardiographic findings in patients with wegener granulomatosis. Mayo Clinic Proc 2005;80(11):1435–40.

110. Luciano N, Valentini V, Calabrò A, et al. One year in review 2015: Sjögren's syndrome. Clin Exp Rheumatol 2015;33(2):259–71.

111. Chiang C-H, Liu C-J, Chen P-J, et al. Primary sjögren's syndrome and the risk of acute myocardial infarction: a nationwide study. Acta Cardiol Sin 2013;29(2): 124–31.

112. Bartoloni E, Baldini C, Schillaci G, et al. Cardiovascular disease risk burden in primary Sjögren's syndrome: results of a population-based multicentre cohort study. J Intern Med 2015;278(2):185–92.

113. Gyöngyösi M, Pokorny G, Jambrik Z, et al. Cardiac manifestations in primary Sjögren's syndrome. Ann Rheum Dis 1996;55(7):450–4.

114. Vassiliou VA, Moyssakis I, Boki KA, et al. Is the heart affected in primary Sjögren's syndrome? An echocardiographic study. Clin Exp Rheumatol 2008;26(1): 109–12.

115. Bayram NA, Cicek OF, Erten S, et al. Assessment of left ventricular functions in patients with Sjögren's syndrome using tissue Doppler echocardiography. Int J Rheum Dis 2013;16(4):425–9.

116. Levin MD, Zoet-Nugteren SK, Markusse HM. Myocarditis and primary Sjögren's syndrome. Lancet 1999;354(9173):128–9.

117. Kau C-K, Hu J-C, Lu L-Y, et al. Primary Sjögren's syndrome complicated with cryoglobulinemic glomerulonephritis, myocarditis, and multi-organ involvement. J Formos Med Assoc 2004;103(9):707–10.

118. Brito-Zerón P, Pasoto SG, Robles-Marhuenda A, et al. Autoimmune congenital heart block and primary Sjögren's syndrome: characterisation and outcomes of 49 cases. Clin Exp Rheumatol 2020;38(Suppl 126):95–102, 4.

119. Caforio ALP, Adler Y, Agostini C, et al. Diagnosis and management of myocardial involvement in systemic immune-mediated diseases: a position statement of the European Society of Cardiology Working Group on Myocardial and Pericardial Disease. Eur Heart J 2017;38(35):2649–62.

120. Hamzeh N, Steckman DA, Sauer WH, et al. Pathophysiology and clinical management of cardiac sarcoidosis. Nat Rev Cardiol 2015;12(5):278–88.

121. Iwai K, Takemura T, Kitaichi M, et al. Pathological studies on sarcoidosis autopsy. II. Early change, mode of progression and death pattern. Acta Pathol Jpn 1993;43(7–8):377–85.

122. Perry A, Vuitch F. Causes of death in patients with sarcoidosis. A morphologic study of 38 autopsies with clinicopathologic correlations. Arch Pathol Lab Med 1995;119(2):167–72.

123. Baughman RP, Teirstein AS, Judson MA, et al. Clinical characteristics of patients in a case control study of sarcoidosis. Am J Respir Crit Care Med 2001;164(10 Pt 1):1885–9.

124. Iwai K, Sekiguti M, Hosoda Y, et al. Racial difference in cardiac sarcoidosis incidence observed at autopsy. Sarcoidosis 1994;11(1):26–31.

125. Kusano KF, Satomi K. Diagnosis and treatment of cardiac sarcoidosis. Heart 2016;102(3):184–90.

126. Uusimaa P, Ylitalo K, Anttonen O, et al. Ventricular tachyarrhythmia as a primary presentation of sarcoidosis. Europace 2008;10(6):760–6.

127. Koplan BA, Soejima K, Baughman K, et al. Refractory ventricular tachycardia secondary to cardiac sarcoid: Electrophysiologic characteristics, mapping, and ablation. Heart Rhythm 2006;3(8):924–9.

128. Zhu TY, Li EK, Tam L-S. Cardiovascular risk in patients with psoriatic arthritis. Int J Rheumatol 2012;2012.

129. Wong K, Gladman DD, Husted J, et al. Mortality studies in psoriatic arthritis: results from a single outpatient clinic. I. Causes and risk of death. Arthritis Rheum 1997;40(10):1868–72.

130. Buckley C, Cavill C, Taylor G, et al. Mortality in psoriatic arthritis – a single-center study from the UK. J Rheumatol 2010;37(10):2141–4.

131. Liew JW, Ramiro S, Gensler LS. Cardiovascular morbidity and mortality in ankylosing spondylitis and psoriatic arthritis. Best Pract Res Clin Rheumatol 2018; 32(3):369–89.

132. Haroon NN, Paterson JM, Li P, et al. Patients with ankylosing spondylitis have increased cardiovascular and cerebrovascular mortality. Ann Intern Med 2015;163(6):409–16.

133. Husted JA, Thavaneswaran A, Chandran V, et al. Cardiovascular and other co-morbidities in patients with psoriatic arthritis: a comparison with patients with psoriasis. Arthritis Care Res (Hoboken) 2011;63(12):1729–35.
134. Atluri RB. Inflammatory myopathies. Mo Med 2016;113(2):127–30.
135. Zhang L, Wang G, Ma L, et al. Cardiac involvement in adult polymyositis or dermatomyositis: a systematic review. Clin Cardiol 2012;35(11):686–91.
136. Gonzalez-Lopez L, Gamez-Nava JI, Sanchez L, et al. Cardiac manifestations in dermato-polymyositis. Clin Exp Rheumatol 1996;14(4):373–9.
137. Allanore Y, Vignaux O, Arnaud L, et al. Effects of corticosteroids and immunosuppressors on idiopathic inflammatory myopathy related myocarditis evaluated by magnetic resonance imaging. Ann Rheum Dis 2006;65(2):249–52.
138. Garg V, Tan W, Ardehali R, et al. Giant cell myocarditis masquerading as orbital myositis with a rapid, fulminant course necessitating mechanical support and heart transplantation. ESC Heart Fail 2017;4(3):371–5.
139. Dalakas MC. Inflammatory muscle diseases. N Engl J Med 2015;372(18):1734–47.
140. Dankó K, Ponyi A, Constantin T, et al. Long-term survival of patients with idiopathic inflammatory myopathies according to clinical features: a longitudinal study of 162 cases. Medicine (Baltimore) 2004;83(1):35–42.
141. Schrezenmeier E, Dörner T. Mechanisms of action of hydroxychloroquine and chloroquine: implications for rheumatology. Nat Rev Rheumatol 2020;16(3):155–66.
142. Chatre C, Roubille F, Vernhet H, et al. Cardiac complications attributed to chloroquine and hydroxychloroquine: a systematic review of the literature. Drug Saf 2018;41(10):919–31.
143. Nadeem U, Raafey M, Kim G, et al. Chloroquine- and hydroxychloroquine-induced cardiomyopathy: a case report and brief literature review. Am J Clin Pathol 2021;155(6):793–801.
144. Jang D-I, Lee A-H, Shin H-Y, et al. The role of tumor necrosis factor alpha (TNF-α) in autoimmune disease and current TNF-α inhibitors in therapeutics. Int J Mol Sci 2021;22(5):2719.
145. Chung ES, Packer M, Lo KH, et al. Anti-TNF Therapy Against Congestive Heart Failure Investigators. Randomized, double-blind, placebo-controlled, pilot trial of infliximab, a chimeric monoclonal antibody to tumor necrosis factor-alpha, in patients with moderate-to-severe heart failure: results of the anti-TNF Therapy Against Congestive Heart Failure (ATTACH) trial. Circulation 2003;107(25):3133–40.
146. Sinagra E, Perricone G, Romano C, et al. Heart failure and anti tumor necrosis factor-alpha in systemic chronic inflammatory diseases. Eur J Intern Med 2013;24(5):385–92.
147. Coletta AP, Clark AL, Banarjee P, et al. Clinical trials update: RENEWAL (RENAISSANCE and RECOVER) and ATTACH. Eur J Heart Fail 2002;4(4):559–61.
148. Iqubal A, Iqubal MK, Sharma S, et al. Molecular mechanism involved in cyclophosphamide-induced cardiotoxicity: Old drug with a new vision. Life Sci 2019;218:112–31.
149. Kurauchi K, Nishikawa T, Miyahara E, et al. Role of metabolites of cyclophosphamide in cardiotoxicity. BMC Res Notes 2017;10(1):406.
150. Higgins AY, O'Halloran TD, Chang JD. Chemotherapy-induced cardiomyopathy. Heart Fail Rev 2015;20(6):721–30.
151. Caforio ALP, Pankuweit S, Arbustini E, et al. Current state of knowledge on aetiology, diagnosis, management, and therapy of myocarditis: a position statement

of the European Society of Cardiology Working Group on Myocardial and Pericardial Diseases. Eur Heart J 2013;34(33):2636–48, 2648a-2648d.

152. Bissell L-A, Anderson M, Burgess M, et al. Consensus best practice pathway of the UK Systemic Sclerosis Study group: management of cardiac disease in systemic sclerosis. Rheumatology (Oxford) 2017;56(6):912–21.

153. Hamzeh NY, Wamboldt FS, Weinberger HD. Management of cardiac sarcoidosis in the United States: a Delphi study. Chest 2012;141(1):154–62.

154. Baker MC, Sheth K, Witteles R, et al. TNF-alpha inhibition for the treatment of cardiac sarcoidosis. Semin Arthritis Rheum 2020;50(3):546–52.

Heart Failure in Rheumatic Disease
Secular Trends and Novel Insights

Brian Bridal Løgstrup, MD, PhD, DMSc

KEYWORDS

- Heart failure • Cardiovascular disease • Rheumatic disease • Rheumatoid arthritis
- Systemic lupus erythematosus • Ankylosing spondylitis • Psoriatic arthritis
- Hyperuricemia

KEY POINTS

- Patients with chronic rheumatic diseases are at increased risk of heart failure.
- Common risk factors and inflammatory processes overlap in rheumatic diseases and heart failure.
- The opportunities for using immune-based strategies to fight development of heart failure in rheumatic diseases are developing.

INTRODUCTION

Cardiovascular diseases (CVDs) are the leading cause of death in chronic inflammatory and autoimmune rheumatic diseases such as rheumatoid arthritis (RA), systemic lupus erythematosus (SLE), ankylosing spondylitis (AS), psoriatic arthritis (PsA), and hyperuricemia. This excess mortality cannot be explained solely by the increased prevalence of cardiovascular (CV) risk factors. The underlying mechanisms leading to such an increased CV risk are not yet clearly understood. Heart failure (HF) is one of the substantial contributors to the increased morbidity and mortality in the rheumatic disease spectrum.

HF can present as a chronic disease or in an acute setting with rapidly decreasing myocardial function either as the primary presentation or as acute decompensation of preexisting HF disease. HF has a rising prevalence in the general population of now 11.8% in people aged 60 years or older.[1] Approximately 50% of all HF patients suffer from HF with reduced ejection fraction (HFrEF; typically considered as EF <40%), whereas the other half suffers from HF with preserved EF (HFpEF; ≥50%). Patients with EF in the range of 41% to 49% present a "gray zone," which is defined as HF

Department of Cardiology, Institute of Clinical Medicine, Aarhus University Hospital, Palle Juul Jensens Boulevard 99, Aarhus N 8200, Denmark
E-mail address: bbl@skejby.rm.dk

Rheum Dis Clin N Am 49 (2023) 67–79
https://doi.org/10.1016/j.rdc.2022.08.003
0889-857X/23/© 2022 Elsevier Inc. All rights reserved.

rheumatic.theclinics.com

with mildly reduced EF. This group of patients also contains HFrEF patients with recovery of EF.[2,3]

This paper gives an overview of HF in the most common types of rheumatic diseases and goes through the common quantities of rheumatic diseases and HF. Furthermore, it eludes on the inflammatory processes and possible treatments.

Heart Failure in Rheumatoid Arthritis

HF is the second highest cause of death in RA patients after myocardial infarction (MI), with studies suggesting up to a 2-fold increase in the incidence of HF in the RA population[4-7] (**Fig. 1**). HF can arise as a result of ischemic or nonischemic heart disease, and both types are increasingly found in RA patients.[4,5,8] There are however some differences in susceptibility, which may be due to differences in the underlying pathogenesis. Ischemic HF was found to be increased in rheumatoid factor positive patients, whereas nonischemic HF was found to increase rapidly following diagnosis and was associated with inflammatory activity and disease activity but not rheumatoid factor positivity.[4]

HF is underdiagnosed in the RA population with subclinical and asymptomatic changes occurring over many years. A recent cohort study of 355 RA patients by Ferreira and colleagues found that almost one-third of the patients met the study characteristics for HF, but only 7% of the cohort had a diagnosis of HF before study enrollment.[9] RA patients, especially with ischemic HF, also present a higher prevalence of traditional CV risk factors such as diabetes and dyslipidemia as well as higher concentrations of markers of inflammation and fibrosis; findings in line with those of HF patients without RA. Importantly, in patients with RA, HF symptoms are often difficult to ascertain (due to concomitant osteoarticular disease and functional limitations), and the HF clinical presentation may be atypical.[10,11] The evidence accumulating in the literature suggests that RA should be considered a risk factor for HF, especially in newly diagnosed patients with high disease activity.[12]

Many of the commonly prescribed therapies for RA carry a risk of cardiotoxicity.[13] Chronic and high-dose corticosteroid use has been independently associated with

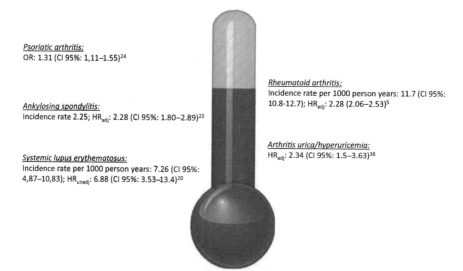

Psoriatic arthritis:
OR: 1.31 (CI 95%: 1,11–1.55)[24]

Rheumatoid arthritis:
Incidence rate per 1000 person years: 11.7 (CI 95%: 10.8-12.7); HR_{adj}: 2.28 (2.06–2.53)[5]

Ankylosing spondylitis:
Incidence rate 2.25; HR_{adj}: 2.28 (CI 95%: 1.80–2.89)[23]

Arthritis urica/hyperuricemia:
HR_{adj}: 2.34 (CI 95%: 1.5–3.63)[38]

Systemic lupus erythematosus:
Incidence rate per 1000 person years: 7.26 (CI 95%: 4,87–10,83); HR_{unadj}: 6.88 (CI 95%: 3.53–13.4)[20]

Fig. 1. Incidence/risk of heart failure in rheumatic diseases.

increased risk of CVD.[14] Similarly, the use of nonsteroidal anti-inflammatory drugs, including cyclooxygenase inhibitors, used to treat joint pain is associated with 2 times increased CV risk. Furthermore, these medications can counteract the antiplatelet effects of aspirin and increase the risk of ischemic heart disease and HF.[15]

Heart Failure in SLE

The prevalence of CV involvement in SLE is estimated to be more than 50%, but estimates vary substantially, possibly because of differences in patient selection.[16] HF is prevalent in SLE; however, data eluding the long-term follow-up are sparse.[17–19] Recently, Yafasova and colleagues investigated the long-term risk and prognosis and found SLE patients to have a higher long-term risk of incident HF than matched control subjects.[20] Second, a history of SLE was associated with higher all-cause mortality among patients developing HF. And finally, the authors observed that SLE patients had a higher long-term risk of other adverse CV outcomes[20] (see **Fig. 1**). The risks of coronary artery disease (CAD) and MI in SLE patients are estimated to be 9 times higher than those in the general population and as much as 50 times higher than those in matched women without SLE.[21,22]

Heart Failure in AS

Not much data regarding the risk of HF in AS exist. A study by Bae and colleagues found that the incidence rates of HF and death were increased in AS patients (hazard ratio: 2.28 and 1.66, respectively)[23] (see **Fig. 1**). Some other small studies have confirmed these observations.[24,25] These data are supported by the increased observation of increased risk of HFpEF in these patients.[26]

Heart Failure in PsA

PsA carries an increased risk of MI, peripheral vascular disease, and HF.[27] Increased risk of HF is associated with a combination of known CV risk factors and measures of disease activity, particularly in nonischemic HF.[28] The overall incidence rates of new-onset HF is associated to the severity of the disease, with and without joint involvement.[29–31] Few studies have reported the risk of overt HF in PsA; however, it has been reported to have a 31% increase in the risk of HF in patients with PsA compared with the general population[24,32,33] (see **Fig. 1**).

Heart Failure in Hyperuricemia

Patients with gout have a higher burden of traditional CV risk factors despite this gout has been shown to be an independent risk factor for CV mortality.[34] More recently, increased focus has been placed on the relationship between hyperuricemia and HF. In a recent study by Colantonio and colleagues,[35] 5713 patients without a history of HF, congenital heart defects, or stroke between 2003 and 2007 were analyzed. With regard to HF hospitalizations, the incidence rates for patients with and without gout were 13.1 and 4.4, per 1000 person-years, respectively.[35] It has been estimated that approximately 10% of patients with gout will develop HF versus 2% in the general population. A linear relationship between the risk of HF and serum urate concentrations has been observed.[36,37] However, based on the aforementioned results, it is difficult to tell if elevated levels of uric acid alone led to an increased risk of HF or if other comorbid conditions are contributing to the development of HF. The study by Wu and colleagues excluded all patients with known risk factors for CVD and HF development and observed 6.5% of patients over the age of 65 years with hyperuricemia to develop an HF event while 3.1% of patients without hyperuricemia developed an HF event.[38]

The authors concluded a 2.34 fold increase in risk of HF events in patients with hyperuricemia (see **Fig. 1**).

Common Quantity of Rheumatic Diseases and Heart Failure

Individuals with underlying chronic inflammatory conditions, despite different patterns of inflammatory pathophysiology, are at increased risk of developing CVD, including CAD and HF. These patients are often undertreated in terms of prevention of CVD, probably because these patients have lower rate of screening for traditional CV risk factors than the general population, including routine lipid testing, diabetic screening, and screening for tobacco abuse.[39,40] Furthermore, prophylaxis and treatment of other risk factors such as hypertension, obesity, and sedentary lifestyle are also highly underutilized.

When addressing the CV risk, traditional risk assessment tools clearly underestimate CV risk in this population with underlying inflammatory disorders.[41,42] The European League Against Rheumatism and the American Heart Association suggest multiplying the traditional risk score by a correction factor (eg, RA by 1.5) to adjust for this underestimation. Despite these initiatives and several guidelines for CVD risk management, implementation of appropriate preventive therapies in clinical practice remains suboptimal.[40,43]

Effort has now been taken to investigate these issues with respect to modifications to risk factors in total.[44]

Inflammation: Cause of Heart Failure?

Besides the previously mentioned shared risk factors, another common quantity linking rheumatic diseases and HF exists: the inflammatory process. However, how inflammation contributes to the pathogenesis of the different forms of HF is diverse and clearly, to a certain extent, not fully understood. For patients suffering from HFpEF, a novel paradigm was postulated which identifies a systematic proinflammatory state induced by comorbidities such as the origin of microvascular endothelial cell inflammation, which triggers HFpEF-specific events, that is, hypertrophy of cardiomyocytes, cardiac remodeling, stiffening of the left ventricle, and cardiac dysfunction.[45] The high-grade enduring systemic inflammation exerted by the rheumatic diseases impacts the accelerating development of heart disease. With respect to patients with HFrEF, the direct impact of myocardial infection, ischemia, or regular MI might trigger eccentric cardiac remodeling and dysfunction. MI associated with inflammatory diseases can cause the whole spectrum of HF.[45,46]

The possible mediators of the bidirectional connection between inflammation and HF are multiple. Inflammation and HF are strongly interconnected and mutually reinforce each other.[47] The shared risk factors (eg, smoking, obesity, sedentary lifestyle, diet), clonal hematopoiesis of independent potential, angiogenesis, extracellular environment, several secreted or circulating factors, and finally the inflammation caused by the rheumatic disease add to the growing evidence connecting inflammation and HF. Several factors regarding the immune contexture in the heart repair process contribute to the decremental effects of the immunologic impact on the heart. The immune system plays a key role in aspects of cardiac biology, pathophysiology, regeneration, and therapeutics.[48–52] The systemic inflammation and tissue fibrosis, mediated by both the innate and adaptive immune systems, contribute to CVD through multiple mechanisms. Increased levels of activated neutrophils, reactive oxygen species, and proinflammatory cytokines lead to endothelial dysfunction, atherosclerosis, and thrombosis.

HF itself has been demonstrated to be driven at least in part by inflammatory pathways that might be turned on by stress responses. The secreted or circulating inflammatory factors such as tumor necrosis factor alfa (TNF-α) levels are associated with disease severity and progression of HF. In addition, several cytokines (eg, interleukin [IL]-1β, IL-6) are involved in deteriorating left ventricular function, and cytokines and cytokine receptors are independent predictors of mortality in patients with advanced HF.[53,54] They have also been found to increase the risk of CAD by causing atherosclerosis, plaque instability, and plaque rupture.[55,56]

Systemic inflammation can induce autonomic nervous system dysfunction. Inflammatory cytokines increase the sympathetic outflow by targeting the autonomic centers in the brain, which in turn inhibits cytokine production and immune-inflammatory activation by stimulating the β2 adrenoreceptors in circulating lympho-monocytes.[57] This self-controlling loop, so-called inflammatory reflex and sympathetic activation, consequently damps excessive immune-inflammatory activation but also affects the heart, potentially favoring the onset of arrhythmias and HF.[58,59]

Immunomodulatory Therapies for Heart Failure and Rheumatic Diseases

Several attempts have been made to direct immunomodulatory therapies to treat HF, including therapies used for rheumatic diseases (**Table 1**). One of the cytokines indicted in inflammation with HF as well as rheumatic disease is TNF-α. Contrary to the promising animal experiments, the use of infliximab, a TNF-α antibody, resulted in a reduced cardiac output in patients with RA without known HF.[60] The anti-TNF therapy against congestive heart failure (ATTACH) trial used infliximab in patients with at least moderate HF, as well as the Randomized Etanercept Worldwide Evaluation (RENEWAL) study (a combined analysis of the randomised etanercept north american stategy to study antagonism of cytokines (RENAISSANCE) research into etanercept cytokine antagonism in ventricular dysfunction trial (RECOVER) trials that used etanercept), and both demonstrated that blocking TNF-α in HF patients does not yield a clinical benefit but exerts adverse effects at higher doses.[61,62] Numerous studies have examined the effect of monoclonal and polyclonal antibodies against TNF-α in septic patients. Both reduce overall mortality in patients with severe sepsis. Monoclonal anti-TNF-α-antibodies improve survival of patients in septic shock.[63] In COVID-19, the use of adalimumab, a TNF-α-antibody, did not reduce mortality or beneficially alter the course of the disease.[64] These results suggest that even though TNF-α is upregulated in HF, as well as in other infections, blocking it by using antibodies has negative effects on HF despite positive effects on some selected infectious diseases.

In the canakinumab antiinflammatory thombosis outcome study (CANTOS) trial, the use of canakinumab, an IL-1β antibody, in patients with MI and active inflammation resulted in less all-cause mortality and a lower rate of HF hospitalization.[65,66] Anakinra, the IL-1β receptor antagonist, proved effective in reducing adverse myocardial remodeling in mice and successfully improved left ventricular function after MI in humans.[67]

A positive effect of the anti-IL-6 antibody tocilizumab has been seen for the cardiac function of patients without HF.[68,69] Until now, no studies have been performed on the use of tocilizumab or other IL-6 inhibitors in HF patients, but a case report of a patient with HF after MI who received tocilizumab, because of a large vessel arteritis, has shown an improvement of myocardial function after the treatment.[70] In the interleukin-6 receptor antibodies for modulating the systemic inflammatory response after out-of-hospital cardiac arrest (IMICA) trial, tocilizumab has shown reduced inflammation as well as myocardial damage in postcardiac arrest syndrome.[71]

In a broader attempt to address the immunologic aspects of HF, the advanced chronic heart failure clinical assessment of immune modulation therapy (ACCLAIM)

Table 1
Inflammatory targets in heart failure

Target	Compound	Patients	Follow-up	Results
Immunomodulation	Pentoxifylline	221 HFrEF	1–6 mo	4-Fold reduction in mortality[79]
	Immunoglobulin i.v	102 HFrEF	6–12 mo	Increased LVEF and symptom relief[80]
	Celacade	2426 HFrEF	10 mo	No effect[72]
	Methotrexate	50 HFrEF	3 mo	No effect[81]
IL-1 receptor	Anakinra	60 HFrEF; 12 HFpEF	2–12 wk	Increase in peak VO_2[82,83]
IL-1β	Canakinumab	HFrEF	3 mo	Increase in LVEF and peak Vo_2[84]
TNF-α	Etanercept	1500 HFrEF	6–12 mo	No effect[61]
	Infliximab	150 HFrEF	7 mo	Harmful?[85]
Xanthine oxidase	Allopurinol	253 HFrEF	6 mo	No effect[86]
	Oxypurinol	405 HFrEF	6 mo	No effect[87]
NOS	NOS inhibitors	HFrEF, shock	<6 mo	No effect[88]
Nonspecific	Rosuvastatin	5000 HFrEF	32–46 mo	No effects[89,90]
NLRP3	Colchicine	HFrEF	6 mo	Reduced CRP and IL-6, no effects on functional status or prognosis[91]
	Dapansutrile	HFrEF	2–4 wk	Increased LVEF and time of exercise[92]

Abbreviations: CRP, C-reactive protein; IL, interleukin; i.v, intravenous; LVEF, left ventricular ejection fraction; NLRP3, NOD-like receptor family pyrin domain containing 3; NOS, nitric oxide synthase; TNF, tumor necrosis factor.

study showed better overall survival in the patients with mildly impaired left ventricular function after using a nonspecific immunomodulatory therapy.[72] Surprisingly, follow-up studies revealed that the circulating antibody amount is the same with or without receiving nonspecific immune modulation.[73] In HF, the use of corticosteroids is controversial and debated; while it may decrease chronic inflammation, it also affects the neurohormonal renin-angiotensin system by inducing angiotensin-converting enzyme inhibitor (ACE).[74] Modulation of the renin-angiotensin-aldosterone system (RASS) by using ACE inhibitors or angiotensin receptor neprilysin inhibitors (ARNIs) is one of the main therapeutic components in HF. It reduces mortality and morbidity with the ARNI valsartan in combination with sacubitril, showing superiority over enalapril in the prospective comparison of angiotensin receptor-neprilysin inhibitor with angiotensin-converting-enzyme inhibitor to dtermine impact on global mortality and mortality in heart failure trial (PARADIGM-HF) study.[75,76] However, the effect on outcomes of systemic sorticosteroid therapy during early management acute heart failure (CORT-AHF) study did not show a difference in adverse events for patients with or without HF after corticosteroid treatment, and this result was independent from the use of ACE inhibitors or ARNI.[77]

Finally, TLR4 is involved in the development of various diseases connected to inflammation. To date, TLR4 signaling cannot be therapeutically targeted; however, this may be a promising avenue to improve cardiac function in HF patients, as well as to reduce myocardial dysfunction in infectious diseases.[78]

Definitely, the characterization of the systemic and/or cardiac immune profile will be a part of precision medicine in the future both in rheumatology and cardiology.

SUMMARY AND PERSPECTIVES

The aim of this paper was to delineate the amount and common quantities linking HF and rheumatic diseases and to shed light on the common risk factor profiles and common immunologic processes in HF and rheumatic diseases. The opportunities for using immune-based strategies to fight development of HF in rheumatic diseases are of interest. The diversity of inflammation further addresses the need for a tailored characterization of inflammation, enabling differentiation of inflammation and subsequent target-specific strategies. The questions raised are which proinflammatory pathways, which patient, which phenotype, which methods, when and how long, and finally which novel therapies will be defined?

This leads the way for introduction of precision medicine in the common field of rheuma-cardiology. An interesting starting point for this therapeutic approach is to influence the release and circulation of cytokines. Inhibition of IL-6 signaling seems to be one of the more promising strategies for the treatment of HF; however, there are a lot of contradictory data, and a clear recommendation for immunomodulatory therapy in patients with rheumatic diseases, at high risk of HF development, cannot be given yet.

CLINICS CARE POINTS

- It is of great importance to acknowledge the increased risk of heart failure in rheumatic diseases
- Heart failure is of utmost importance to acknowledge as early as possible since evidence-based medical treatment decrease morbidity and mortality
- Heart failure is a devasting disease which adds to a poorer prognosis in rheumatic disease

DISCLOSURE

The author has nothing to disclose.

REFERENCES

1. van Riet EES, Hoes AW, Wagenaar KP, et al. Comment on "Epidemiology of heart failure: the prevalence of heart failure and ventricular dysfunction in older adults over time. A systematic review. Eur J Heart Fail 2016;18:242–52.
2. Heidenreich PA, Bozkurt B, Aguilar D, et al. 2022 AHA/ACC/HFSA Guideline for the Management of Heart Failure. J Am Coll Cardiol 2022;79(17). https://doi.org/10.1016/j.jacc.2021.12.012.
3. McDonagh TA, Metra M, Adamo M, et al. 2021 ESC Guidelines for the diagnosis and treatment of acute and chronic heart failure. Eur Heart J 2021;42(36): 3599–726.
4. Mantel Ä, Holmqvist M, Andersson DC, et al. Association Between Rheumatoid Arthritis and Risk of Ischemic and Nonischemic Heart Failure. J Am Coll Cardiol 2017;69(10):1275–85.
5. Løgstrup BB, Ellingsen T, Pedersen AB, et al. Development of heart failure in patients with rheumatoid arthritis: A Danish population-based study. Eur J Clin Invest 2018;48(5):1–8.
6. Crowson CS, Nicola PJ, Kremers HM, et al. How much of the increased incidence of heart failure in rheumatoid arthritis is attributable to traditional cardiovascular risk factors and ischemic heart disease? Arthritis Rheum 2005;52(10):3039–44.
7. Nicola PJ, Maradit-Kremers H, Roger VL, et al. The risk of congestive heart failure in rheumatoid arthritis: A population-based study over 46 years. Arthritis Rheum 2005;52(2):412–20.
8. Løgstrup BB, Ellingsen T, Pedersen AB, et al. Heart Failure and Ischemic Heart Disease in Patients With Rheumatoid Arthritis. J Am Coll Cardiol 2017;70(24): 3069–71.
9. Ferreira MB, Fonseca T, Costa R, et al. Prevalence, risk factors and proteomic bioprofiles associated with heart failure in rheumatoid arthritis: The RA-HF study. Eur J Intern Med 2021;85(September 2020):41–9.
10. Solomon DH, Karlson EW, Rimm EB, et al. Cardiovascular morbidity and mortality in women diagnosed with rheumatoid arthritis. Circulation 2003;107(9):1303–7.
11. Peters MJL, Van Halm VP, Voskuyl AE, et al. Does rheumatoid arthritis equal diabetes mellitus as an independent risk factor for cardiovascular disease? A prospective study. Arthritis Care Res 2009;61(11):1571–9.
12. Khalid Y, Dasu N, Shah A, et al. Incidence of congestive heart failure in rheumatoid arthritis: a review of literature and meta-regression analysis. ESC Hear Fail 2020;7(6):3745–53.
13. Baniaamam M, Paulus WJ, Blanken AB, et al. The effect of biological DMARDs on the risk of congestive heart failure in rheumatoid arthritis: a systematic review. Expert Opin Biol Ther 2018;18(5):585–94.
14. Solomon DH, Greenberg J, Curtis JR, et al. Derivation and internal validation of an expanded cardiovascular risk prediction score for rheumatoid arthritis: A consortium of rheumatology researchers of North America registry study. Arthritis Rheumatol 2015;67(8):1995–2003.
15. Nissen SE, Yeomans ND, Solomon DH, et al. Cardiovascular Safety of Celecoxib, Naproxen, or Ibuprofen for Arthritis. N Engl J Med 2016;375(26):2519–29.
16. Moder KG, Miller TD, Tazelaar HD. Cardiac involvement in systemic lupus erythematosus. Mayo Clin Proc 1999;74(3):275–84.

17. Kim CH, Al-Kindi SG, Jandali B, et al. Incidence and risk of heart failure in systemic lupus erythematosus. Heart 2017;103(3):227–33.
18. Chen SK, Barbhaiya M, Fischer MA, et al. Heart failure risk in systemic lupus erythematosus compared to diabetes mellitus and general medicaid patients. Semin Arthritis Rheum 2019;49(3):389–95.
19. Dhakal BP, Kim CH, Al-Kindi SG, et al. Heart failure in systemic lupus erythematosus. Trends Cardiovasc Med 2018;28(3):187–97.
20. Yafasova A, Fosbøl EL, Schou M, et al. Long-Term Cardiovascular Outcomes in Systemic Lupus Erythematosus. J Am Coll Cardiol 2021;77(14):1717–27.
21. Manzi S, Meilahn EN, Rairie JE, et al. Age-specific incidence rates of myocardial infarction and angina in women with systemic lupus erythematosus: Comparison with the Framingham study. Am J Epidemiol 1997;145(5):408–15.
22. Jonsson H, Nived O, Sturfelt G. Outcome in Systemic Lupus Erythematosus - A prospective Study of Patients from a Defined Population. Medicne 1989;68(3): 141–50.
23. Bae KH, Hong JB, Choi YJ, et al. Association of Congestive Heart Failure and Death with Ankylosing Spondylitis : A Nationwide Longitudinal Cohort Study in Korea. J Korean Neurosurg Soc 2019;62(2):217–24.
24. Han C, Robinson DWJ, Hackett MV, et al. Cardiovascular disease and risk factors in patients with rheumatoid arthritis, psoriatic arthritis, and ankylosing spondylitis. J Rheumatol 2006;33(11):2167–72.
25. Castaneda S, Gonzalez-Juanatey C, Gonzalez-Gay MA. Inflammatory Arthritis and Heart Disease. Curr Pharm Des 2018;24(3):262–80.
26. Heslinga SC, Van Dongen CJ, Konings TC, et al. Diastolic left ventricular dysfunction in ankylosing spondylitis–a systematic review and meta-analysis. Semin Arthritis Rheum 2014;44(1):14–9.
27. Ahlehoff O, Gislason GH, Charlot M, et al. Psoriasis is associated with clinically significant cardiovascular risk: A Danish nationwide cohort study. J Intern Med 2011;270(2):147–57.
28. Koppikar S, Colaco K, Harvey P, et al. Incidence of and Risk Factors for Heart Failure in Patients With Psoriatic Disease: A Cohort Study. Arthritis Care Res (Hoboken) 2021;74(8):1244–53.
29. Khalid U, Ahlehoff O, Gislason GH, et al. Psoriasis and risk of heart failure: a nationwide cohort study. Eur J Heart Fail 2014;16(7):743–8.
30. Kondratiouk S, Udaltsova N, Klatsky AL. Associations of psoriatic arthritis and cardiovascular conditions in a large population. Perm J 2008;12(4):4–8.
31. Gladman DD, Ang M, Su L, et al. Cardiovascular morbidity in psoriatic arthritis. Ann Rheum Dis 2009;68(7):1131–5.
32. Kibari A, Cohen AD, Gazitt T, et al. Cardiac and cardiovascular morbidities in patients with psoriatic arthritis: a population-based case control study. Clin Rheumatol 2019;38(8):2069–75.
33. Polachek A, Touma Z, Anderson M, et al. Risk of Cardiovascular Morbidity in Patients With Psoriatic Arthritis: A Meta-Analysis of Observational Studies. Arthritis Care Res 2017;69(1):67–74.
34. Lottmann K, Chen X, Schädlich PK. Association between gout and all-cause as well as cardiovascular mortality: A systematic review. Curr Rheumatol Rep 2012;14(2):195–203.
35. Colantonio LD, Saag KG, Singh JA, et al. Gout is associated with an increased risk for incident heart failure among older adults: the REasons for Geographic And Racial Differences in Stroke (REGARDS) cohort study. Arthritis Res Ther 2020;22(1):86.

36. Huang H, Huang B, Li Y, et al. Uric acid and risk of heart failure: A systematic review and meta-analysis. Eur J Heart Fail 2014;16(1):15–24.
37. Krishnan E. Gout and the risk for incident heart failure and systolic dysfunction. BMJ Open 2012;2(1):1–8.
38. Wu X, Jian G, Tang Y, et al. Asymptomatic hyperuricemia and incident congestive heart failure in elderly patients without comorbidities. Nutr Metab Cardiovasc Dis 2020;30(4):666–73.
39. Bartels CM, Kind AJH, Everett C, et al. Low frequency of primary lipid screening among Medicare patients with rheumatoid arthritis. Arthritis Rheum 2011;63(5): 1221–30.
40. Toms TE, Panoulas VF, Douglas KMJ, et al. Statin use in rheumatoid arthritis in relation to actual cardiovascular risk: Evidence for substantial undertreatment of lipid-associated cardiovascular risk? Ann Rheum Dis 2010;69(4):683–8.
41. Alemao E, Cawston H, Bourhis F, et al. Comparison of cardiovascular risk algorithms in patients with vs without rheumatoid arthritis and the role of C-reactive protein in predicting cardiovascular outcomes in rheumatoid arthritis. Rheumatol (United Kingdom) 2017;56(5):777–86.
42. Esdaile JM, Abrahamowicz M, Grodzicky T, et al. Traditional Framingham risk factors fail to fully account for accelerated atherosclerosis in systemic lupus erythematosus. Arthritis Rheum 2001;44(10):2331–7.
43. Van Breukelen-van der Stoep DF, Van Zeben D, Klop B, et al. Marked underdiagnosis and undertreatment of hypertension and hypercholesterolaemia in rheumatoid arthritis. Rheumatol (United Kingdom) 2016;55(7):1210–6.
44. Svensson AL, Christensen R, Persson F, et al. Multifactorial intervention to prevent cardiovascular disease in patients with early rheumatoid arthritis: Protocol for a multicentre randomised controlled trial. BMJ Open 2016;6(4). https://doi.org/10.1136/bmjopen-2015-009134.
45. Paulus WJ, Tschöpe C. A novel paradigm for heart failure with preserved ejection fraction: Comorbidities drive myocardial dysfunction and remodeling through coronary microvascular endothelial inflammation. J Am Coll Cardiol 2013;62(4): 263–71.
46. Westermann D, Lindner D, Kasner M, et al. Cardiac inflammation contributes to changes in the extracellular matrix in patients with heart failure and normal ejection fraction. Circ Hear Fail 2011;4(1):44–52.
47. Van Linthout S, Tschöpe C. Inflammation – Cause or Consequence of Heart Failure or Both? Curr Heart Fail Rep 2017;14(4):251–65.
48. Porrello Enzo, Mahmoud Ahmed, Simpson Emma, et al. Transient Regenerative Potential of the Neonatal Mouse Heart. Science 2011;331(6020):1078–80 .Transient.
49. Farache Trajano L, Smart N. Immunomodulation for optimal cardiac regeneration: insights from comparative analyses. Npj Regen Med 2021;6(1):1–11.
50. Bansal Shyam S, Ismahil Mohamad, Goel Mehek, et al. Activated T-Lymphocytes are Essential Drivers of Pathological Remodeling in Ischemic Heart Failure. Circ Hear Fail 2017;10(3):e003688. Activated.
51. Dolejsi T, Delgobo M, Schuetz T, et al. Adult T-cells impair neonatal cardiac regeneration. Eur Heart J 2022. https://doi.org/10.1093/eurheartj/ehac153.
52. Garbern JC, Lee RT. Heart regeneration: 20 years of progress and renewed optimism. Dev Cell 2022;57(4):424–39.
53. Torre-Amione G, Kapadia S, Benedict C, et al. Proinflammatory cytokine levels in patients with depressed left ventricular ejection fraction: A report from the studies of left ventricular dysfunction (SOLVD). J Am Coll Cardiol 1996;27(5):1201–6.

54. Deswal A, Petersen NJ, Feldman AM, et al. Cytokines and cytokine receptors in advanced heart failure: An analysis of the cytokine database from the Vesnarinone Trial (VEST). Circulation 2001;103(16):2055–9.
55. Libby P, Ridker PM, Hansson GK. Inflammation in Atherosclerosis. From Pathophysiology to Practice. J Am Coll Cardiol 2009;54(23):2129–38.
56. Libby P. Role of Inflammation in Atherosclerosis Associated with Rheumatoid Arthritis. Am J Med 2008;121(10 SUPPL.1). https://doi.org/10.1016/j.amjmed.2008.06.014.
57. Elenkov IJ, Wilder RL, Chrousos GP, et al. The sympathetic nerve–an integrative interface between two supersystems: the brain and the immune system. Pharmacol Rev 2000;52(4):595–638.
58. Ahlehoff O, Gislason GH, Jorgensen CH, et al. Psoriasis and risk of atrial fibrillation and ischaemic stroke: A Danish Nationwide Cohort Study. Eur Heart J 2012;33(16):2054–64.
59. Lazzerini PE, Capecchi PL, Laghi-Pasini F. Assessing QT interval in patients with autoimmune chronic inflammatory diseases: Perils and pitfalls. Lupus Sci Med 2016;3(1):1–5.
60. Santos RC, Figueiredo VN, Martins LC, et al. Infliximab reduces cardiac output in rheumatoid arthritis patients without heart failure. Rev Assoc Med Bras 2012;58(6):698–702.
61. Mann DL, McMurray JJV, Packer M, et al. Targeted Anticytokine Therapy in Patients with Chronic Heart Failure: Results of the Randomized Etanercept Worldwide Evaluation (RENEWAL). Circulation 2004;109(13):1594–602.
62. Chung CP, Giles JT, Petri M, et al. Prevalence of traditional modifiable cardiovascular risk factors in patients with rheumatoid arthritis: Comparison with control subjects from the multi-ethnic study of atherosclerosis. Semin Arthritis Rheum 2012;41(4):535–44.
63. Lv S, Han M, Yi R, et al. Anti-TNF-α therapy for patients with sepsis: a systematic meta-analysis. Int J Clin Pract 2014;68(4):520–8.
64. Fakharian A, Barati S, Mirenayat M, et al. Evaluation of adalimumab effects in managing severe cases of COVID-19 : A randomized controlled trial. Int Immunopharmacol 2021;99:107961.
65. Everett BM, Siddiqi HK. Heart Failure, the Inflammasome, and Interleukin-1β: Prognostic and Therapeutic? J Am Coll Cardiol 2019;73(9):1026–8.
66. Ridker PM, Everett BM, Thuren T, et al. Antiinflammatory therapy with canakinumab for atherosclerotic disease. N Engl J Med 2017;377(12):1119–31.
67. Buckley Leo, Carbone Salvatore, Trankle Cory, et al. Effect of Interleukin-1 Blockade on Left Ventricular Systolic Performance and Work: A Post-Hoc Pooled Analysis of Two Clinical Trials. J Cardiovasc Pharmacol 2018;72(1):68–70. Effect.
68. Kobayashi H, Kobayashi Y, Giles JT, et al. Tocilizumab treatment increases left ventricular ejection fraction and decreases left ventricular mass index in patients with rheumatoid arthritis without cardiac symptoms: Assessed using 3.0 tesla cardiac magnetic resonance imaging. J Rheumatol 2014;41(10):1916–21.
69. Yokoe I, Kobayashi H, Kobayashi Y, et al. Impact of tocilizumab on N-terminal pro-brain natriuretic peptide levels in patients with active rheumatoid arthritis without cardiac symptoms. Scand J Rheumatol 2018;47(5):364–70.
70. Yano T, Osanami A, Shimizu M, et al. Utility and safety of tocilizumab in Takayasu arteritis with severe heart failure and muscle wasting. ESC Hear Fail 2019;6(4):894–7.
71. Meyer MAS, Wiberg S, Grand J, et al. Treatment Effects of Interleukin-6 Receptor Antibodies for Modulating the Systemic Inflammatory Response After Out-of-

Hospital Cardiac Arrest (The IMICA Trial): A Double-Blinded, Placebo-Controlled, Single-Center, Randomized, Clinical Trial. Circulation 2021;143(19):1841–51.

72. Torre-Amione G, Anker SD, Bourge RC, et al. Results of a non-specific immuno-modulation therapy in chronic heart failure (ACCLAIM trial): a placebo-controlled randomised trial. Lancet (London, England) 2008;371(9608):228–36.

73. Torre-Amione G, Sestier F, Radovancevic B, et al. Effects of a novel immune modulation therapy in patients with advanced chronic heart failure: results of a randomized, controlled, phase II trial. J Am Coll Cardiol 2004;44(6):1181–6.

74. Fishel RS, Eisenberg S, Shai SY, et al. Glucocorticoids induce angiotensin-converting enzyme expression in vascular smooth muscle. Hypertens (Dallas, Tex 1979) 1995;25(3):343–9.

75. Garg R, Yusuf S. Overview of randomized trials of angiotensin-converting enzyme inhibitors on mortality and morbidity in patients with heart failure. Collaborative Group on ACE Inhibitor Trials. JAMA 1995;273(18):1450–6.

76. McMurray JJV, Packer M, Desai AS, et al. Angiotensin-neprilysin inhibition versus enalapril in heart failure. N Engl J Med 2014;371(11):993–1004.

77. Ò Miró, Takagi K, Gayat E, et al. CORT-AHF Study: Effect on Outcomes of Systemic Corticosteroid Therapy During Early Management Acute Heart Failure. JACC Heart Fail 2019;7(10):834–45.

78. Ain QU, Batool M, Choi S. TLR4-Targeting Therapeutics: Structural Basis and Computer-Aided Drug Discovery Approaches. Molecules 2020;25(3). https://doi.org/10.3390/molecules25030627.

79. Champion S, Lapidus N, Cherié G, et al. Pentoxifylline in heart failure: A meta-analysis of clinical trials. Cardiovasc Ther 2014;32(4):159–62.

80. Aukrust P, Yndestad A, Damås JK, et al. Inflammation and chronic heart failure-potential therapeutic role of intravenous immunoglobulin. Autoimmun Rev 2004;3(3):221–7.

81. Moreira DM, Vieira JL, Mascia Gottschall CA. The Effects of METhotrexate Therapy on the Physical Capacity of Patients With ISchemic Heart Failure: A Randomized Double-Blind, Placebo-Controlled Trial (METIS Trial). J Card Fail 2009;15(10):828–34.

82. Van Tassell BW, Canada J, Carbone S, et al. Interleukin-1 blockade in recently decompensated systolic heart failure: Results from REDHART (Recently Decompensated Heart Failure Anakinra Response Trial). Circ Hear Fail 2017;10(11):1–11.

83. Van Tassell BW, Arena R, Biondi-Zoccai G, et al. Effects of interleukin-1 blockade with anakinra on aerobic exercise capacity in patients with heart failure and preserved ejection fraction (from the D-HART pilot study). Am J Cardiol 2014;113(2):321–7.

84. Trankle CR, Canada JM, Cei L, et al. Usefulness of Canakinumab to Improve Exercise Capacity in Patients With Long-Term Systolic Heart Failure and Elevated C-Reactive Protein. Am J Cardiol 2018;122(8):1366–70.

85. Chung ES, Packer M, Lo KH, et al. Randomized, double-blind, placebo-controlled, pilot trial of infliximab, a chimeric monoclonal antibody to tumor necrosis factor-α, in patients with moderate-to-severe heart failure: Results of the anti-TNF therapy against congestive heart failure (ATTACH. Circulation 2003;107(25):3133–40.

86. Givertz MM, Anstrom KJ, Redfield MM, et al. Effects of Xanthine Oxidase Inhibition in Hyperuricemic Heart Failure Patients: The Xanthine Oxidase Inhibition for Hyperuricemic Heart Failure Patients (EXACT-HF) Study. Circulation 2015;131(20):1763–71.

87. Hare JM, Mangal B, Brown J, et al. Impact of oxypurinol in patients with symptomatic heart failure. Results of the OPT-CHF study. J Am Coll Cardiol 2008;51(24): 2301–9.
88. Tang L, Wang H, Ziolo MT. Targeting NOS as a therapeutic approach for heart failure. Pharmacol Ther 2014;142(3):306–15.
89. Tavazzi L, Maggioni AP, Marchioli R, et al. Effect of rosuvastatin in patients with chronic heart failure (the GISSI-HF trial): a randomised, double-blind, placebo-controlled trial. Lancet (London, England) 2008;372(9645):1231–9.
90. Kjekshus J, Apetrei E, Barrios V, et al. Rosuvastatin in older patients with systolic heart failure. N Engl J Med 2007;357(22):2248–61.
91. Deftereos S, Giannopoulos G, Panagopoulou V, et al. Anti-inflammatory treatment with colchicine in stable chronic heart failure: a prospective, randomized study. JACC Heart Fail 2014;2(2):131–7.
92. Wohlford GF, Van Tassell BW, Billingsley HE, et al. Phase 1B, Randomized, Double-Blinded, Dose Escalation, Single-Center, Repeat Dose Safety and Pharmacodynamics Study of the Oral NLRP3 Inhibitor Dapansutrile in Subjects With NYHA II-III Systolic Heart Failure. J Cardiovasc Pharmacol 2020;77(1):49–60.

Cardiovascular Disease in Large Vessel Vasculitis

Risks, Controversies, and Management Strategies

Alison H. Clifford, MD

KEYWORDS

- Takayasu's arteritis • Giant cell arteritis • Large vessel vasculitis
- Cardiovascular disease • Atherosclerosis • Stroke • Myocardial infarction
- Aortic aneurysm

KEY POINTS

- Cardiovascular events and mortality are increased in patients with TAK and GCA.
- Disease activity, damage, and accelerated atherosclerosis contribute to CV risk.
- Early diagnosis and rapid control of vascular inflammation are critical.
- All patients with LVV, regardless of age, should be counseled re: benefits of:
  o Smoking cessation.
  o Maintenance of healthy body weight.
  o Balanced diet and regular exercise.
- Patients with LVV should be screened for hypertension, dyslipidemia, and hyperglycemia and treated aggressively, if present.

INTRODUCTION

The primary systemic large vessel vasculitides (LVV), Takayasu's arteritis (TAK), and giant cell arteritis (GCA), are rare diseases characterized by the inflammation of blood vessel walls. Typically affected sites include the aorta and its major branch vessels; however, essentially any medium to the large vessel may be involved. Cellular infiltrates damage the blood vessel walls, producing wall thickening, stenoses, occlusions, or aneurysms with potential for dissection or rupture. Cardiovascular disease (CVD) is the leading cause of death in both TAK and GCA.[1–3] Several potential mechanisms, including active vasculitis, vascular damage from prior inflammation, and accelerated atherosclerosis, are postulated to contribute to the increased CV burden

Department of Medicine, Division of Rheumatology, University of Alberta, Edmonton, Alberta T6G 2G3, Canada
E-mail address: alison5@ualberta.ca

Rheum Dis Clin N Am 49 (2023) 81–96
https://doi.org/10.1016/j.rdc.2022.08.004
0889-857X/23/© 2022 Elsevier Inc. All rights reserved.

rheumatic.theclinics.com

observed in these patients. While TAK and GCA share many similarities, including vascular targets, clinical symptoms, and histopathology, significant differences exist in their target demographics, which may allow for insight into the mechanisms underlying CV events. In this review, we will compare and contrast CVD in TAK and GCA, including event rates, hypothesized mechanisms of disease, areas of ongoing uncertainty, and possible risk mitigation strategies.

TAKAYASU'S ARTERITIS AND GIANT CELL ARTERITIS: EPIDEMIOLOGY, VASCULAR TARGETS AND PATHOGENESIS

Although TAK and GCA share many similarities, they target strikingly different patient populations. TAK is a disease of young people, with usual age of onset between 18 and 40 years.[4] Predominantly females are affected, and there is substantial geographical variation, with the highest disease incidence observed in Asia and South America.[1,5] Like TAK, GCA also preferentially affects women, but in contrast, it is a disease of the elderly, by definition affecting those only after the age of 50. The average age of onset in GCA is typically closer to 75–85 years; at a time of life when atherosclerosis is also highly prevalent. GCA is most common in those of Northern European ancestry.[6] Both TAK and GCA target the elastic arteries, most frequently the subclavian arteries and aorta. Additionally, in TAK, the carotid, renal and mesenteric arteries are commonly involved,[4] while GCA prefers the superficial temporal, ophthalmic, posterior ciliary, vertebral, and axillary arteries.[4]

Vascular infiltrates in TAK and GCA consist of macrophages, lymphocytes, and multinucleated giant cells, with resulting hyperplasia of the intima and adventitia, and thinning of the media due to loss of elastic fibers.[6,7] Although in many cases their histopathology is indistinguishable, in comparison to GCA, TAK lesions typically contain more natural killer cells and a lower CD4/CD8 ratio.[4] In both TAK and GCA, treatment consists of high doses of glucocorticoids with slow taper over months to years, in combination with steroid-sparing medications, such as methotrexate (TAK or GCA), anti-TNF alpha agents (TAK only), or anti-IL-6 therapy (TAK and GCA.)[8]

ESTIMATES OF CARDIOVASCULAR RISK IN TAKAYASU'S ARTERITIS AND GIANT CELL ARTERITIS: AN OVERVIEW

A disease of young people, TAK is associated with a significantly increased risk of mortality, with an estimated standardized mortality rate (SMR) of 2.73.[1,9] CVD is the leading cause of death in TAK,[1,9–11] with CV events being about 10 times more common than expected.[12] In contrast, although overall mortality does not appear to be increased in GCA, like TAK, a greater than expected risk of CV death, specifically, has been observed even in these elderly patients, with an SMR of 1.3.[2,3] A comparison of the specific CV risks in TAK and GCA is discussed next (and summarized in **Table 1**).

CORONARY ARTERY DISEASE IN TAKAYASU'S ARTERITIS

Multiple observational studies have demonstrated an increased prevalence of coronary artery disease in patients with TAK.[10–15] In a 2018 systematic review and meta-analysis of 35 studies, including 3262 patients, the pooled prevalence of MI was noted to be 3.4% at any time during the course of TAK. MI's were most prevalent in patients from Central and South America (18.8%) as compared to those in Asia (1.2–1.3%), and less common in childhood onset versus adult-onset disease (5.8% vs 13.5%).[12]

Table 1
Comparison of epidemiology, CV risks, and mechanisms in TAK and GCA

	TAK	GCA
Epidemiology		
Typical age of onset (years)	18–40	75–85
Sex	F > M	F > M
Highest geographical prevalence	Asia	N. Europe
Overall mortality	↑	No difference
Cardiovascular risk		
CV death	↑	↑
MI	↑	Unclear
CVA	↑	↑
Ao aneurysm	↑	↑
VTE	No data	↑
Evidence for CVD mechanism		
Systemic inflammation	+	+
Active vasculitis	+	+
Vascular damage from prior inflammation	+	+
Accelerated atherosclerosis	+	No

Abbreviations: Ao, aortic; CVA, cerebrovascular accident; F, female; M, male; MI, myocardial infarction; N. Europe, Northern Europe; PAD, peripheral arterial disease; VTE, venous thromboembolism.

In terms of mechanism, the reported frequency of coronary artery vasculitis in TAK varies widely, reported in between 3 and 50% of patients.[16–19] The lowest prevalence of coronary vasculitis (3–5%) comes from series including childhood onset TAK,[19,20] while involvement in adults is typically estimated around 10%.[17] In a retrospective review of 130 adult patients with TAK (mean age 32 years) who systematically underwent coronary angiography due to symptoms, abnormal ECG's or echocardiograms; however, over 50% of patients were found to have coronary artery involvement, of whom 35% were asymptomatic, suggesting that this manifestation is likely to be under-estimated.[18] In this series, the presence of coronary artery involvement by angiography independently predicted subsequent major CV event and CV death.[18]

Autopsy data also confirm that coronary vasculitis is present in 11–45% patients with TAK.[21] Histopathologically, coronary lesions most commonly appear as ostial or proximal artery stenoses resulting from an extension of the inflammatory process in the ascending aorta, however diffuse or focal coronary arteritis in skip lesions, or more rarely coronary aneurysms, may be seen.[22] Concomittant coronary vasculitis and early atherosclerosis has also been observed.[21,23]

CORONARY ARTERY DISEASE IN GIANT CELL ARTERITIS

In contrast, conflicting evidence exists with respect to whether the incidence of MI is greater than that which would be expected for age in GCA. Although several cohort studies suggested increased risk,[24,25] a 2015 systematic review and meta-analysis identified a nonsignificant trend only toward increased coronary artery events in patients with GCA.[26] Subsequently, a very large study of 9778 patients with GCA matched to nonvasculitis controls by age, sex, and number years of history, found that postdiagnosis, patients with GCA were significantly more likely to have incident MI's, with an adjusted HR of 1.57.[27]

Unlike in TAK, no studies have systematically imaged the coronary arteries of patients with GCA using angiography, and therefore the relative contributions of active coronary vasculitis, vascular damage from prior vasculitis, or accelerated atherosclerosis to the incidence of coronary events in GCA remains unclear. In several reports, the risk of coronary events appears highest in first 1 month to 1 year after diagnosis, supporting the role of active systemic inflammation in MI.[24,25] Small case series describing histopathological proof of coronary vasculitis in GCA,[28-30] and an association between anticardiolipin antibodies and acute coronary thrombosis in GCA have rarely been reported.[31]

Using noncontrast CT to assess for vascular calcification, Bannerjee and colleagues assessed the coronaries, as well as aorta and branch vessels of patients with GCA, TAK, and control patients with hyperlipidemia (HLD). Interestingly, although total Agatston scores (summed vascular calcification score) were significantly higher in patients with GCA than HLD controls, calcification in the coronary arteries, specifically, occurred less often (35% GCA vs 67% HLD group, $p < 0.01$), suggesting that coronary events in GCA and LVV may relate moreso to disease-specific events rather than traditional cardiovascular risk factors.[32]

CEREBROVASCULAR DISEASE IN TAKAYASU'S ARTERITIS

Stroke or transient ischemic attacks (TIA) are common in TAK.[12,14,33,34] With an adjusted odds ratio of 4.66 compared to the general population, stroke is the third most common reason for hospitalization among US patients with TAK.[35] In 2 large systematic reviews and meta-analyses on this subject, including over 3000 patients with TAK each, the prevalence of stroke and TIA was identified to be between 11.7% and 15.8%.[12,36]

Stroke in TAK typically occurs due to extracranial vasculitis affecting the carotid and subclavian arteries;[37] however, small studies also suggest that intracranial vascular involvement may occasionally be seen.[37,38] Accelerated atherosclerosis also appears to play a role. In a study by Seyahi and colleagues using B mode ultrasound of the carotid arteries in 30 patients with TAK (mean age 35.4 years), carotid intimal-media thickness (cIMT) was found to be significantly increased in patients with TAK as compared to systemic lupus erythematosus (SLE) patients and controls. Although cIMT had a diffuse, homogenous appearance most suggestive of vasculitic involvement in patients with TAK, atherosclerotic plaques were also significantly more common, visualized in 27% TAK and only 2% controls, $p = 0.005$. Interestingly, plaques in patients with TAK almost exclusively formed within vasculitic carotid arteries, suggesting a direct association between vasculitis and accelerated atherosclerosis.[39] Similar findings were observed by Hatri and colleagues,[40] who found a high prevalence of plaque in patients with TAK (45% of patients with mean age 41), as compared to controls (4%, mean age 44, $p < 0.001$), despite a low prevalence of traditional cardiovascular risk factors.

CEREBROVASCULAR DISEASE IN GIANT CELL ARTERITIS

Patients with GCA are also at increased risk of CVA.[24,25,27] In a large systematic review and meta-analysis including over 17,000 patients with GCA, the pooled risk ratio of stroke was 1.40.[41] In addition, patients with GCA who experience stroke have a significantly poorer survival.[42] Stroke in GCA is notable for preferentially affecting the posterior circulation,[43-45] with ischemic vision loss being the most consistent clinical predictor (OR 5, $p = 0.0002$)[42,46,47] The risk of stroke is consistently reported to be highest in the early phase of the disease (first 1 to 4 weeks.)[46,47]

In keeping with the above observations, active vasculitis appears to be the main mechanism contributing to stroke risk in GCA. In a detailed report of 12 autopsies performed on patients with GCA who died during the acute phase of disease of stroke, active vasculitis of the vertebral arteries was observed in 100% of patients. Vertebral artery inflammation was bilateral and diffuse, starting from the vessel origin and continuing to a point 5 mm past the perforation of the dura before abruptly normalizing. Given the striking consistencies observed in this pattern, it was hypothesized that the inflammatory reaction in GCA may represent a targeted response to the presence and degree of elastic tissue in particular vessel walls.[29]

Like TAK, intracranial involvement in GCA occurs, but is less common. Among 20 patients with GCA who underwent magnetic resonance angiography (MRA) of the head and neck, 10 (50%) were noted to have uptake in the intradural carotids;[43] however, in a larger study of 51 patients, only 10% had probable/definite involvement of intracranial vessels.[44] Accelerated atherosclerosis does not appear to be a major contributor to elevated stroke risk in GCA. In 40 biopsy-proven patients with GCA, carotid ultrasonography actually revealed reduced cIMT as compared to controls (p = 0.005), with no difference in presence of atherosclerotic plaque.[48]

AORTIC DISEASE IN TAKAYASU'S ARTERITIS

Aortic involvement is typical in TAK, present in 90% patients.[4] Although any segment of the aorta may be targeted, abdominal aortic involvement is more common in those of Asian ethnicity or childhood onset, while thoracic aortic involvement is more frequent in patients from North America and Europe.[7,9,20,34] Patients with TAK are at markedly increased risk of aortic aneurysm compared to their age-matched counterparts, with an adjusted OR 40.76.[35] In these patients, thoracic aortic aneurysm is especially important to recognize, as an independent predictor of death.[9] Aortic regurgitation due to aneurysmal change in the ascending aorta is also observed.[7]

AORTIC DISEASE IN GIANT CELL ARTERITIS

Thoracic aortic involvement is also common in GCA.[49–52] Prospective imaging studies confirm that between 50 and 65% of patients with GCA have aortic inflammation[53,54] and 8–15% have aortic structural damage (ASD), such as dilatation or aneurysm, present at diagnosis.[54,55] The risk of ASD increases over time, affecting nearly 30% of patients by 10 years. Overall, the adjusted HR for aortic aneurysm in GCA is significantly elevated at 1.92–1.98.[27,56]

Development of aortic disease in GCA appears to be influenced by both traditional risk factors, such as male sex,[56,57] hypertension or use of antihypertensives,[49,52,56,57] smoking,[55,56] dyslipidemia,[58] and coronary artery disease,[58] as well as disease-specific factors, such as the presence of polymyalgia rheumatica,[49] and baseline aortic fluorodeoxyglucose (FDG) uptake on positron emission tomography (PET). Aortic FDG uptake is one of the most important predictors of future aortic dilatation,[57,59] suggesting that aneurysmal change most likely develops as a consequence of damage from prior inflammation. In support of this theory, aortic tissue specimens from GCA patients with ASD are most notable for the striking loss of elastic fibers in the aortic wall.[51]

THROMBOSIS IN TAKAYASUS ARTERITIS (TAK) AND GIANT CELL ARTERITIS

To date, there are little data evaluating the risk of venous thromboembolism (VTE) in TAK. In a single study, VTE was reported to be responsible for 6% of admissions to hospital in patients with TAK, but no further details were available.[35]

In GCA, however, the risk of VTE is clearly increased above baseline. Among Canadian patients with GCA, the HR for VTE was measured to be 2.44, with the highest risk of thrombosis observed during the 1st year of diagnosis.[60] Similarly, a large study evaluating U.K. health records between 1990 and 2013 found an overall incidence rate of VTE of 5.9 per 1000 person-years in patients with GCA, producing an adjusted RR of 2.25 for PE, and 1.96 for DVT. The risk of any VTE was significantly increased even 1 year prior to diagnosis of GCA, rose progressively up to the point of diagnosis (HR 9.9), then gradually declined over subsequent months to years, strongly suggesting a role for inflammation-induced thrombosis.[61]

RISK FACTORS FOR CARDIOVASCULAR DISEASES IN TAKAYASUS ARTERITIS (TAK) AND GIANT CELL ARTERITIS

Susceptibility to CV events in LVV appears to be influenced by a number of nonmodifiable and modifiable factors, as summarized in **Fig. 1**, and discussed in detail later in discussion.

Genetics and Cardiovascular Risk

In patients with TAK, the presence of HLA Bw52, previously identified to correlate with systemic inflammation and disease progression,[62,63] also significantly correlates with myocardial disease. Specifically, this haplotype confers an increased risk of echocardiographic abnormality, aortic regurgitation, and perfusion abnormality by myocardial scintigraphy.[64] In addition, a synergistic role between HLA-B (which encodes for MHC class I) and non-HLA genes in TAK susceptibility has been identified, with the presence of an IL12b variant correlating with both the development and severity of aortic regurgitation in these patients.[65]

In contrast, genes encoding the HLA class II region have the strongest association with GCA disease susceptibility.[66,67] In addition, PLG (plasminogen), a known shared risk for atherosclerosis and periodontitis,[68] has recently been identified as a GCA risk

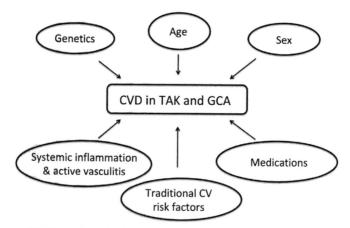

Fig. 1. Nonmodifiable and modifiable contributors to CV events in LVV. Modifiable contributors to CVD in LVV, including systemic inflammation, active vasculitis, and traditional CV risk factors (smoking, obesity, physical inactivity, hypertension, dyslipidemia, hyperglycemia) should be treated early to minimize CV risk in LVV. Judicious use of medications, including the minimization of glucocorticoids where possible, and increased use of adjunctive immunosuppressive agents, may ameliorate outcomes.

gene.[67] With roles in angiogenesis and lymphocyte recruitment, whether *PLG* may have an overlapping role in CVD predisposition in GCA requires further study.

Age and Sex

The prevalence of serious CV events like MI and stroke increases with increasing age in TAK.[12] Age independently predicts coronary artery involvement (OR of 1.537 for every 10 year increase in age, p = 0.002),[18] and is significantly associated with the presence of carotid artery plaque in these patients.[38] Similarly, in GCA increased age appears associated with higher risk of CVD,[42,69] and in both forms of LVV, age correlates with worsening vascular calcification.[32] While in GCA, male sex appears to be a particular risk for aortic aneurysm,[52,56] similar findings have not been identified in TAK.

Traditional Cardiovascular Risk Factors

Controversy exists surrounding the contribution of traditional risk factors to high CV event rates observed in LVV. While several studies have found increased prevalence of hypertension,[13,33,70,71] metabolic syndrome,[71] hypertriglyceridemia,[71] and Framingham risk scores[13] in patients with TAK, their presence does not appear to correlate with the degree of atherosclerotic plaque[39] or sufficiently explain the observed increased events experienced by these young patients.[18,39,40,70]

In GCA, conflicting evidence exists as to whether traditional CV risk factors are more prevalent prior to a vasculitis diagnosis.[27,72,73] Postdiagnosis, however, rates of diabetes, hypertension, and dyslipidemia are clearly increased,[27,74] likely due to glucocorticoid therapy. Although traditional CV risk factors, particularly hypertension and current or former smoking increase the risk of CV events in patients with GCA,[3,52,55–57,75] these do not adequately explain the excess risk of stroke or VTE observed.

Systemic Inflammation

Systemic inflammation appears to play a key role in CV events in LVV. In TAK, baseline active disease correlates with increased risk of major CV event (HR 7.084),[18] and type V angiographic disease (most extensive) conveys highest risk for coronary artery involvement[18,76] and events.[15] Low body mass index and anemia, surrogate markers of chronic inflammation, correlate with CV risk,[14] and CRP predicts the presence of carotid plaque.[40] Similarly, in GCA the risk of particular events (namely stroke and VTE) appear to peak at the time of diagnosis, suggesting a definite role for acute inflammation in these events.[25,46,60,61,72] In both TAK and GCA, active disease is associated with endothelial dysfunction, which improves with glucocorticoid treatment and resolution of disease activity.[77,78]

MANAGEMENT STRATEGIES TO MINIMIZE CARDIOVASCULAR DISEASES IN LARGE VESSEL VASCULITIDES: CONTROVERSIES AND PRACTICAL SUGGESTIONS

To date, there is a paucity of prospective data addressing the CV benefits and risks of immunosuppressive and cardioprotective drugs in patients with LVV. Existing evidence is discussed in the following sections (**Table 2** for summary.)

Immunosuppressive Agents

In TAK, the absence of immunosuppressive therapy is associated with a significantly increased risk of CV event;[18] however, teasing apart the effects of specific therapies is challenging. Corticosteroids, with known potent antiinflammatory and proatherogenic properties, appear overall neutral with respect to CV risk in TAK.[15,40,79] On the contrary, methotrexate use seems protective.[15] In addition to steroid-sparing benefits,

Table 2
CV benefits and risks of immunosuppressive and cardiovascular drugs in LVV

Drug	TAK	GCA
Prednisone		
Benefits	Improved endothelial function,[a] rapid control of vasculitis	Improved endothelial function,[a] rapid control of vasculitis[b]
Risks	HTN, hyperglycemia, dyslipidemia, weight gain, vascular calcification[a]	HTN, hyperglycemia, dyslipidemia, weight gain, vascular calcification[a]
Methotrexate		
Benefits	Modest steroid-sparing evidence[a] 60% reduced risk ischemic events[a]	Modest steroid-sparing evidence[b] No data re: reduction in CV events
Risks	None identified	None identified
Tocilizumab		
Benefits	Steroid-sparing evidence.[b] Improvement in vasculitic coronary artery stenoses.[a]	Strong steroid-sparing evidence.[b] Reduced visual manifestations.[a]
Risks	Dyslipidemia	Dyslipidemia
Anti-TNF therapy		
Benefits	Steroid-sparing evidence[a]	Not indicated
Risks	Exacerbation of moderate to severe CHF[b]	Not indicated
Antiplatelet or anticoagulant		
Benefits	Conflicting data[a]	Conflicting data[a] Meta-analysis: reduced risk of severe ischemic events[a]
Risks	Rare bleeding[a]	No increased bleeding risk noted[a]
Statin		
Benefits	No evidence of routine benefit[a]	Conflicting data[a]
Risks	None identified	Triggered vasculitis[a]

Abbreviations: anti-TNF therapy, anti-tumour necrosis factor therapy; HTN, hypertension.
[a] Observational data available (retrospective, prospective or cross-sectional).
[b] Randomized control trial data available.

in a retrospective review of 207 patients with TAK, the use of methotrexate was associated with a 60% reduced risk of ischemic event, while no such association was observed in those receiving glucocorticoids or azathioprine.[15] Potential cardioprotective mechanisms of methotrexate include the inhibition of foam cell formation, reversal of cholesterol transport,[80] and promotion of healthy endothelial cell function through the reduction of free radicals and oxidative stress.[81] In addition to methotrexate, both tocilizumab (TCZ) and anti-TNF therapy have demonstrated steroid-sparing benefits in TAK.[82,83] While case reports and small retrospective series suggest TCZ may significantly ameliorate coronary artery stenoses,[84,85] no specific data on CVD reduction with anti-TNF's are available. Given potential for exacerbation, anti-TNF therapy is usually avoided in patients with known moderate to severe CHF.[86]

In GCA, although high dose glucocorticoids may help acutely with endothelial cell dysfunction and vasculitis control,[78,87] long-term use is associated with worsening vascular calcification[32] and numerous toxicities.[88] For every 1 g of cumulative glucocorticoid exposure, patients with GCA experience an associated 3–8% increased risk of adverse event, including hypertension or glucose intolerance.[89] The addition of TCZ, an IL-6 receptor antibody, to GCA therapy results in significant steroid sparing,[90] reduction in disease flare and new visual manifestations, but with some risk of dyslipidemia.[91] Thus far, data suggest that rates of MI and stroke are similar in TCZ-treated and TCZ–naïve patients with GCA.[92]

Antiplatelet Use

The use of antiplatelet agents in TAK remains controversial. While a small retrospective cohort study of 41 patients with TAK suggested a significant protective effect of antiplatelet on the risk of ischemic event (HR 0.055, p = 0.001)[33] this finding could not be confirmed in subsequent larger studies.[15,79]

Likewise, most[93,94] but not all[95] retrospective studies found the concomitant use of low-dose acetylsalicylic acid (ASA) to be associated with reduced risk of ischemic events in GCA. Subsequently, a cumulative meta-analysis of 6 studies (all retrospective) including 914 patients with GCA found antiplatelet or anticoagulant use to be associated with a reduced risk of severe ischemic events (OR 0.318, p = 0.049) without increasing bleeding risk.[96] Although some major societies endorse the use of low-dose ASA (75–300 mg daily) in patients with GCA with ocular involvement,[97] others advise this be considered on a case-by-case basis only, due to the lack of high-quality evidence.[98,99] Taken together, existing retrospective data favor a possible beneficial effect of antiplatelet use in GCA, but prospective confirmation is needed.

Statin Use

Statins, with dual lipid-lowering and anti-inflammatory effects, are of high interest in the prevention of CVD in LVV. Prior studies have confirmed the ability of statins to reduce the risk of major CV events in patients with elevated CRP despite normal LDL levels.[100–102] Postulated mechanisms for this include the inhibition of macrophage activation, reduction of TNF-alpha and IL-6 levels, and improved endothelial cell function.[100,103,104]

Despite the above, however, the benefits of routine statin use in patients with LVV are still unclear. Although one study found a nonstatistically significant trend toward reduced glucocorticoid requirements with statin use in GCA,[105] rarely, statins may also trigger new vasculitis.[106] Data with respect to CVD prevention in LVV are conflicting. In one retrospective study of 103 patients with GCA, cumulative daily dose of statin independently predicted the need for subsequent hospitalization for CVD,[107] while another study with a similar number of subjects and follow-up, found no benefit.[108] Similarly, although statin use is more common among patients with TAK than their age-matched counterparts,[13] routine use has not yet been proven to reduce their risk of CV event.[15,79] Currently, best evidence based on recommendations from major societies, such as the Canadian Cardiovascular Society, are that all patients with inflammatory diseases like LVV be actively screened for dyslipidemia, and a validated score, such as Framingham risk score, be used to guide subsequent treatment decisions.[109]

SUMMARY

Both TAK and GCA are associated with an increased risk of CVD and CV mortality. The relative increased risk is particularly striking in young patients with TAK in whom such events would otherwise be uncommon, but even in elderly patients with GCA, the increased risk is appreciated for particular events such as stroke, aortic aneurysm, and VTE's. In TAK, active vasculitis, vascular damage from prior inflammation and accelerated atherosclerosis all contribute to CVD, while in GCA, systemic inflammation and active vasculitis appear to be the main drivers. Given the recognized increased risk of CV death, all patients with LVV, regardless of age, should be counseled at diagnosis regarding the benefits of lifestyle modifications, including smoking cessation, maintenance of healthy body weight, diet, and regular exercise. Early vasculitis diagnosis and rapid and sustained control of active vascular inflammation are critical to minimize damage and reduce early events, while increased use of adjunctive immunosuppressive medications to minimize glucocorticoid exposure will likely yield improved outcomes and deserves future study. Lastly, all patients with LVV should be actively screened for the presence of hypertension, dyslipidemia, and hyperglycemia, and treated aggressively for these if present. Although there is no international consensus regarding the routine use of ASA in LVV, a low threshold for its addition should be considered based on patients' history of CV events, risk factors, and degree and territory of vascular stenoses.

CLINICS CARE POINTS

- CV events and mortality are increased in patients with TAK and GCA
- Disease activity, damage, and accelerated atherosclerosis contribute to CV risk
- Early diagnosis and rapid control of vascular inflammation are critical
- All patients with LVV, regardless of age, should be counseled re: benefits of:
  o Smoking cessation
  o Maintenance of healthy body weight
  o Balanced diet and regular exercise
- Patients with LVV should be screened for hypertension, dyslipidemia, and hyperglycemia and treated aggressively, if present

DISCLOSURE

A.H. Clifford is a site principal investigator for an industry-initiated clinical trial (Abbvie) and has received honoraria from UCB and Hoffman La-Roche.

REFERENCES

1. Egebjerg K, Baslund B, Obel N, et al. Mortality and cardiovascular morbidity among patients diagnosed with Takayasu's arteritis: a Danish nationwide cohort study. Clin Exp Rheumatol 2020;38 Suppl 124(2):91–4.
2. Lee YH, Song GG. Overall and cause-specific mortality in giant cell arteritis : a meta-analysis. Z Rheumatol 2018;77(10):946–51.
3. Uddhammar A, Eriksson A-L, Nyström L, et al. Increased mortality due to cardiovascular disease in patients with giant cell arteritis in northern Sweden. J Rheumatol 2002;29(4):737–42.
4. Watanabe R, Berry GJ, Liang DH, et al. Pathogenesis of giant cell arteritis and takayasu arteritis-similarities and differences. Curr Rheumatol Rep 2020; 22(10):68.
5. Onen F, Akkoc N. Epidemiology of Takayasu arteritis. Presse Médicale 2017; 46(7, Part 2):e197–203.
6. Weyand CM, Goronzy JJ. Medium- and large-vessel vasculitis. N Engl J Med 2003;349(2):160–9.
7. Kerr GS, Hallahan CW, Giordano J, et al. Takayasu arteritis. Ann Intern Med 1994;120(11):919–29.

8. Saadoun D, Vautier M, Cacoub P. Medium- and large-vessel vasculitis. Circulation 2021;143(3):267–82.
9. Mirouse A, Biard L, Comarmond C, et al. Overall survival and mortality risk factors in Takayasu's arteritis: a multicenter study of 318 patients. J Autoimmun 2019;96:35–9.
10. Lupi-Herrera E, Sánchez-Torres G, Marcushamer J, et al. Takayasu's arteritis. Clinical study of 107 cases. Am Heart J 1977;93(1):94–103.
11. Ishikawa K, Maetani S. Long-term outcome for 120 Japanese patients with Takayasu's disease. Clinical and statistical analyses of related prognostic factors. Circulation 1994;90(4):1855–60.
12. Kim H, Barra L. Ischemic complications in Takayasu's arteritis: a meta-analysis. Semin Arthritis Rheum 2018;47(6):900–6.
13. Alibaz-Oner F, Koster MJ, Unal AU, et al. Assessment of the frequency of cardiovascular risk factors in patients with Takayasu's arteritis. Rheumatol Oxf Engl 2017;56(11):1939–44.
14. Liu Q, Dang A, Lv N, et al. Anaemia and low body mass index are associated with increased cardiovascular disease in patients with Takayasu arteritis. Clin Exp Rheumatol 2016;34(3 Suppl 97):S16–20.
15. Kwon OC, Park JH, Park Y-B, et al. Disease-specific factors associated with cardiovascular events in patients with Takayasu arteritis. Arthritis Res Ther 2020; 22(1):180.
16. Rav-Acha M, Plot L, Peled N, et al. Coronary involvement in Takayasu's arteritis. Autoimmun Rev 2007;6(8):566–71.
17. Endo M, Tomizawa Y, Nishida H, et al. Angiographic findings and surgical treatments of coronary artery involvement in Takayasu arteritis. J Thorac Cardiovasc Surg 2003;125(3):570–7.
18. Wang H, Liu Z, Shen Z, et al. Impact of coronary involvement on long-term outcomes in patients with Takayasu's arteritis. Clin Exp Rheumatol 2020;38(6): 1118–26.
19. Lei C, Huang Y, Yuan S, et al. Takayasu arteritis with coronary artery involvement: differences between pediatric and adult patients. Can J Cardiol 2020; 36(4):535–42.
20. Fan L, Zhang H, Cai J, et al. Clinical course and prognostic factors of childhood Takayasu's arteritis: over 15-year comprehensive analysis of 101 patients. Arthritis Res Ther 2019;21(1):31.
21. Hotchi M. Pathological studies on Takayasu arteritis. Heart Vessels Suppl 1992; 7:11–7.
22. Matsubara O, Kuwata T, Nemoto T, et al. Coronary artery lesions in Takayasu arteritis: pathological considerations. Heart Vessels Suppl 1992;7:26–31.
23. Filer A, Nicholls D, Corston R, et al. Takayasu arteritis and atherosclerosis: illustrating the consequences of endothelial damage. J Rheumatol 2001;28(12): 2752–3.
24. Tomasson G, Peloquin C, Mohammad A, et al. Risk for cardiovascular disease early and late after a diagnosis of giant-cell arteritis: a cohort study. Ann Intern Med 2014;160(2):73–80.
25. Amiri N, De Vera M, Choi HK, et al. Increased risk of cardiovascular disease in giant cell arteritis: a general population-based study. Rheumatol Oxf Engl 2016; 55(1):33–40.
26. Ungprasert P, Koster MJ, Warrington KJ. Coronary artery disease in giant cell arteritis: a systematic review and meta-analysis. Semin Arthritis Rheum 2015; 44(5):586–91.

27. Li L, Neogi T, Jick S. Giant cell arteritis and vascular disease-risk factors and outcomes: a cohort study using UK Clinical Practice Research Datalink. Rheumatol Oxf Engl 2017;56(5):753–62.
28. Lie JT. Aortic and extracranial large vessel giant cell arteritis: a review of 72 cases with histopathologic documentation. Semin Arthritis Rheum 1995;24(6): 422–31.
29. Wilkinson IM, Russell RW. Arteries of the head and neck in giant cell arteritis. A pathological study to show the pattern of arterial involvement. Arch Neurol 1972; 27(5):378–91.
30. Morris CR, Scheib JS. Fatal myocardial infarction resulting from coronary arteritis in a patient with polymyalgia rheumatica and biopsy-proved temporal arteritis. A case report and review of the literature. Arch Intern Med 1994;154(10): 1158–60.
31. Shan KS, Zhang Q, Bisaria S, et al. A rare case of coronary artery thrombosis in a patient with recently diagnosed giant cell arteritis: is anticardiolipin antibody involved? Cureus 2020;12(5):e8077.
32. Banerjee S, Bagheri M, Sandfort V, et al. Vascular calcification in patients with large-vessel vasculitis compared to patients with hyperlipidemia. Semin Arthritis Rheum 2019;48(6):1068–73.
33. de Souza AWS, Machado NP, Pereira VM, et al. Antiplatelet therapy for the prevention of arterial ischemic events in takayasu arteritis. Circ J Off J Jpn Circ Soc 2010;74(6):1236–41.
34. Lee GY, Jang SY, Ko SM, et al. Cardiovascular manifestations of Takayasu arteritis and their relationship to the disease activity: analysis of 204 Korean patients at a single center. Int J Cardiol 2012;159(1):14–20.
35. Ungprasert P, Wijarnpreecha K, Cheungpasitporn W, et al. Inpatient prevalence, burden and comorbidity of Takayasu's arteritis: Nationwide inpatient sample 2013-2014. Semin Arthritis Rheum 2019;49(1):136–9.
36. Duarte MM, Geraldes R, Sousa R, et al. Stroke and transient ischemic attack in takayasu's arteritis: a systematic review and meta-analysis. J Stroke Cerebrovasc Dis 2016;25(4):781–91.
37. Ringleb PA, Strittmatter EI, Loewer M, et al. Cerebrovascular manifestations of Takayasu arteritis in Europe. Rheumatol Oxf Engl 2005;44(8):1012–5.
38. Bond KM, Nasr D, Lehman V, et al. Intracranial and extracranial neurovascular manifestations of takayasu arteritis. AJNR Am J Neuroradiol 2017;38(4):766–72.
39. Seyahi E, Ugurlu S, Cumali R, et al. Atherosclerosis in takayasu arteritis. Ann Rheum Dis 2006;65(9):1202–7.
40. Hatri A, Guermaz R, Laroche J-P, et al. [Takayasu's arteritis and atherosclerosis]. J Med Vasc 2019;44(5):311–7.
41. Ungprasert P, Wijarnpreecha K, Koster MJ, et al. Cerebrovascular accident in patients with giant cell arteritis: A systematic review and meta-analysis of cohort studies. Semin Arthritis Rheum 2016;46(3):361–6.
42. Pariente A, Guédon A, Alamowitch S, et al. Ischemic stroke in giant-cell arteritis: French retrospective study. J Autoimmun 2019;99:48–51.
43. Siemonsen S, Brekenfeld C, Holst B, et al. 3T MRI reveals extra- and intracranial involvement in giant cell arteritis. AJNR Am J Neuroradiol 2015;36(1):91–7.
44. Laura D, Keean N, Rebello R, et al. Involvement of the intracranial circulation in giant cell arteritis. Can J Ophthalmol J Can Ophtalmol 2020;55(5). https://doi.org/10.1016/j.jcjo.2020.04.002.
45. Samson M, Jacquin A, Audia S, et al. Stroke associated with giant cell arteritis: a population-based study. J Neurol Neurosurg Psychiatr 2015;86(2):216–21.

46. Gonzalez-Gay MA, Vazquez-Rodriguez TR, Gomez-Acebo I, et al. Strokes at time of disease diagnosis in a series of 287 patients with biopsy-proven giant cell arteritis. Medicine (Baltimore) 2009;88(4):227–35.
47. de Boysson H, Liozon E, Larivière D, et al. Giant cell arteritis-related stroke: a retrospective multicenter case-control study. J Rheumatol 2017;44(3):297–303.
48. Gonzalez-Juanatey C, Lopez-Diaz MJ, Martin J, et al. Atherosclerosis in patients with biopsy-proven giant cell arteritis. Arthritis Rheum 2007;57(8):1481–6.
49. Nuenninghoff DM, Hunder GG, Christianson TJH, et al. Incidence and predictors of large-artery complication (aortic aneurysm, aortic dissection, and/or large-artery stenosis) in patients with giant cell arteritis: a population-based study over 50 years. Arthritis Rheum 2003;48(12):3522–31.
50. Nuenninghoff DM, Hunder GG, Christianson TJH, et al. Mortality of large-artery complication (aortic aneurysm, aortic dissection, and/or large-artery stenosis) in patients with giant cell arteritis: a population-based study over 50 years. Arthritis Rheum 2003;48(12):3532–7.
51. García-Martínez A, Arguis P, Prieto-González S, et al. Prospective long term follow-up of a cohort of patients with giant cell arteritis screened for aortic structural damage (aneurysm or dilatation). Ann Rheum Dis 2014;73(10):1826–32.
52. Gonzalez-Gay MA, Garcia-Porrua C, Piñeiro A, et al. Aortic aneurysm and dissection in patients with biopsy-proven giant cell arteritis from northwestern Spain: a population-based study. Medicine (Baltimore) 2004;83(6):335–41.
53. Blockmans D, de Ceuninck L, Vanderschueren S, et al. Repetitive 18F-fluorodeoxyglucose positron emission tomography in giant cell arteritis: a prospective study of 35 patients. Arthritis Rheum 2006;55(1):131–7.
54. Prieto-González S, Arguis P, García-Martínez A, et al. Large vessel involvement in biopsy-proven giant cell arteritis: prospective study in 40 newly diagnosed patients using CT angiography. Ann Rheum Dis 2012;71(7):1170–6.
55. Koster MJ, Crowson CS, Labarca C, et al. Incidence and predictors of thoracic aortic damage in biopsy-proven giant cell arteritis. Scand J Rheumatol 2021;50(3):239–42.
56. Robson JC, Kiran A, Maskell J, et al. The relative risk of aortic aneurysm in patients with giant cell arteritis compared with the general population of the UK. Ann Rheum Dis 2015;74(1):129–35.
57. Muratore F, Crescentini F, Spaggiari L, et al. Aortic dilatation in patients with large vessel vasculitis: A longitudinal case control study using PET/CT. Semin Arthritis Rheum 2019;48(6):1074–82.
58. Schmidt WA, Blockmans D. Investigations in systemic vasculitis - The role of imaging. Best Pract Res Clin Rheumatol 2018;32(1):63–82.
59. Blockmans D, Coudyzer W, Vanderschueren S, et al. Relationship between fluorodeoxyglucose uptake in the large vessels and late aortic diameter in giant cell arteritis. Rheumatol Oxf Engl 2008;47(8):1179–84.
60. Aviña-Zubieta JA, Bhole VM, Amiri N, et al. The risk of deep venous thrombosis and pulmonary embolism in giant cell arteritis: a general population-based study. Ann Rheum Dis 2016;75(1):148–54.
61. Unizony S, Lu N, Tomasson G, et al. Temporal trends of venous thromboembolism risk before and after diagnosis of giant cell arteritis. Arthritis Rheumatol Hoboken NJ 2017;69(1):176–84.
62. Numano F, Isohisa I, Kishi U, et al. Takayasu's disease in twin sisters. Possible genetic factors. Circulation 1978;58(1):173–7.
63. Numano F, Ohta N, Sasazuki T. HLA and clinical manifestations in Takayasu disease. Jpn Circ J 1982;46(2):184–9.

64. Kasuya K, Hashimoto Y, Numano F. Left ventricular dysfunction and HLA Bw52 antigen in Takayasu arteritis. Heart Vessels Suppl 1992;7:116–9.
65. Terao C, Yoshifuji H, Kimura A, et al. Two susceptibility loci to takayasu arteritis reveal a synergistic role of the IL12B and HLA-B regions in a japanese population. Am J Hum Genet 2013;93(2):289–97.
66. Carmona FD, Mackie SL, Martín J-E, et al. A large-scale genetic analysis reveals a strong contribution of the HLA class II region to giant cell arteritis susceptibility. Am J Hum Genet 2015;96(4):565–80.
67. Carmona FD, Vaglio A, Mackie SL, et al. A Genome-wide Association Study Identifies Risk Alleles in Plasminogen and P4HA2 Associated with Giant Cell Arteritis. Am J Hum Genet 2017;100(1):64–74.
68. Schaefer AS, Bochenek G, Jochens A, et al. Genetic evidence for PLASMINOGEN as a shared genetic risk factor of coronary artery disease and periodontitis. Circ Cardiovasc Genet 2015;8(1):159–67.
69. Robson JC, Kiran A, Maskell J, et al. Which patients with giant cell arteritis will develop cardiovascular or cerebrovascular disease? A clinical practice research datalink study. J Rheumatol 2016;43(6):1085–92.
70. Comarmond C, Cluzel P, Toledano D, et al. Findings of cardiac magnetic resonance imaging in asymptomatic myocardial ischemic disease in Takayasu arteritis. Am J Cardiol 2014;113(5):881–7.
71. da Silva TF, Levy-Neto M, Bonfá E, et al. High prevalence of metabolic syndrome in Takayasu arteritis: increased cardiovascular risk and lower adiponectin serum levels. J Rheumatol 2013;40(11):1897–904.
72. Tomasson G, Bjornsson J, Zhang Y, et al. Cardiovascular risk factors and incident giant cell arteritis: a population-based cohort study. Scand J Rheumatol 2019;48(3):213–7.
73. Udayakumar PD, Chandran AK, Crowson CS, et al. Cardiovascular risk and acute coronary syndrome in giant cell arteritis: a population-based retrospective cohort study. Arthritis Care Res 2015;67(3):396–402.
74. Monti S, Robson J, Klersy C, et al. Early development of new cardiovascular risk factors in the systemic vasculitides. Clin Exp Rheumatol 2020;38 Suppl 124(2): 126–34.
75. de Mornac D, Agard C, Hardouin J-B, et al. Risk factors for symptomatic vascular events in giant cell arteritis: a study of 254 patients with large-vessel imaging at diagnosis. Ther Adv Musculoskelet Dis 2021;13. 1759720X211006967.
76. Li T, Du J, Gao N, et al. Numano type V Takayasu arteritis patients are more prone to have coronary artery involvement. Clin Rheumatol 2020;39(11): 3439–47.
77. Wang Z, Dang A, Lv N. Brachial-ankle pulse wave velocity is increased and associated with disease activity in patients with takayasu arteritis. J Atheroscler Thromb 2020;27(2):172–82.
78. Gonzalez-Juanatey C, Llorca J, Garcia-Porrua C, et al. Steroid therapy improves endothelial function in patients with biopsy-proven giant cell arteritis. J Rheumatol 2006;33(1):74–8.
79. Laurent C, Prieto-González S, Belnou P, et al. Prevalence of cardiovascular risk factors, the use of statins and of aspirin in Takayasu Arteritis. Sci Rep 2021; 11(1):14404.
80. Reiss AB, Carsons SE, Anwar K, et al. Atheroprotective effects of methotrexate on reverse cholesterol transport proteins and foam cell transformation in human THP-1 monocyte/macrophages. Arthritis Rheum 2008;58(12):3675–83.

81. Zimmerman MC, Clemens DL, Duryee MJ, et al. Direct antioxidant properties of methotrexate: Inhibition of malondialdehyde-acetaldehyde-protein adduct formation and superoxide scavenging. Redox Biol 2017;13:588–93.
82. Shuai Z-Q, Zhang C-X, Shuai Z-W, et al. Efficacy and safety of biological agents in the treatment of patients with Takayasu arteritis: a systematic review and meta-analysis. Eur Rev Med Pharmacol Sci 2021;25(1):250–62.
83. Nakaoka Y, Isobe M, Tanaka Y, et al. Long-term efficacy and safety of tocilizumab in refractory Takayasu arteritis: final results of the randomized controlled phase 3 TAKT study. Rheumatol Oxf Engl 2020;59(9):2427–34.
84. Yokokawa T, Kunii H, Kaneshiro T, et al. Regressed coronary ostial stenosis in a young female with Takayasu arteritis: a case report. BMC Cardiovasc Disord 2019;19(1):79.
85. Pan L, Du J, Liu J, et al. Tocilizumab treatment effectively improves coronary artery involvement in patients with Takayasu arteritis. Clin Rheumatol 2020;39(8):2369–78.
86. Chung ES, Packer M, Lo KH, et al. Anti-TNF Therapy Against Congestive Heart Failure Investigators. Randomized, double-blind, placebo-controlled, pilot trial of infliximab, a chimeric monoclonal antibody to tumor necrosis factor-alpha, in patients with moderate-to-severe heart failure: results of the anti-TNF Therapy Against Congestive Heart Failure (ATTACH) trial. Circulation 2003;107(25):3133–40.
87. Mazlumzadeh M, Hunder GG, Easley KA, et al. Treatment of giant cell arteritis using induction therapy with high-dose glucocorticoids: a double-blind, placebo-controlled, randomized prospective clinical trial. Arthritis Rheum 2006;54(10):3310–8.
88. Broder MS, Sarsour K, Chang E, et al. Corticosteroid-related adverse events in patients with giant cell arteritis: a claims-based analysis. Semin Arthritis Rheum 2016;46(2):246–52.
89. Gale S, Wilson JC, Chia J, et al. Risk associated with cumulative oral glucocorticoid use in patients with giant cell arteritis in real-world databases from the USA and UK. Rheumatol Ther 2018;5(2):327–40.
90. Stone JH, Tuckwell K, Dimonaco S, et al. Trial of tocilizumab in giant-cell arteritis. N Engl J Med 2017;377(4):317–28.
91. Unizony S, McCulley TJ, Spiera R, et al. Clinical outcomes of patients with giant cell arteritis treated with tocilizumab in real-world clinical practice: decreased incidence of new visual manifestations. Arthritis Res Ther 2021;23(1):8.
92. Gale S, Trinh H, Tuckwell K, et al. Adverse events in giant cell arteritis and rheumatoid arthritis patient populations: analyses of tocilizumab clinical trials and claims data. Rheumatol Ther 2019;6(1):77–88.
93. Nesher G, Berkun Y, Mates M, et al. Low-dose aspirin and prevention of cranial ischemic complications in giant cell arteritis. Arthritis Rheum 2004;50(4):1332–7.
94. Lee MS, Smith SD, Galor A, et al. Antiplatelet and anticoagulant therapy in patients with giant cell arteritis. Arthritis Rheum 2006;54(10):3306–9.
95. Narváez J, Bernad B, Gómez-Vaquero C, et al. Impact of antiplatelet therapy in the development of severe ischemic complications and in the outcome of patients with giant cell arteritis. Clin Exp Rheumatol 2008;26(3 Suppl 49):S57–62.
96. Martínez-Taboada VM, López-Hoyos M, Narvaez J, et al. Effect of antiplatelet/anticoagulant therapy on severe ischemic complications in patients with giant cell arteritis: a cumulative meta-analysis. Autoimmun Rev 2014;13(8):788–94.

97. Bienvenu B, Ly KH, Lambert M, et al. Management of giant cell arteritis: recommendations of the french study group for large vessel vasculitis (GEFA). Rev Med Interne 2016;37(3):154–65.
98. Mackie SL, Dejaco C, Appenzeller S, et al. British society for rheumatology guideline on diagnosis and treatment of giant cell arteritis. Rheumatol Oxf Engl 2020;59(3):e1–23.
99. Hellmich B, Agueda A, Monti S, et al. 2018 Update of the EULAR recommendations for the management of large vessel vasculitis. Ann Rheum Dis 2020;79(1): 19–30.
100. Ridker PM, Rifai N, Pfeffer MA, et al. Long-term effects of pravastatin on plasma concentration of C-reactive protein. The Cholesterol and Recurrent Events (CARE) Investigators. Circulation 1999;100(3):230–5.
101. Kent SM, Flaherty PJ, Coyle LC, et al. Effect of atorvastatin and pravastatin on serum C-reactive protein. Am Heart J 2003;145(2):e8.
102. Ridker PM, Danielson E, Fonseca FAH, et al. Rosuvastatin to prevent vascular events in men and women with elevated C-reactive protein. N Engl J Med 2008;359(21):2195–207.
103. Devaraj S, Siegel D, Jialal I. Statin therapy in metabolic syndrome and hypertension post-JUPITER: what is the value of CRP? Curr Atheroscler Rep 2011;13(1): 31–42.
104. Mora S, Ridker PM. Justification for the Use of Statins in Primary Prevention: an Intervention Trial Evaluating Rosuvastatin (JUPITER)–can C-reactive protein be used to target statin therapy in primary prevention? Am J Cardiol 2006; 97(2A):33A–41A.
105. Pugnet G, Sailler L, Bourrel R, et al. Is statin exposure associated with occurrence or better outcome in giant cell arteritis? Results from a French population-based study. J Rheumatol 2015;42(2):316–22.
106. de Jong HJI, Meyboom RHB, Helle MJ, et al. Giant cell arteritis and polymyalgia rheumatica after reexposure to a statin: a case report. Ann Intern Med 2014; 161(8):614–5.
107. Pugnet G, Sailler L, Fournier J-P, et al. Predictors of Cardiovascular Hospitalization in Giant Cell Arteritis: Effect of Statin Exposure. A French Population-based Study. J Rheumatol 2016;43(12):2162–70.
108. Narváez J, Bernad B, Nolla JM, et al. Statin therapy does not seem to benefit giant cell arteritis. Semin Arthritis Rheum 2007;36(5):322–7.
109. Pearson GJ, Thanassoulis G, Anderson TJ, et al. 2021 Canadian Cardiovascular Society Guidelines for the Management of Dyslipidemia for the Prevention of Cardiovascular Disease in Adults. Can J Cardiol 2021. https://doi.org/10.1016/j.cjca.2021.03.016. S0828-282X(21)00165-3.

Venous Thromboembolism in the Inflammatory Rheumatic Diseases

Durga Prasanna Misra, DM, MRCP(UK), FRCP(Edin)[a],*,
Sakir Ahmed, DM[b], Mohit Goyal, MD, FRCP(Edin)[c],
Aman Sharma, MD, FRCP(London)[d], Vikas Agarwal, DM, FRCP(Edin)[a]

KEYWORDS

- Venous thromboembolism • Deep venous thrombosis • Pulmonary embolism
- Cardiovascular diseases • Systemic lupus erythematosus
- Antiphospholipid antibody syndrome • Rheumatoid arthritis • Vasculitis

KEY POINTS

- Risk of venous thromboembolism is increased in most inflammatory rheumatic diseases.
- Underlying antiphospholipid antibody syndrome or high-risk antiphospholipid antibody profile increases venous thromboembolism risk.
- A careful assessment of cardiovascular risk, including the risk of venous thromboembolism, is recommended before the initiation of Janus kinase inhibitors.

INTRODUCTION

Venous thromboembolism (VTE), which generally refers to either deep venous thrombosis (DVT) or pulmonary embolism (PE), is an important cardiovascular comorbidity in chronic diseases. Overall, patients with immune-mediated inflammatory diseases (IMIDs) are at a greater risk of VTE than the general population,[1] nearly 10% of which recur.[2] Hospitalized patients with an IMID are at an increased risk of VTE.[3] The recent black box warning from the United States Food and Drug Administration (US FDA) in

[a] Department of Clinical Immunology and Rheumatology, C block, Sanjay Gandhi Postgraduate Institute of Medical Sciences (SGPGIMS), Rae Bareli Road, Lucknow 226014, India; [b] Department of Clinical Immunology and Rheumatology, Kalinga Institute of Medical Sciences (KIMS), Bhubaneswar 751024, India; [c] Department of Rheumatology and Clinical Immunology, CARE Pain and Arthritis Centre, Udaipur 313002, Rajasthan, India; [d] Department of Internal Medicine, Postgraduate Institute of Medical Education and Research (PGIMER), Chandigarh 160012, India
* Corresponding author. Department of Clinical Immunology and Rheumatology, C block, Sanjay Gandhi Postgraduate Institute of Medical Sciences (SGPGIMS), Rae Bareli Road, Lucknow 226014, India.
E-mail addresses: durgapmisra@gmail.com; dpmisra@sgpgi.ac.in
Twitter: @DurgaPrasannaM1 (D.P.M.); @sakir_rheum (S.A.); @drmohitgoyal (M.G.); @Amansharmapgi (A.S.); @vikasagrIMMUNO (V.A.)

Rheum Dis Clin N Am 49 (2023) 97–127
https://doi.org/10.1016/j.rdc.2022.08.001
0889-857X/23/© 2022 Elsevier Inc. All rights reserved.

rheumatic.theclinics.com

relation to an increased VTE risk along with other major cardiovascular events and malignancies with Janus kinase inhibitors has brought these comorbidities into sharp focus in IMIDs.[4] In this article, we take an overview of the risk for VTE in different inflammatory rheumatic diseases (IRDs), delineate the risk factors for VTE in specific diseases, elucidate the mechanisms driving such VTE risk and analyze therapeutic considerations for VTE in different IRDs.

Discussion of Venous Thromboembolism in Individual Inflammatory Rheumatic Diseases

Rheumatoid arthritis

A recent systematic review of 10 observational studies confirmed that rheumatoid arthritis (RA) is associated with a greater risk of VTE (pooled odds ratio [OR] 2.23 with 95% confidence interval [95%CI]: 1.80–2.77).[5] Recent cohort studies have confirmed an increased VTE risk in RA, particularly in those with active disease and in the first year following diagnosis.[6,7] Different risk factors contribute toward VTE and atherosclerotic cardiovascular disease (ASCVD) risk; prior VTE increases the subsequent risk of ASCVD in RA.[8] Adipokines are associated with ASCVD but not with VTE risk in RA[9] (**Table 1**).

Spondyloarthropathies

A systematic review reported increased risk of VTE with ankylosing spondylitis (AS) [Risk ratio - RR 1.60 (95%CI 1.05–2.44)],[10] confirmed in subsequent cohort studies.[11–13] On the contrary, VTE risk does not appear to be increased in psoriatic arthritis (PsA).[14,15] Whenever VTE events occur in PsA, they associate with older age, prior VTE event,[15] corticosteroid use, and diabetes mellitus[16] (see **Table 1**). Shared genetic risk factors for AS and for VTE associated with polymorphisms in *MTHFR, SH2B3, PON1,* and *ERAP1* genes have been proposed.[17]

Systemic Lupus Erythematosus

Patients with systemic lupus erythematosus (SLE) have an increased risk of VTE, highest in the year following diagnosis,[18,19] associated with antiphospholipid antibodies (APL),[20] male sex,[21] and greater comorbidity burden.[22] VTE can even precede SLE diagnosis.[23] VTE can occur even in SLE in drug-free remission.[24] Incidence of VTE has remained similar over time[20] whereas, mortality due to VTE in SLE has progressively reduced.[25] APL profiles as risk factors for VTE differ with ethnicity.[26] About one-tenth of lupus nephritis patients develop VTE.[27] Association of class of lupus nephritis with VTE risk differs with the age of onset.[27] VTE in SLE associates with a greater risk of dying[25,28] or disability,[25] as well as higher hospital costs.[25] VTE might also contribute toward chronic thromboembolic pulmonary hypertension (CTEPH) in SLE[29] (**Table 2**).

Antiphospholipid antibodies (APL), namely, anticardiolipin antibodies (ACLA), anti-beta2glycoprotein I antibodies (anti-β2GPI), antiprothrombin antibodies (anti-PT), antiphosphatidyl serine antibodies (anti-PS), and lupus anticoagulant (LAC), increase VTE risk in lupus, with a greater risk in those with two or more APLs, particularly with triple APL positivity (ACLA, anti-β2GPI & LAC).[21,30–32] APLs or antibodies to activated protein C increase thrombotic risk in SLE by inducing resistance to activated protein C.[33,34] Complement 4 deposition on platelets[35] and serum galectin-3 binding protein are other biomarkers of VTE risk in SLE[36] (see **Table 2**).

Antiphospholipid Antibody Syndrome

Antiphospholipid antibody syndrome (APS) is a well-recognized autoimmune cause of unprovoked venous and arterial thromboses. APS could be primary or secondary (ie,

Table 1
Venous thromboembolism in rheumatoid arthritis and spondyloarthritis

Disease	Reference, Location	Type of Study	Participants	Key Findings
Rheumatoid arthritis	Li, et al[6] 2021, Canada	Population-based health care database	39,142 RA, 78,078 controls (adjusted for age, sex, VTE risk factors	HR for VTE 1.28 (95%CI 1.20–1.36) in RA vs controls Highest in the first year following diagnosis
	Molander, et al[7] 2021, Sweden	National database	46,316 RA, 5 population-based controls per case	RR for VTE 1.88 (95%CI 1.65–2.15) in RA vs controls (adjusted for age, sex, geographic location) VTE risk increased with increasing disease activity state [RR for low 1.12(95%CI 0.96–1.31), moderate 1.48 (95%CI 1.30–1.68), and high disease activity 2.03(95%CI 1.73–2.38) VTE risk higher than controls at any disease activity state, including those in remission
	Ozen, et al[8] 2021, USA	Prospective registry	31,366 RA	Compared VTE and ASCVD risk factors ↑age, male sex, ↑comorbidities, previous fracture, ↑disability, ↑disease activity, GC use ↑risk, and HCQ ↓risk of both VTE and ASCVD DM, HTN, CKD ↑ ASCVD risk but not VTE risk Obesity ↑VTE but with ↓ASCVD risk Prior VTE ↑ risk of subsequent ASCVD [adjusted HR 2.05(95%CI 1.43–2.95)]
	Federico, et al [9] 2022, USA	Prospective registry	2598 RA	Serum adiponectin, leptin, and fibroblast growth factor 21 associated with ASCVD or CVD death but not with VTE risk
Spondyloarthritis	Bengtsson, et al[11] 2017, Sweden	Population-based prospective cohort study	6448 AS 5190 USpA 16,063 PsA 266,435 population-based controls	↑ age- and sex-adjusted HR of VTE with AS [1.53(95%CI 1.25–1.87)], USpA [1.55(95%CI 1.19–2.02)] and PsA [95% CI 1.46(1.29–1.65)] vs controls

(continued on next page)

Table 1
(continued)

Disease	Reference, Location	Type of Study	Participants	Key Findings
	Eriksson, et al[12] 2017, Sweden	Retrospective analysis of health care databases	5358 AS 25006 age- and sex-matched controls	Higher risk in women than in men (1.29, 1.07 and 1.59 times ↑ risk in AS, USpA and PsA, respectively) ↑ risk of DVT or PE (ie, VTE) in AS [HR 1.4(95%CI 1.1–1.9)]. Similar risk across age groups 1.33 times ↑ risk in men
	Aviña-Zubieta, et al[13] 2019, Canada	Population-based health care database	7190 AS, 71,900 controls	VTE HR with AS 1.53(95%CI 1.16–2.01) (adjusted for age, sex, time of cohort entry, GC use, and prior health care visits)
	Ogdie, et al[14] 2018, UK	Primary health care database	12,084 PsA, 1,225,571 controls	No ↑ risk of VTE in PsA [on DMARDs, HR 1.10 (95%CI 0.92–1.31); not on DMARDs, HR 1.07 (95%CI 0.88–1.29)] (adjusted for age, sex, comorbidities, prior medications, and prior arthroplasties)
	Gazitt, et al[15] 2022, Israel	Retrospective analysis of health care database	5275 PsA, 21,011 controls	Similar risk of VTE in PsA and controls [adjusted HR 1.27 (95%CI 0.91–1.80)] Among those with PsA, ↑ age [HR 1.08 (95%CI 1.05–1.11)] & prior documented VTE [HR 19.60(95%CI 8.37–45.94)] ↑ VTE risk
	Damian, et al 2021,[16] Canada	Multicentric prospective cohort	1639 PsA, 794 PsO	26 VTE episodes over mean 8.9 y follow-up After multivariable adjustment, ↑ age [HR 1.04 (95%CI 1.01–1.07)], GC use [HR 11.02 (95%CI 4.48–26.84)], and DM [HR 4.35 (95%CI 1.82–10.27)] ↑ VTE risk (in PsA and PsO taken together)

Abbreviations: 95%CI, 95% confidence intervals; AS, ankylosing spondylitis; ASCVD, atherosclerotic cardiovascular disease; CKD, chronic kidney disease; CVD, cardiovascular disease; DM, diabetes mellitus; DMARDs, Disease-modifying antirheumatic drugs; DVT, deep venous thrombosis; GC, glucocorticoid; HCQ, hydroxychloroquine; HR, hazard ratio; HTN, hypertension; PE, pulmonary embolism; PsA, psoriatic arthritis; PsO, psoriasis; RA, rheumatoid arthritis; RR, risk ratio; SpA, spondyloarthritis; UK, United Kingdom; USA, United States of America; USpA, Undifferentiated spondyloarthritis; VTE, venous

Table 2
Venous thromboembolism in systemic lupus erythematosus

Type of Study	Reference, Location	Type of Study	Participants	Key Findings
Risk evaluation	Yafasova, et al 2021,[18] Denmark	Registry of hospital visits	3411 SLE, 13,644 population controls (matched for age, sex, time of hospital visit, prevalent comorbidities	SLE associated with ↑ VTE risk, highest in the year following diagnosis [HR for first year 15.6 (95%CI 8.33–29.10] and thereafter [HR 3.46 (95%CI 2.79–4.29)]
	Aviña-Zubieta, et al[19] 2015, Canada	Population-based database	4863 SLE, 49,838 population controls (matched for age, sex, time of database entry)	Overall VTE risk [HR 5.50 (95%CI 4.35–6.94)] as well as individually for DVT [HR 6.69 (95%CI 4.92–9.09)] and PE [HR 4.46 (95%CI 3.23–6.14)] ↑ in SLE Risks highest in the first year after diagnosis and gradually decreased thereafter although remained higher than the general population
	Mok, et al[20] 2010, Hong Kong	Retrospective hospital-based cohort	516 SLE	↑ VTE risk in SLE [overall SIR 11.9 (95%CI 7.3–19.6), highest in <30 y, decreasing with increasing age] APL ↑ VTE risk [adjusted HR 4.36(95%CI 1.67–11.40)]
	Mok, et al[21] 2005, USA and Hong Kong	Prospective hospital-based cohort study	625 SLE	Similar incidence of VTE over time Female sex, Chinese ethnicity, diabetes and leukopenia ↓ risk of VTE Obesity, hemolytic anemia, and renal involvement ↑ VTE risk
	Ahlehoff, et al[22] 2017, Denmark	Population-based registry	3627 SLE, 5,590,070 population controls	↑VTE risk in SLE [HR 3.32(95%CI 2.73–4.03), adjusted for age, sex, socioeconomic status, prevalent comorbidities and medications] ↑VTE risk in cutaneous lupus erythematosus [adjusted HR 1.39(95% CI 1.10–1.78)] Male sex, ↑age, and ↑ comorbidities associated with higher VTE risk

(continued on next page)

Table 2
(continued)

Type of Study	Reference, Location	Type of Study	Participants	Key Findings
	Chang, et al[23] 2018, USA	Retrospective analysis of insurance database	682 SLE, 1364 age & sex matched controls	Young patients (10–24 y) with newly-diagnosed SLE had more hospital visits in the preceding year. VTE was a major cause for hospital visits. VTE preceded SLE diagnosis by median 10 mo
	Jakez-Ocampo, et al[24] 2020, Mexico	Retrospective hospital-based cohort	44 SLE in remission, 88 SLE with persistent disease activity	VTE risk increased even in SLE in remission [RR for SLE in remission vs active SLE 7.42 (95%CI 0.85–64.51)]
	Kishore, et al[25] 2019, USA	Retrospective analysis of a national in-patient database	299,595 SLE admissions (VTE in 3.06%)	Greater odds of in-hospital mortality in SLE with VTE when compared with those without [OR 2.35 (95%CI 2.10–2.62)] as well as higher disability [OR for moderate or severe disability 1.53(95% CI 1.46–1.62)] ↑ in median 3.57 d of hospitalization and ↑ median cost of hospitalization of 25,400 USD in SLE with VTE Mortality due to VTE in SLE reduced over time from 2003 to 2011
	Gkrouzman, et al[26] 2022, USA	Retrospective hospital-based cohort	97 SLE with DVT (59 White, 38 African American)	African American individuals ↓ odds of classical thrombotic APL risk profile than white individuals [adjusted OR 0.34(95%CI 0.12–0.96)] LAC positivity ↑ in African American patients Triple positivity (ACLA, anti-β2GPI and LAC) ↑ in white patients.
	Cooley, et al[27] 2021, USA	Retrospective database of renal biopsies	534 SLE with LN	1 in 10 LN develop VTE Similar overall odds of VTE for class III/IV vs V LN Stratified for age at diagnosis of LN, younger class III/IV lupus nephritis have ↑ VTE risk than class V LN

	Study	Study type	N	Findings
	Cervera, et al[28] 2003, Europe	Prospective, multicentric registry	1000 SLE	Older class V LN have ↑ VTE risk than class III/IV LN; 6% deaths due to PE
	Akdogan, et al[29] 2013, Turkey	Prospective cohort	122 SLE	CTEPH in 4/9 SLE with PH diagnosed by right-heart catheterization
Biomarkers	Brouwer, et al[30] 2004, Netherlands	Prospective hospital-based cohort study	144 SLE	VTE events in 10% at 12.7 y median follow-up; Univariable analyses - ↑ VTE risk with LAC, ACLA, Factor V Leiden and Prothrombin G20210 A mutation. Presence of one of these factors ↑ VTE risk by 5.1 times (95%CI 1.64–15.86); presence of any two factors ↑ VTE risk 8.2-fold (2.04–32.90) (comparisons with those lacking any of these risk factors)
	Mok, et al[21] 2005, USA and Hong Kong	Prospective hospital-based cohort study	625 SLE	HDL-C≤1 mmol/L and APL ↑VTE risk in SLE
	Sallai, et al[31] 2007, Hungary	Cross-sectional study	105 SLE	↑ risk of VTE with ACLA (RR 8.18, 95%CI 2.44–27.49), anti-β2GPI (RR 7.41, 95%CI 2.21–24.78), anti-PT (RR 4.44, 95%CI 1.09–18.05) anti-PS (RR 7.27, 95%CI 2.12–24.97) or LAC (RR 6.49, 95%CI 1.96–21.47); Triple APL positivity (ACLA, anti-β2GPI and LAC) ↑↑ VTE risk (RR 7.50, 95%CI 2.10–26.75); Inherited thrombophilia, viz., Factor V Leiden, ↑ factor VIII and ↑homocysteine did not incrementally ↑ thromboembolic event risk in SLE significantly beyond that with APLs
	Elbagir, et al[32] 2021, Sweden	Cross-sectional study	332 SLE	LAC ↑ VTE risk after adjustment for ACLA or anti-β2GPI

(continued on next page)

Table 2
(continued)

Type of Study	Reference, Location	Type of Study	Participants	Key Findings
	Nojima, et al[33] 2005, Japan	Cross-sectional study	87 SLE (21 with VTE)	Anti-PS/PT ↑ VTE risk after adjustment for all 3 APLs (LAC, ACLA or anti-β2GPI) or for ACLA and anti-β2GPI alone IgG anti-PS/PT and IgM anti-PS/PT individually ↑ VTE risk after adjustment for IgA anti-PS/PT antibodies Presence of ACLA or anti-β2GPI, or anti-PS or anti-PT correlated significantly with LAC.
	Ramirez, et al[34] 2021, UK	Cross-sectional study	156 SLE	ACLA/anti-β2GPI [OR 4.98(1.51–16.40)] or anti-PS/PT [OR 7.54 (95%CI 2.30–24.70)] ↑ odds of VTE in lupus on multivariable-adjusted analyses Mechanistically, adsorbing out ACLA/anti-β2GPI or anti-PS/PT reduced activated protein C resistance in vitro Prevalence of anti-PC 54.5% Prevalence of high-avidity anti-PC 26.3% High-avidity anti-PC ↑ thromboembolism risk (both arterial and venous together, separate data NA for VTE) Mechanistically, anti-PC contributed toward activated protein C resistance
	Svenungsson, et al[35] 2020, Sweden	Cross-sectional study	308 SLE (46 with VTE)	Complement 4 deposition on platelets identified by flow cytometry ↑ odds of VTE [OR 2.9 (95%CI 1.5–5.8)], about one-half that observed with LAC in the same cohort [OR 5.2 (95%CI 2.6–10.5)]
	Peretz, et al[36] 2021, Sweden	Prospective cohort study	162 SLE	14 VTE events at study enrollment, 10 incident VTE events over median 5 y follow-up.

	Serum galectin-3 binding protein ↑ VTE risk [HR 1.18(95%CI 1.05–1.33).
	No ↑ or ↓ VTE risk with interferon gamma induced protein 10, TNF-like weak inducer of apoptosis, soluble CD163 or leptin.

Abbreviations: 95%CI, 95% confidence intervals; ACLA, anticardiolipin antibodies; anti-PC, anti-protein C antibodies; anti-PS, antiphosphatidylserine antibodies; anti-PS/PT, antiphosphatidylserine or antiprothrombin antibodies; anti-PT, antiprothrombin antibodies; APL, antiphospholipid antibodies; anti-β2GPI, anti-beta 2 glycoprotein I antibody; CTEPH, chronic thromboembolic pulmonary hypertension; DVT, deep venous thrombosis; HDL-C, high-density lipoprotein cholesterol; HR, hazard ratio; LAC, lupus anticoagulant; LN, lupus nephritis; NA, not available; OR, odds ratio; PE, pulmonary embolism; PH, pulmonary hypertension; RR; risk ratio, SIR; standardized incidence ratio, SLE; systemic lupus erythematosus, USD; United States dollars, VTE; venous thromboembolism.

associated with other IRD such as SLE). APS accounts for nearly one-tenth of VTE events.[37] Uncommonly, APS might result in florid multiorgan or multisystem thrombosis occurring in rapid succession (within a week or a month). This life-threatening entity of catastrophic APS requires histopathological demonstration of thrombus from some of the involved organs for definitive classification.[38] Three distinct clusters of APS phenotypes have been identified, two of which associate with VTE.[39] Higher levels of D-dimer increase VTE risk in APS.[40] Chronic VTE in APS can predispose toward CTEPH[41] (**Table 3**).

The associations of APL subtypes with VTE had already been discussed in the section on SLE. Thrombosis in APS results from endothelial injury, platelet activation, and the formation of platelet–leukocyte complexes, activation of neutrophils resulting in neutrophil extracellular traps (NETs), complement activation, and aberrant triggering of the coagulation cascade and decreased fibrinolysis.[38] Antibodies to complement factor H (anti-CFH) increase the risk as well as recurrence of VTE in APS.[42] The APS clot has a distinct composition[43] and is resistant to fibrinolysis[44] (see **Table 3**).

Systemic Vasculitis

Risk of DVT (but not of PE or overall VTE) is increased in antineutrophil cytoplasmic antibody (ANCA)-associated vasculitis (AAV).[45] The risk of recurrent VTE in AAV remains high[46] (**Table 4**). Higher disease activity, antimyeloperoxidase antibodies,[46] cardiac, lung (diffuse alveolar hemorrhage), renal, gastrointestinal, or cutaneous involvement, erythrocyturia, or elevated C-reactive protein[47] associate with higher VTE risk, whereas anti-proteinase-3 antibodies associate with lower VTE risk.[46] This risk is highest in the first 2 years following diagnosis.[47] Neutrophil activation resulting in the formation of NETs, associated APLA, microparticles containing thrombogenic tissue factor, and impaired fibrinolysis (partly driven by anti-plasminogen antibodies) are mechanistic explanations of increased VTE risk in AAV.[47] VTE risk is not increased with IgA vasculitis.[48] Risk of DVT or PE is increased in polyarteritis nodosa[49] (see **Table 4**).

A meta-analysis of 3 observational studies revealed an increased VTE risk in giant cell arteritis (GCA) than in controls [pooled RR 2.26 (95%CI 1.38–3.71)],[50] highest in the 3 months after diagnosis.[51] Cohort studies have confirmed a higher risk of DVT and PE in GCA and its counterpart, polymyalgia rheumatica[52]; greater risk has been observed in hospitalized patients[53] (see **Table 4**). VTE is reported in Takayasu arteritis, but the magnitude of risk is unknown.[54] VTE risk is increased in Behcet's disease (BD),[55] associates with erythema nodosum and fever.[56] Immunosuppressive therapy decreases VTE risk in BD[56] (see **Table 4**). Resistance to activated protein C or decreased circulating levels of activated protein C might confer VTE risk in BD.[57,58] VTE occurs in nearly 40% patients with the recently diagnosed vacuoles, E1 enzyme, X-linked, autoinflammatory, somatic (VEXAS) syndrome that mimics vasculitis.[59,60] VTE in VEXAS is driven by LAC, NETs, complement activation, monocyte activation and endothelial injury.[59,60]

Sjogren's Syndrome

A systematic review and meta-analysis of 4 observational studies reported increased VTE risk in Sjogren's syndrome (SS) when compared with controls [RR 2.05 (95%CI 1.86–2.27)],[61] confirmed in subsequent cohort studies.[62,63] VTE risk is higher in the initial years following diagnosis,[62,63] varies with age,[63] and is higher when both antibodies to Ro and La are present[63] (**Table 5**).

Inflammatory Myositis

A systematic review reported an increased risk for VTE [OR 4.31 (95%CI 2.55–7.29, 5 studies)], DVT [OR 4.85 (95%CI 1.38–17.12, 3 studies)], and PE [OR 4.74 (95%CI 2.18–

Table 3
Venous thromboembolism in antiphospholipid antibody syndrome

Type of Study	Reference, Location	Type of Study	Participants	Key Findings
Risk evaluation	Miranda, et al[37] 2020, Canada	Retrospective analysis of a hospital-based database	Incident VTEs from 2002-2011	9 (95%CI 6.7–11.8)% could be classified as APS
	Zuily, et al[39] 2020, multiple centers across the globe	Prospective registry	497 APS	Three distinct clusters of APS • Female patients without any other IRD with triple APL positivity (ACLA, anti-β2GPI and LAC) and VTEs • Female patients with serology suggestive of lupus, LAC positivity, VTEs, renal and hematological manifestations (hemolytic anemia and thrombocytopenia) • Older males associated with arterial thrombotic events and cutaneous (livedo rash or ulcers), endocarditis, and neurologic manifestations along with CVD risk factors
	Bucci, et al[40] 2022, Italy	Prospective cohort study	100 APS (60 with VTE, 40 with ATE)	Different risk factors for ATE and VTE Risk factors for ATE: diabetes mellitus, hypertension and ↑ platelet counts Risk factors for VTE: ↑ D-dimer
	Rosen, et al[41] 2022, Israel	Case-control study	504 APS; 19 APS with CTEPH compared with 50 APS without CTEPH	3.8% had CTEPH Risk factors associated with CTEPH • Primary APS • History of PE • History of recurrent VTE • CAPS • ↑ IgG ACLA • ↑ IgG anti-β2GPI • ↑ Russell's viper venom time ratio • ↑ PTT or PTT ratio

(continued on next page)

Table 3
(continued)

Type of Study	Reference, Location	Type of Study	Participants	Key Findings
				• Triple APL positivity • ↓ Lower platelet counts
Biomarkers	Foltyn Zadura, et al[42] 2015, Europe	Cross-sectional study	146 APS, 266 VTE	Anti-CFH associate with ↑ VTE risk in both primary and secondary APS Anti-CFH ↑ risk of recurrent VTE [HR 2.0 (95%CI 1.2–3.3)]
	Stachowicz, et al[43] 2018, Poland	Cross-sectional study	23 APS with VTE, 19 non-APS with VTE, 20 healthy controls	APS clots have ↑ bone marrow proteoglycan, immunoglobulins, terminal complement complexes, thrombospondin 1, apolipoprotein B-100 and platelet-derived proteins, and ↓ prothrombin, anti-thrombin III, apolipoprotein A-1 and histidine-rich glycoprotein
	Celinska-Löwenhoff, et al[44] 2018, Poland	Prospective cohort study	126 APS with thrombotic events, 105 controls	↓ clot permeability and increased clot lysis time in-vitro in clots from APS with VTE or ATE than without ↓ clot permeability/increased clot lysis time predict future thrombotic events

Abbreviations: 95%CI, 95% confidence intervals; ACLA, anticardiolipin antibodies; anti-CFH, antibodies to complement factor H; anti-β2GPI, anti-beta 2 glycoprotein I antibody; APL, antiphospholipid antibodies; APS, antiphospholipid antibody syndrome; ATE, arterial thrombotic events; CAPS, Catastrophic APS; CTEPH, chronic thromboembolic pulmonary hypertension; CVD, cardiovascular disease; DVT, deep venous thrombosis; HR, hazard ratio; IRD, inflammatory rheumatic diseases, LAC; lupus anticoagulant, PE; pulmonary embolism, PTT; partial thromboplastin time, VTE; venous thromboembolism.

10.30, 4 studies)] in polymyositis or dermatomyositis.[64] The risk of PE is highest in the initial years after diagnosis,[65] increases with age, in female patients, and with greater burden of comorbidities[66] (see **Table 5**). Corticosteroid use has been hypothesized but is not yet proven as a risk factor for VTE in inflammatory myositis.[67]

Systemic Sclerosis

A systematic review of 5 observational studies identified a higher VTE risk in systemic sclerosis (SSc) than controls [RR 2.51 (95%CI 1.79–3.54)],[68] confirmed in subsequent

Table 4
Venous thromboembolism in systemic vasculitis

Disease	Reference, Location	Type of Study	Participants	Key Findings
ANCA vasculitis	Berti, et al[45] 2018, USA	Population-based cohort study	58 AAV, 174 controls	Significantly ↑ risk of DVT [adjusted HR 6.25 (95%CI 1.16–33.60)] in AAV vs controls; nonsignificant ↑ VTE risk in AAV [HR 3.26 (95%CI 0.84–12.60) adjusted for age, sex and time of cohort entry] or of PE [adjusted HR 1.33 (95%CI 0.23–7.54)] in AAV vs controls
	Hansrivijit, et al[46] 2021	Systematic review	4442 AAV	12.4 (95%CI 8.8–17.2)% AAV develop VTE; recurrent VTE in 10 (95%CI 5.2–18.6)% with prior VTE
IgA vasculitis	Tracy, et al[48] 2019, UK	Retrospective analysis of a health care database	2828 adult-onset IgAV (vs 5655 controls) and 10,405 pediatric-onset IgAV (vs 20,810 controls)	Adjusted HR of VTE in adult-onset IgAV vs controls 1.21 (95%CI 0.76–1.95) Adjusted HR of VTE in pediatric-onset IgAV vs controls 1.10 (95%CI 0.68–1.79)
Polyarteritis nodosa	Ungprasert, et al[49] 2020, USA	Retrospective analysis of national database for hospitalizations	4110 PAN, 4110 controls without PAN (matched for ethnicity)	↑ risk of DVT [adjusted OR 1.97 (95%CI 1.47–2.63] or PE [adjusted OR 1.93 (95%CI 1.41–2.65)] with PAN vs controls

(continued on next page)

Table 4
(continued)

Disease	Reference, Location	Type of Study	Participants	Key Findings
Giant cell arteritis	Unizony, et al[51] 2017, UK	Population-based database of electronic medical records	6441 GCA, 63,985 controls	Patients with GCA had an increasing risk of VTE in the year preceding diagnosis, highest in the first 3 mo after GCA diagnosis and declining thereafter
	Michailidou, et al[52] 2022, USA	Retrospective analysis of a health care database of army veterans	1535 GCA, 10,265 PMR, 1203 with overlapping GCA/PMR, 39,009 OA of similar age & sex as controls	↑ risk of DVT [adjusted HR for GCA 3.88 (95%CI 3.11–4.86) and PMR 2.04 (95%CI 1.78–2.36) vs OA] ↑ risk of PE [adjusted HR for GCA 4.21 (95%CI 3.04–5.85) and for PMR 2.71 (95%CI 2.23–3.29) vs OA]
	Unizony, et al[53] 2015, USA	Retrospective analysis of national database for hospitalizations	9311 GCA, 8,194,136 non-GCA controls	↑ risk of DVT [adjusted OR 2.08 (95%CI 1.76–2.45)] or PE [adjusted OR 1.58(95%CI 1.27–1.96)] in hospitalized patients with GCA
Behcet's disease	Thomas, et al[55] 2020, UK	Retrospective analysis of primary care database	1281 BD, 5124 controls (age and sex matched)	↑ VTE risk with BD [adjusted HR 4.80 (95%CI 2.42–9.54)]
	Toledo-Samaniego, et al[56] 2020, Spain	Case-control study	12 BD with VTE, 45 BD with VTE	Erythema nodosum (OR 4.62), fever (OR 8.23), and the lack of immunosuppressive therapy (OR 20, 95%CI 19.2–166.6) ↑ VTE risk

Abbreviations: 95%CI, 95% confidence intervals; AAV, ANCA, associated vasculitis; ANCA, antineutrophil cytoplasmic antibody; BD, Behcet's disease; DVT, deep venous thrombosis; GC, Glucocorticoid; GCA, giant cell arteritis; HR, hazard ratio; IgAV, IgA vasculitis, JIA, juvenile idiopathic arthritis, OA, osteoarthritis, OR, odds ratio, PAN, polyarteritis nodosa, PE, pulmonary embolism, PMR, polymyalgia rheumatica, VTE, venous thromboembolism.

Table 5
Venous thromboembolism in Sjogren's syndrome, systemic sclerosis, inflammatory myositis, juvenile idiopathic arthritis, sarcoidosis and gout

Disease	Reference, Location	Type of Study	Participants	Key Findings
Sjogren's syndrome	Aviña-Zubieta, et al[62] 2017, Canada	Population-based cohort study	1175 SS, 11,947 controls (matched for age, sex, time of cohort entry)	MVA HR for incident PE (4.07, 95%CI 2.04–8.09), DVT (2.80, 95%CI 1.27–6.17), and overall VTE (2.92, 95%CI 1.66–5.16) ↑ in SS vs controls; greatest ↑ in risk of PE, DVT, VTE observed in first year after diagnosis of SS
	Mofors, et al[63] 2019, Sweden	Population-based cohort study	960 SS, 9035 controls (matched for age, sex, geographic location of residence)	VTE risk ↑ with SS vs controls [HR 2.1 (95%CI 1.6–2.9)] at median 9.5 y follow-up Stratifying risk based on double positivity for antibodies against Ro and Lo, single positivity for either antibody, or negativity for both antibodies, VTE risk ↑ in double positive (HR 3.1, 95%CI 1.9–4.8) but not in single positive (HR 1.7, 95%CI 0.9–3.0) or double negative patients with SS (HR 1.6, 95%CI 0.9–3.0) vs controls Overall VTE risk did not vary much with duration of disease. In subset double-positive for anti-Ro and anti-La, VTE risk ↑↑ in the first 5 y and decreased thereafter

(continued on next page)

Table 5
(continued)

Disease	Reference, Location	Type of Study	Participants	Key Findings
Inflammatory myositis	Carruthers, et al [65] 2016, Canada	Retrospective cohort study	443 PM, 355 DM	In PM, ↑ IRR for VTE and PE in first year and similar IRR for DVT over first 5 years following diagnosis In DM, similar IRR of VTE and DVT over first 5 years following diagnosis; IRR for PE ↑↑ in the 2 years following diagnosis
	Chung, et al [66] 2014, Taiwan	Retrospective analysis of health care insurance databases	2031 PM or DM	Female subjects had 1.2 times ↑ VTE risk than males. VTE risk ↑ 3-times in age > 65 y than ≤ 65 y Comorbid conditions doubled VTE risk
Systemic sclerosis	Butt, et al [69] 2019, Denmark	Retrospective analysis of a population-based database	2778 SSc, 13,520 controls (age and sex matched)	↑ risk of prevalent VTE [OR 3.07 (95%CI 2.36–3.99)] & incident VTE [HR 2.10 (95%CI 1.65–2.67)] in SSc vs controls
	Schoenfeld, et al [70] 2016, Canada	Population-based cohort study	1245 SSc, 12,670 controls (matched for age, sex, time of cohort entry)	↑ VTE risk [HR 3.47(95%CI 2.14–5.64)] in SSc vs controls (adjusted for prior healthcare visits and GC use) VTE risk ↑↑ in the year following diagnosis and declined thereafter

Key findings (top): VTE risk ↑ overall in < 50 year old; in double antibody positive, VTE risk highest between 50–70 y

	Johnson, et al [71] 2018, Canada	Multicentric hospital-based cohort	1181 SSc	VTE prevalence 2.7 (95%CI 1.9–3.7) per 1000 person-years (compared to 2 per 1000 person-years in the general population) PAH, PAD, ACLA or anti-Scl-70 antibodies ↑↑ VTE risk in SSc VTE did not confer ↑ risk of dying ↑ D-dimer did not confer a greater risk of VTE in SSc
	Furtado, et al [72] 2021, France	Retrospective hospital-based cohort study	214 SSc	
Juvenile idiopathic arthritis	Johannesdottir, et al [73] 2012, Denmark	Population-based case-control study	13 JIA, 33 controls (for any VTE); 11 JIA, 17 controls (for unprovoked VTE)	MVA IRR for any VTE 3.0 (95%CI 1.4–6.4), for unprovoked VTE 4.2 (95%CI 1.8–10.0) in JIA vs controls. All VTE episodes in JIA occurred after a year following diagnosis (occurred earlier in other autoimmune diseases)
	Horton, et al [74] 2021, USA	Population-based insurance database	7500 JIA on GC, 10,790 JIA not on GC	Incidence of anti-thrombotic therapy (surrogate of VTE) 7.3 (95%CI 5.9–8.8) per 1 million person-days Incidence of anti-thrombotic therapy with VTE requiring hospitalization (1.6, 95% CI 1.0–2.4). Both events were highest in those currently receiving GC when compared with those not on GC.

(continued on next page)

Table 5
(continued)

Disease	Reference, Location	Type of Study	Participants	Key Findings
Sarcoidosis	Ungprasert, et al [76,77]2017, 2017, USA	Population-based cohort study	345 sarcoidosis, 345 controls (age and sex matched)	Cumulative VTE incidence at 10 y of 4.0 (95%CI 1.6–6.3) % Unadjusted HR for VTE, 3.04 (95%CI 1.47–6.29), DVT 3.14 (95%CI 1.32–7.48), and PE 4.29 (95%CI 1.21–15.23) for sarcoidosis vs controls After adjusting for CVD risk factors, HR for VTE 3.09 (95%CI 1.27–7.53), DVT 3.04 (95% CI 1.06–8.71) and 4.38 (95%CI 1.15–16.74) for sarcoidosis vs controls
	Parrish, et al [78]2018, USA	Retrospective analysis of military personnel healthcare database	9908 sarcoidosis	2.5 fold ↑ VTE risk in the 6 mo following a diagnosis of sarcoidosis
	Kolluri, et al[79] 2021, USA	Retrospective hospital-based cohort study	323 cardiac (with or without extracardiac) and 91 extracardiac sarcoidosis, 235 controls without sarcoidosis	Over median 3.1 y follow-up, 12% PE, 14% DVT in cardiac sarcoidosis, 7.6% PE, 3.3% DVT in extracardiac sarcoidosis, 4% PE, 8% DVT in non-sarcoidosis On MVA, prior VTE ↑ risk of PE (HR 11.75, 95%CI 5.14–26.82) and DVT (HR 13.22, 95%CI 5.56–31.39)

Gout				
				GC use ↑ risk of PE (HR 3.06, 95%CI 1.36–6.91) and DVT (HR 6.21, 95%CI 2.69–14.34) History of malignancy ↑ risk of DVT (HR 2.23, 95%CI 1.12–4.24) but not PE
	Li, et al[81] 2020, Canada	Population-based cohort study	130,708 gout, 131,349 non-gout controls	↑ risk of VTE (HR 1.22, 95% CI 1.13–1.32), DVT (HR 1.28, 95%CI 1.17–1.41) and PE (HR 1.16, 95%CI 1.05–1.29) in gout vs controls ↑ VTE risk evident in the 3 y preceding diagnosis and in the 5 y following the diagnosis of gout
	Sultan, et al 2019,[82] UK	Primary healthcare database	62,234 gout, 62,234 controls	MVA HR for VTE 1.25 (95% CI 1.15–1.35) in gout vs controls; risk of VTE similar in males and females, or in those receiving ULT vs those not on ULT. VTE risk ↑ in those <50 y age, belonging to more affluent socioeconomic status, in the first year after diagnosis, in outpatients (but not in admitted patients)

Abbreviations: 95%CI, 95% confidence intervals; ACLA, anticardiolipin antibodies; CVD, cardiovascular disease; DM, dermatomyositis; DVT, deep venous thrombosis; GC, glucocorticoid; HR, hazard ratio; IRR, incidence risk ratio; JIA, juvenile idiopathic arthritis; MVA, multivariable adjusted analyses; OR, odds ratio; PAD, peripheral arterial disease; PAH, pulmonary arterial hypertension; PE, pulmonary embolism; PM, polymyositis; RR, risk ratio; SS, Sjogren's syndrome; SSc, Systemic sclerosis; UK, united kingdom; ULT, Urate-lowering therapy; USA, United States of America; VTE, venous thromboembolism.

cohort studies.[69,70] VTE risk is highest in the year following diagnosis of SSc,[70] associates with pulmonary arterial hypertension, peripheral vascular disease, ACLA or anti-Scl-70 antibodies,[71] but not with elevated D-dimer.[72] VTE in SSc does not confer a greater mortality risk[71] (see **Table 5**).

Juvenile Idiopathic Arthritis

Few cohort studies have observed increased VTE risk in JIA,[73] highest after a year of diagnosis (contrary to other IRDs),[73] and associated with ongoing glucocorticoid use[74] (see **Table 5**).

Sarcoidosis

A systematic review of 3 observational studies (29,270 patients with sarcoidosis) reported an increased risk of VTE in sarcoidosis [pooled RR 1.42 (95%CI 1.12–1.79) versus population-based controls],[75] confirmed in subsequent cohort studies.[76,77] Such VTE risk is higher in the 6 months following diagnosis when compared with the time period preceding diagnosis of sarcoidosis.[78] Prior VTE, corticosteroid use and malignancy increase VTE risk in sarcoidosis[79] (see **Table 5**).

Gout

A systematic review identified a pooled prevalence of 2.05 (95%CI 1.22–3.43) in gout as well as an increased risk of VTE in gout compared with controls (HR from different studies ranged from 1.22-1.66).[80] Increased VTE risk precedes the diagnosis of gout by as much as 3 years,[81] higher in patients younger than 50 years, in the first year after diagnosis, in outpatients (compared with inpatients) and in those belonging to more affluent socioeconomic strata[82] (see **Table 5**).

Therapeutic Considerations in Patients with Inflammatory Rheumatic Disease in Relation to Venous Thromboembolism

Specific therapeutic considerations in IRDs from a viewpoint of VTE are summarized in **Table 6**, and detailed below.

Anticoagulation Therapy

Patients with IRD with an identifiable trigger for the VTE should receive anticoagulation for 3 months.[83] For those with VTE and a definitive trigger, a high-risk APL profile (such as triple APL positivity) should bring into consideration a longer duration of antithrombotic therapy.[83,84] Unprovoked VTE or the presence of associated APS merits long-term anticoagulation therapy (possibly lifelong).[84] In APS with the first episode of VTE, therapy with vitamin K antagonists (VKA) with target prothrombin time international normalized ratio (INR) between 2 to 3 is recommended.[84] If recurrent VTE occur despite attaining this target INR and ensuring drug compliance, then a higher INR target (3–4), the addition of antiplatelet agents or substitution of VKA with low-molecular weight heparin are therapeutic options.[84] Although directly-acting oral anticoagulants (DOACs) such as rivaroxaban or dabigatran do not associate with an increased recurrence of VTE, their use is not recommended in APS because of increased arterial thrombotic events observed in patients treated with these drugs.[84–86] This risk is particularly higher in those with triple APL positivity and male subjects.[84–86] Limited evidence favors lesser recurrent thrombotic events in APS treated with monthly infusions of intravenous immunoglobulin along with anticoagulation or anti-platelets, a strategy that might be useful in refractory, recurrent thromboses with APS.[87]

Table 6
Management considerations for patients with inflammatory rheumatic diseases from the viewpoint of risk for venous thromboembolism

Issue	Considerations
Anticoagulation	Provoked VTE without high-risk APL profile – 3–6 mo of anticoagulation Provoked VTE with high-risk APL profile – long-term anticoagulation Unprovoked VTE/VTE with APS – long-term anticoagulation First VTE episode – VKA with INR 2–3 Recurrent VTE despite target INR achieved – Increase target INR to 3–4 • Addition of antiplatelet agents • Substitute with low molecular weight heparin in prophylactic doses Avoid DOACs when there is associated APS
DMARD therapy	Glucocorticoid use increases VTE risk Hydroxychloroquine decreases VTE risk Little evidence to suggest biologic DMARDs increase VTE risk in comparison to conventional DMARDs Anti-drug antibodies might increase the risk of thrombotic events in patients on biologic DMARDs Avoid JAKinibs in those with prior VTE risk factors or prior VTE
Peri-operative VTE risk	Prophylactic dose of heparin/low-molecular weight heparin in those with ↑ age • ↑ Disability • Prior thrombotic events. • Presence of APLs/high risk APL profile.
VTE in Behcet's disease	Immunosuppression is the treatment of choice Anticoagulation is not preferred
Pulmonary hypertension in CTDs	If the cause is CTEPH, then anticoagulation or pulmonary artery endarterectomy might be required
Other considerations	Screen for underlying malignancy when there is no obvious reason to explain VTE in patients with IRDs Counseling regarding smoking cessation should be offered The use of estrogen-containing oral contraceptive pills should be avoided in female patients at a high risk of VTE

Abbreviations: APL, antiphospholipid antibody; APS, antiphospholipid antibody syndrome; CTD, connective tissue diseases; CTEPH, chronic thromboembolic pulmonary hypertension; DMARD, Disease-modifying antirheumatic drugs; DOACs, Direct oral anticoagulants; INR, international normalized ratio for prothrombin time; IRDs, Inflammatory rheumatic diseases; JAKinibs, Janus kinase inhibitors; VKA, Vitamin K antagonists; VTE, venous thromboembolism.

DMARD Therapy (Other than Janus Kinase Inhibitors)

Glucocorticoid use increases [adjusted HR 1.99 (95%CI 1.66–2.40)] and hydroxychloroquine decreases [adjusted HR 0.79 (95%CI 0.62–0.98)] VTE risk in RA.[8] Analysis of the Medicare insurance database from the USA comparing 26,534 propensity-score matched patients each with RA treated with methotrexate or hydroxychloroquine as the first DMARD reported a greater risk of VTE with methotrexate compared with hydroxychloroquine [HR 2.26 (95%CI 1.75–2.91)].[88] Other studies have also suggested decreased risk of VTE with hydroxychloroquine in RA and SLE.[89] Overall biologic DMARD use does not appear to be a risk factor for VTE. A propensity-matched RA cohort from Taiwan of 7062 patients on biologics compared with 14,124 on conventional DMARDs reported similar risk of VTE in both groups [HR for biologic vs conventional DMARD 1.11 (95%CI 0.79–1.55)].[90] However, anti-drug antibodies might portend a greater VTE risk. A retrospective analysis of 272 RA patients from the Netherlands treated with adalimumab reported a significantly higher risk of vascular thrombotic events (both venous and arterial) with antiadalimumab antibodies [adjusted HR 7.6 (95%CI 1.3–45.1)].[91]

Janus Kinase Inhibitors

Janus kinase inhibitors (JAKinibs, viz., tofacitinib, baricitinib, upadacitinib, filgotinib, peficitinib) have emerged as effective orally administered therapies with comparable effects to biologic DMARDs. Effective amelioration of inflammatory mechanisms such as interleukin-6, interleukin-1 β, and TNF-α with JAKinibs, which are shared pathways in IRDs and CVD, resulted in the hypothesis that JAKinibs might actually ameliorate CVD risk in IRDs.[92] A recent phase 3b-4 post-marketing trial in RA with inadequate response to methotrexate (MTX-IR) older than 50 years with CVD risk factors compared the safety of tofacitinib at doses 5 mg bd ($n = 1455$) or 10 mg bd ($n = 1456$) with TNFi (adalimumab or etanercept, $n = 1451$).[93] The risk of VTE, DVT, and PE were considerably higher for tofacitinib 10 mg bd, and not significantly higher for the 5 mg bd dose, when compared with TNFi.[93] Risks for cancer and major adverse cardiovascular events were also similarly increased with tofacitinib.[93] All risks were amplified for the 10 mg bd (a dose rarely used in clinical practice).[93] This prompted a "black box" warning from the US FDA regarding the use of JAKinibs in inflammatory diseases and stated that patients should be clearly informed of the risks of CVD events, VTE and malignancies, as well as that the use of JAKinibs should be preferably only after TNFi failure[4,94] (**Fig. 1**).

Other studies offer contrary viewpoints. An analysis of patients with RA and PsA treated with tofacitinib in different clinical trials (including long-term follow-ups) reported similar VTE risk with tofacitinib 5 mg bd or 10 mg bd compared to placebo.[95] Incidence rates were higher in those with prior VTE risk factors (see **Fig 1**).[95] Similar findings were observed from a registry of RA patients from the USA in active RA with comparable VTE risk to biologic DMARDs.[95] Analysis of three population-based cohorts of RA from the USA comparing matched patients initiated on tofacitinib or on TNFi identified no increase in VTE risk with tofacitinib (see **Fig 1**).[96] A 2-year open label extension of the SELECT-COMPARE trial comparing upadacitinib with adalimumab in MTX-IR RA patients reported similar VTE event rates with upadacitinib or adalimumab.[97] A systematic review of 42 trials of tofacitinib, baricitinib, upadacitinib or filgotinib in immune-mediated inflammatory diseases reported similar or decreased VTE risk with JAKinibs compared to placebo.[98]

Recently published post-hoc analyses of the ORAL Surveillance study revealed that a significant VTE risk with tofacitinib vs TNFi was only evident in those receiving tofacitinib at 10 mg bd dose who had high baseline cardiovascular risk.[99] Multivariable-adjusted clinical predictors of increased VTE risk included male sex, age ≥ 65 years, body mass index ≥ 30 kg/m^2 prior VTE, concomitant use of antidepressants, glucocorticoids, oral contraceptive pills, or hormone replacement therapy, whereas proton pump inhibitor use was protective.[100] **Fig. 1** summarizes current controversies in VTE risk with JAKinibs. Ongoing postmarketing surveillance studies of JAKinibs in IRDs shall help to further clarify this impasse.[4,94] Until then, from the viewpoint of

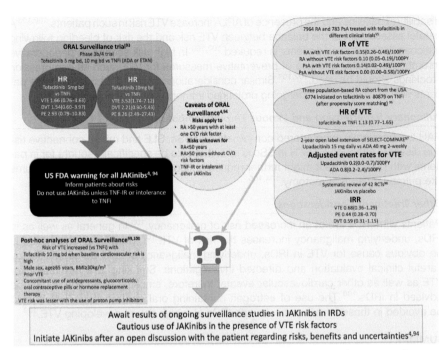

Fig. 1. Controversies regarding JAKinibs and VTE risk. ADA, adalimumab; CVD, cardiovascular disease; DVT, deep venous thrombosis; ETAN, etanercept; HR, hazard ratio; IRR, Incidence risk ratio; JAKinibs, Janus kinase inhibitors; PE, Pulmonary embolism; PsA, Psoriatic arthritis; PY, person-years; R, Incidence rate; RA, Rheumatoid arthritis; RCT, Randomized controlled trial; TNF-IR, Inadequate response to TNFi; TNFi, Tumor necrosis factor-α inhibitors; VTE, venous thromboembolism.

VTE risk, it might be prudent to avoid JAKinibs in older patients with risk factors for VTE.[4,94]

Venous Thromboembolism in Behcet's Disease

Endothelial injury due to immune activation might lead on to VTE in vascular BD. Immunosuppressive therapy associates with lesser risk of VTE in BD.[56] The inflammatory thrombus in BD is best treated with immunosuppressive therapy (which limits endothelial injury and prevents further progression of the thrombus).[101] The venous thrombus in BD is less likely to embolize.[101] Underlying undetected pulmonary artery aneurysms might rupture in BD on anticoagulation and result in catastrophic pulmonary haemorrhage.[101] Based on observational data, the use of immunosuppressive therapy (but not anticoagulation) reduces recurrence of VTE and postphlebitic syndrome in the affected extremity in BD.[101] Therefore, anticoagulation is contraindicated in VTE due to BD.[101]

Perioperative Anticoagulation During Arthroplasty in Inflammatory Rheumatic Disease

As seen earlier, patients with IRDs hospitalized for any cause are at increased risk of VTE.[25] Such risk is amplified when patients with IRD such as RA, SLE, SpA or PsA require replacement of major joints such as knee, hip, and shoulder due to joint damage resulting in significant disability. History of prior thrombotic events, increasing age, greater disability at baseline and the presence of APLA increase VTE risk in such patients.[102,103] A careful assessment of the balance between VTE risk and the risk of bleeding following anticoagulation in such patients is required.[102,103] In high-risk scenarios, perioperative thromboprophylaxis and use of preventative measures for VTE such as compression stockings should be used.[102,103] Similar considerations should hold true for those patients with IRDs who are undergoing prolonged immobilization for any cause.

Pulmonary Hypertension and Venous Thromboembolism

PAH is a frequently encountered complication of SSc, SLE and mixed connective tissue disease. Although CTEPH in SSc is rare, it should be specifically sought for in patients with prior VTE as it might further require anticoagulation or surgical procedures like pulmonary endarterectomy.[104,105]

Other Treatment Considerations

Patients with IRDs are at an increased risk of malignancy.[106] In general as well as in IRDs, underlying malignancy increases the risk of VTE.[107] Therefore, when there is no obvious cause for VTE in IRDs, underlying malignancy should be sought for by careful clinical evaluation and directed investigations. Smoking is a risk factor for VTE as well as other cardiovascular events, therefore, smoking cessation should be advised in IRDs.[108] The use of estrogen-containing oral contraceptive pills should be avoided in those female patients with IRDs at a high risk of developing VTE.[109]

SUMMARY

VTE risk is increased in most IRDs, based on data from systematic reviews or from individual observational studies. Various factors drive VTE risk in IRDs, particularly a high-risk triple positive APL profile. Duration of anticoagulation following VTE is determined by whether the event was provoked on unprovoked, and whether there exist underlying thrombophilic states such as APLs. VTE associated with BD requires immunosuppression rather than anticoagulation. JAKinibs should be used with caution in those with prior VTE events. Results of ongoing post-marketing surveillance studies of various JAKinibs should help to further clarify VTE risk with this group of medications.

CLINICS CARE POINTS

- The risk of venous thromboembolism is increased in most inflammatory rheumatic diseases.
- Venous thromboembolism risk is particularly increased in systemic lupus erythematosus and antiphospholipid antibody syndrome.
- Long-term anticoagulation should be considered following venous thromboembolism in the presence of unprovoked venous thrombosis, underlying antiphospholipid antibody syndrome or high-risk antiphospholipid antibody profile.
- Patients with inflammatory rheumatic diseases undergoing major surgeries (such as large joint replacement) or who have prolonged immobilization should be assessed for risk of venous thromboembolism and managed as per the assessed risk.
- Careful assessment of venous thromboembolism risk should precede the initiation of Janus kinase inhibitors in inflammatory rheumatic diseases, preferably using alternative treatment strategies in those with high risk.
- Unlike other rheumatic diseases, venous thromboembolism in Behcet's disease requires immunosuppressive therapy instead of anticoagulation.

FUNDING

D.P. Misra acknowledges support from the Indian Council of Medical Research (Grant No 5/4/1-2/2019-NCD-II) for his research on Takayasu arteritis (not related to this work).

DISCLOSURE

The authors have nothing to disclose.

REFERENCES

1. Galloway J, Barrett K, Irving P, et al. Risk of venous thromboembolism in immune-mediated inflammatory diseases: a UK matched cohort study. RMD Open 2020;6(3):e001392.
2. Ruiz-Sada P, Mazzolai L, Braester A, et al. Venous thromboembolism in patients with autoimmune disorders: a comparison between bleeding complications during anticoagulation and recurrences after its discontinuation. Br J Haematol 2022;197(4):489–96.
3. Yusuf HR, Hooper WC, Beckman MG, et al. Risk of venous thromboembolism among hospitalizations of adults with selected autoimmune diseases. J Thromb Thrombolysis 2014;38(3):306–13.
4. Kragstrup TW, Glintborg B, Svensson AL, et al. Waiting for JAK inhibitor safety data. RMD Open 2022;8(1):e002236.
5. Hu LJ, Ji B, Fan HX. Venous thromboembolism risk in rheumatoid arthritis patients: a systematic review and updated meta-analysis. Eur Rev Med Pharmacol Sci 2021;25(22):7005–13.
6. Li L, Lu N, Avina-Galindo AM, et al. The risk and trend of pulmonary embolism and deep vein thrombosis in rheumatoid arthritis: a general population-based study. Rheumatology (Oxford) 2021;60(1):188–95.
7. Molander V, Bower H, Frisell T, et al. Risk of venous thromboembolism in rheumatoid arthritis, and its association with disease activity: a nationwide cohort study from Sweden. Ann Rheum Dis 2021;80(2):169–75.
8. Ozen G, Pedro S, Schumacher R, et al. Risk factors for venous thromboembolism and atherosclerotic cardiovascular disease: do they differ in patients with rheumatoid arthritis? RMD Open 2021;7(2):e001618.
9. Federico LE, Johnson TM, England BR, et al. Circulating Adipokines and Associations with Incident Cardiovascular Disease in Rheumatoid Arthritis. Arthritis Care Res (Hoboken) 2022. https://doi.org/10.1002/acr.24885. In press.
10. Ungprasert P, Srivali N, Kittanamongkolchai W. Ankylosing spondylitis and risk of venous thromboembolism: A systematic review and meta-analysis. Lung India 2016;33(6):642–5.
11. Bengtsson K, Forsblad-d'Elia H, Lie E, et al. Are ankylosing spondylitis, psoriatic arthritis and undifferentiated spondyloarthritis associated with an increased risk of cardiovascular events? A prospective nationwide population-based cohort study. Arthritis Res Ther 2017;19(1):102.
12. Eriksson JK, Jacobsson L, Bengtsson K, et al. Is ankylosing spondylitis a risk factor for cardiovascular disease, and how do these risks compare with those in rheumatoid arthritis? Ann Rheum Dis 2017;76(2):364–70.
13. Aviña-Zubieta JA, Chan J, De Vera M, et al. Risk of venous thromboembolism in ankylosing spondylitis: a general population-based study. Ann Rheum Dis 2019; 78(4):480–5.

14. Ogdie A, Kay McGill N, Shin DB, et al. Risk of venous thromboembolism in patients with psoriatic arthritis, psoriasis and rheumatoid arthritis: a general population-based cohort study. Eur Heart J 2018;39(39):3608–14.
15. Gazitt T, Pesachov J, Lavi I, et al. The association between psoriatic arthritis and venous thromboembolism: a population-based cohort study. Arthritis Res Ther 2022;24(1):16.
16. Damian AC, Colaco K, Rohekar S, et al. The incidence and risk factors for venous thromboembolic events in patients with psoriasis and psoriatic arthritis. Semin Arthritis Rheum 2021;51(3):547–52.
17. Goulielmos GN, Zervou MI. Risk of Venous Thromboembolism in Ankylosing Spondylitis and Rheumatoid Arthritis: Genetic Aspects. J Rheumatol 2021;48(9):1492–3.
18. Yafasova A, Fosbøl EL, Schou M, et al. Long-Term Cardiovascular Outcomes in Systemic Lupus Erythematosus. J Am Coll Cardiol 2021;77(14):1717–27.
19. Aviña-Zubieta JA, Vostretsova K, De Vera MA, et al. The risk of pulmonary embolism and deep venous thrombosis in systemic lupus erythematosus: A general population-based study. Semin Arthritis Rheum 2015;45(2):195–201.
20. Mok CC, Ho LY, Yu KL, et al. Venous thromboembolism in southern Chinese patients with systemic lupus erythematosus. Clin Rheumatol 2010;29(6):599–604.
21. Mok CC, Tang SS, To CH, et al. Incidence and risk factors of thromboembolism in systemic lupus erythematosus: a comparison of three ethnic groups. Arthritis Rheum 2005;52(9):2774–82.
22. Ahlehoff O, Wu JJ, Raunsø J, et al. Cutaneous lupus erythematosus and the risk of deep venous thrombosis and pulmonary embolism: A Danish nationwide cohort study. Lupus 2017;26(13):1435–9.
23. Chang JC, Mandell DS, Knight AM. High Health Care Utilization Preceding Diagnosis of Systemic Lupus Erythematosus in Youth. Arthritis Care Res (Hoboken) 2018;70(9):1303–11.
24. Jakez-Ocampo J, Rodriguez-Armida M, Fragoso-Loyo H, et al. Clinical characteristics of systemic lupus erythematosus patients in long-term remission without treatment. Clin Rheumatol 2020;39(11):3365–71.
25. Kishore S, Jatwani S, Malhotra B, et al. Systemic Lupus Erythematosus Is Associated With a High Risk of Venous Thromboembolism in Hospitalized Patients Leading to Poor Outcomes and a Higher Cost: Results From Nationwide Inpatient Sample Database 2003-2011. ACR Open Rheumatol 2019;1(3):194–200.
26. Gkrouzman E, Peng M, Davis-Porada J, et al. Venous Thromboembolic Events in African American Lupus Patients in Association With Antiphospholipid Antibodies Compared to White Patients. Arthritis Care Res (Hoboken) 2022;74(4):656–64.
27. Cooley I, Derebail VK, Gibson KL, et al. Association of Lupus Nephritis Histopathologic Classification With Venous Thromboembolism-Modification by Age at Biopsy. Kidney Int Rep 2021;6(6):1653–60.
28. Cervera R, Khamashta MA, Font J, et al. Morbidity and Mortality in Systemic Lupus Erythematosus During a 10-Year Period: A Comparison of Early and Late Manifestations in a Cohort of 1,000 Patients. Medicine 2003;82(5):299–308.
29. Akdogan A, Kilic L, Dogan I, et al. Pulmonary hypertension in systemic lupus erythematosus: pulmonary thromboembolism is the leading cause. J Clin Rheumatol 2013;19(8):421–5.
30. Brouwer JL, Bijl M, Veeger NJ, et al. The contribution of inherited and acquired thrombophilic defects, alone or combined with antiphospholipid antibodies, to

venous and arterial thromboembolism in patients with systemic lupus erythematosus. Blood 2004;104(1):143–8.

31. Sallai KK, Nagy E, Bodó I, et al. Thrombosis risk in systemic lupus erythematosus: the role of thrombophilic risk factors. Scand J Rheumatol 2007;36(3): 198–205.

32. Elbagir S, Grosso G, Mohammed NA, et al. Associations with thrombosis are stronger for antiphosphatidylserine/prothrombin antibodies than for the Sydney criteria antiphospholipid antibody tests in SLE. Lupus 2021;30(8):1289–99.

33. Nojima J, Kuratsune H, Suehisa E, et al. Acquired activated protein C resistance associated with IgG antibodies against beta2-glycoprotein I and prothrombin as a strong risk factor for venous thromboembolism. Clin Chem 2005;51(3):545–52.

34. Ramirez GA, Mackie I, Nallamilli S, et al. Anti-protein C antibodies and acquired protein C resistance in SLE: novel markers for thromboembolic events and disease activity? Rheumatology (Oxford) 2021;60(3):1376–86.

35. Svenungsson E, Gustafsson JT, Grosso G, et al. Complement deposition, C4d, on platelets is associated with vascular events in systemic lupus erythematosus. Rheumatology (Oxford) 2020;59(11):3264–74.

36. Peretz ASR, Rasmussen NS, Jacobsen S, et al. Galectin-3-binding protein is a novel predictor of venous thromboembolism in systemic lupus erythematosus. Clin Exp Rheumatol 2021;39(6):1360–8.

37. Miranda S, Park J, Le Gal G, et al. Prevalence of confirmed antiphospholipid syndrome in 18-50 years unselected patients with first unprovoked venous thromboembolism. J Thromb Haemost 2020;18(4):926–30.

38. Knight JS, Kanthi Y. Mechanisms of immunothrombosis and vasculopathy in antiphospholipid syndrome. Semin Immunopathol 2022;44(3):347–62.

39. Zuily S, Clerc-Urmès I, Bauman C, et al. Cluster analysis for the identification of clinical phenotypes among antiphospholipid antibody-positive patients from the APS ACTION Registry. Lupus 2020. https://doi.org/10.1177/0961203320940776. In press.

40. Bucci T, Ames PRJ, Triggiani M, et al. Cardiac and vascular features of arterial and venous primary antiphospholipid syndrome. The multicenter ATHERO-APS study. Thromb Res 2022;209:69–74.

41. Rosen K, Raanani E, Kogan A, et al. Chronic thromboembolic pulmonary hypertension in patients with antiphospholipid syndrome: Risk factors and management. J Heart Lung Transpl 2022;41(2):208–16.

42. Foltyn Zadura A, Memon AA, Stojanovich L, et al. Factor H Autoantibodies in Patients with Antiphospholipid Syndrome and Thrombosis. J Rheumatol 2015; 42(10):1786–93.

43. Stachowicz A, Zabczyk M, Natorska J, et al. Differences in plasma fibrin clot composition in patients with thrombotic antiphospholipid syndrome compared with venous thromboembolism. Sci Rep 2018;8(1):17301.

44. Celinska-Löwenhoff M, Zabczyk M, Iwaniec T, et al. Reduced plasma fibrin clot permeability is associated with recurrent thromboembolic events in patients with antiphospholipid syndrome. Rheumatology (Oxford) 2018;57(8):1340–9.

45. Berti A, Matteson EL, Crowson CS, et al. Risk of Cardiovascular Disease and Venous Thromboembolism Among Patients With Incident ANCA-Associated Vasculitis: A 20-Year Population-Based Cohort Study. Mayo Clin Proc 2018; 93(5):597–606.

46. Hansrivijit P, Trongtorsak A, Gadhiya KP, et al. Incidence and risk factors of venous thromboembolism in ANCA-associated vasculitis: a metaanalysis and metaregression. Clin Rheumatol 2021;40(7):2843–53.

47. Misra DP, Thomas KN, Gasparyan AY, et al. Mechanisms of thrombosis in ANCA-associated vasculitis. Clin Rheumatol 2021;40(12):4807–15.
48. Tracy A, Subramanian A, Adderley NJ, et al. Cardiovascular, thromboembolic and renal outcomes in IgA vasculitis (Henoch-Schönlein purpura): a retrospective cohort study using routinely collected primary care data. Ann Rheum Dis 2019;78(2):261–9.
49. Ungprasert P, Koster MJ, Cheungpasitporn W, et al. Inpatient burden and association with comorbidities of polyarteritis nodosa: National Inpatient Sample 2014. Semin Arthritis Rheum 2020;50(1):66–70.
50. Ungprasert P, Koster MJ, Thongprayoon C, et al. Risk of venous thromboembolism among patients with vasculitis: a systematic review and meta-analysis. Clin Rheumatol 2016;35(11):2741–7.
51. Unizony S, Lu N, Tomasson G, et al. Temporal Trends of Venous Thromboembolism Risk Before and After Diagnosis of Giant Cell Arteritis. Arthritis Rheumatol 2017;69(1):176–84.
52. Michailidou D, Zhang T, Stamatis P, et al. Risk of venous and arterial thromboembolism in patients with giant cell arteritis and/or polymyalgia rheumatica: A Veterans Health Administration population-based study in the United States. J Intern Med 2022;291(5):665–75.
53. Unizony S, Menendez ME, Rastalsky N, et al. Inpatient complications in patients with giant cell arteritis: decreased mortality and increased risk of thromboembolism, delirium and adrenal insufficiency. Rheumatology (Oxford) 2015;54(8): 1360–8.
54. Tshifularo N, Arnold M, Moore SW. Thromboembolism and venous thrombosis of the deep veins in surgical children–an increasing challenge? J Pediatr Surg 2011;46(3):433–6.
55. Thomas T, Chandan JS, Subramanian A, et al. Epidemiology, morbidity and mortality in Behçet's disease: a cohort study using The Health Improvement Network (THIN). Rheumatology (Oxford) 2020;59(10):2785–95.
56. Toledo-Samaniego N, Galeano-Valle F, Pinilla-Llorente B, et al. Clinical features and management of venous thromboembolism in patients with Behçet's syndrome: a single-center case-control study. Intern Emerg Med 2020;15(4): 635–44.
57. Navarro S, Ricart JM, Medina P, et al. Activated protein C levels in Behçet's disease and risk of venous thrombosis. Br J Haematol 2004;126(4):550–6.
58. Abdel Badaee H, Edrees A, Amin S, et al. Activated protein C resistance in Behcet's disease. Thromb J 2013;11(1):17.
59. Obiorah IE, Patel BA, Groarke EM, et al. Benign and malignant hematologic manifestations in patients with VEXAS syndrome due to somatic mutations in UBA1. Blood Adv 2021;5(16):3203–15.
60. Groarke EM, Dulau-Florea AE, Kanthi Y. Thrombotic manifestations of VEXAS syndrome. Semin Hematol 2021;58(4):230–8.
61. Ungprasert P, Srivali N, Kittanamongkolchai W. Risk of venous thromboembolism in patients with Sjögren's syndrome: a systematic review and meta-analysis. Clin Exp Rheumatol 2015;33(5):746–50.
62. Aviña-Zubieta JA, Jansz M, Sayre EC, et al. The Risk of Deep Venous Thrombosis and Pulmonary Embolism in Primary Sjögren Syndrome: A General Population-based Study. J Rheumatol 2017;44(8):1184–9.
63. Mofors J, Holmqvist M, Westermark L, et al. Concomitant Ro/SSA and La/SSB antibodies are biomarkers for the risk of venous thromboembolism and cerebral infarction in primary Sjögren's syndrome. J Intern Med 2019;286(4):458–68.

64. Li Y, Wang P, Li L, et al. Increased risk of venous thromboembolism associated with polymyositis and dermatomyositis: a meta-analysis. Ther Clin Risk Manag 2018;14:157–65.
65. Carruthers EC, Choi HK, Sayre EC, et al. Risk of deep venous thrombosis and pulmonary embolism in individuals with polymyositis and dermatomyositis: a general population-based study. Ann Rheum Dis 2016;75(1):110–6.
66. Chung WS, Lin CL, Sung FC, et al. Increased risk of venous thromboembolism in patients with dermatomyositis/polymyositis: a nationwide cohort study. Thromb Res 2014;134(3):622–6.
67. Parperis K. Idiopathic Inflammatory Myopathy and Venous Thromboembolic Events: Comment on the Article by Antovic et al. Arthritis Care Res (Hoboken) 2019;71(10):1396.
68. Ungprasert P, Srivali N, Kittanamongkolchai W. Systemic sclerosis and risk of venous thromboembolism: A systematic review and meta-analysis. Mod Rheumatol 2015;25(6):893–7.
69. Butt SA, Jeppesen JL, Torp-Pedersen C, et al. Cardiovascular Manifestations of Systemic Sclerosis: A Danish Nationwide Cohort Study. J Am Heart Assoc 2019; 8(17):e013405.
70. Schoenfeld SR, Choi HK, Sayre EC, et al. Risk of Pulmonary Embolism and Deep Venous Thrombosis in Systemic Sclerosis: A General Population-Based Study. Arthritis Care Res (Hoboken) 2016;68(2):246–53.
71. Johnson SR, Hakami N, Ahmad Z, et al. Venous Thromboembolism in Systemic Sclerosis: Prevalence, Risk Factors, and Effect on Survival. J Rheumatol 2018; 45(7):942–6.
72. Furtado S, Dunogué B, Jourdi G, et al. High D-dimer plasma concentration in systemic sclerosis patients: Prevalence and association with vascular complications. J Scleroderma Relat Disord 2021;6(2):178–86.
73. Johannesdottir SA, Schmidt M, Horváth-Puhó E, et al. Autoimmune skin and connective tissue diseases and risk of venous thromboembolism: a population-based case-control study. J Thromb Haemost 2012;10(5):815–21.
74. Horton DB, Xie F, Chen L, et al. Oral Glucocorticoids and Incident Treatment of Diabetes Mellitus, Hypertension, and Venous Thromboembolism in Children. Am J Epidemiol 2021;190(3):403–12.
75. Ungprasert P, Srivali N, Wijarnpreecha K, et al. Sarcoidosis and risk of venous thromboembolism: A systematic review and meta-analysis. Sarcoidosis Vasc Diffuse Lung Dis 2015;32(3):182–7.
76. Ungprasert P, Crowson CS, Matteson EL. Epidemiology and clinical characteristics of sarcoidosis: an update from a population-based cohort study from Olmsted County, Minnesota. Reumatismo 2017;69(1):16–22.
77. Ungprasert P, Crowson CS, Matteson EL. Association of Sarcoidosis With Increased Risk of VTE: A Population-Based Study, 1976 to 2013. Chest 2017; 151(2):425–30.
78. Parrish SC, Lin TK, Sicignano NM, et al. Sarcoidosis in the United States Military Health System. Sarcoidosis Vasc Diffuse Lung Dis 2018;35(3):261–7.
79. Kolluri N, Elwazir MY, Rosenbaum AN, et al. Effect of Corticosteroid Therapy in Patients With Cardiac Sarcoidosis on Frequency of Venous Thromboembolism. Am J Cardiol 2021;149:112–8.
80. Cox P, Gupta S, Zhao SS, et al. The incidence and prevalence of cardiovascular diseases in gout: a systematic review and meta-analysis. Rheumatol Int 2021; 41(7):1209–19.

81. Li L, McCormick N, Sayre EC, et al. Trends of venous thromboembolism risk before and after diagnosis of gout: a general population-based study. Rheumatology (Oxford) 2020;59(5):1099–107.

82. Sultan AA, Muller S, Whittle R, et al. Venous thromboembolism in patients with gout and the impact of hospital admission, disease duration and urate-lowering therapy. CMAJ 2019;191(22):E597–603.

83. Kearon C, Akl EA, Ornelas J, et al. Antithrombotic Therapy for VTE Disease: CHEST Guideline and Expert Panel Report. Chest 2016;149(2):315–52.

84. Tektonidou MG, Andreoli L, Limper M, et al. EULAR recommendations for the management of antiphospholipid syndrome in adults. Ann Rheum Dis 2019; 78(10):1296–304.

85. Cerdà P, Becattini C, Iriarte A, et al. Direct oral anticoagulants versus vitamin K antagonists in antiphospholipid syndrome: A meta-analysis. Eur J Intern Med 2020;79:43–50.

86. Dufrost V, Wahl D, Zuily S. Direct oral anticoagulants in antiphospholipid syndrome: Meta-analysis of randomized controlled trials. Autoimmun Rev 2021; 20(1):102711.

87. Tenti S, Guidelli GM, Bellisai F, et al. Long-term treatment of antiphospholipid syndrome with intravenous immunoglobulin in addition to conventional therapy. Clin Exp Rheumatol 2013;31(6):877–82.

88. He M, Pawar A, Desai RJ, et al. Risk of venous thromboembolism associated with methotrexate versus hydroxychloroquine for rheumatoid arthritis: A propensity score-matched cohort study. Semin Arthritis Rheum 2021;51(6):1242–50.

89. Jorge A, Lu N, Choi H, et al. Hydroxychloroquine Use and Cardiovascular Events Among Patients with Systemic Lupus Erythematosus and Rheumatoid Arthritis. Arthritis Care Res (Hoboken) 2021. https://doi.org/10.1002/acr.24850. In press.

90. Chen CP, Kung PT, Chou WY, et al. Effect of introducing biologics to patients with rheumatoid arthritis on the risk of venous thromboembolism: a nationwide cohort study. Sci Rep 2021;11(1):17009.

91. Korswagen LA, Bartelds GM, Krieckaert CL, et al. Venous and arterial thromboembolic events in adalimumab-treated patients with antiadalimumab antibodies: a case series and cohort study. Arthritis Rheum 2011;63(4):877–83.

92. Baldini C, Moriconi FR, Galimberti S, et al. The JAK-STAT pathway: an emerging target for cardiovascular disease in rheumatoid arthritis and myeloproliferative neoplasms. Eur Heart J 2021;42(42):4389–400.

93. Ytterberg SR, Bhatt DL, Mikuls TR, et al. Cardiovascular and Cancer Risk with Tofacitinib in Rheumatoid Arthritis. N Engl J Med 2022;386(4):316–26.

94. Singh JA. Risks and Benefits of Janus Kinase Inhibitors in Rheumatoid Arthritis - Past, Present, and Future. N Engl J Med 2022;386(4):387–9.

95. Mease P, Charles-Schoeman C, Cohen S, et al. Incidence of venous and arterial thromboembolic events reported in the tofacitinib rheumatoid arthritis, psoriasis and psoriatic arthritis development programmes and from real-world data. Ann Rheum Dis 2020;79(11):1400–13.

96. Desai RJ, Pawar A, Khosrow-Khavar F, et al. Risk of venous thromboembolism associated with tofacitinib in patients with rheumatoid arthritis: a population-based cohort study. Rheumatology (Oxford) 2021;61(1):121–30.

97. Fleischmann R, Mysler E, Bessette L, et al. Long-term safety and efficacy of upadacitinib or adalimumab in patients with rheumatoid arthritis: results through 3 years from the SELECT-COMPARE study. RMD Open 2022;8(1):e002012.

98. Yates M, Mootoo A, Adas M, et al. Venous Thromboembolism Risk With JAK Inhibitors: A Meta-Analysis. Arthritis Rheumatol 2021;73(5):779–88.
99. Buch MH, Charles-Schoeman C, Curtis J, et al. POS0237 major adverse cardiovascular events, malignancies and venous thromboembolism by baseline cardiovascular risk: a post hoc analysis of oral surveillance. Ann Rheum Dis 2022;81(Suppl 1):356.
100. Charles-Schoeman C, Fleischmann RM, Mysler E, et al. POS0239 risk of venous thromboembolic events in patients with rheumatoid arthritis aged ≥50 years with ≥1 cardiovascular risk factor: results from a phase 3b/4 randomised study of tofacitinib vs tumour necrosis factor inhibitors. Ann Rheum Dis 2022;81(Suppl 1):358.
101. Seyahi E, Yurdakul S. Behçet's Syndrome and Thrombosis. Mediterr J Hematol Infect Dis 2011;3(1):e2011026.
102. Goodman SM, Bass AR. Perioperative medical management for patients with RA, SPA, and SLE undergoing total hip and total knee replacement: a narrative review. BMC Rheumatol 2018;2:2.
103. Gualtierotti R, Parisi M, Ingegnoli F. Perioperative Management of Patients with Inflammatory Rheumatic Diseases Undergoing Major Orthopaedic Surgery: A Practical Overview. Adv Ther 2018;35(4):439–56.
104. Martinez C, Wallenhorst C, Teal S, et al. Incidence and risk factors of chronic thromboembolic pulmonary hypertension following venous thromboembolism, a population-based cohort study in England. Pulm Circ 2018;8(3). 2045894018791358.
105. Almaaitah S, Highland KB, Tonelli AR. Management of Pulmonary Arterial Hypertension in Patients with Systemic Sclerosis. Integr Blood Press Control 2020;13: 15–29.
106. Chang SH, Park JK, Lee YJ, et al. Comparison of cancer incidence among patients with rheumatic disease: a retrospective cohort study. Arthritis Res Ther 2014;16(4):428.
107. Kim SC, Schneeweiss S, Liu J, et al. Risk of venous thromboembolism in patients with rheumatoid arthritis. Arthritis Care Res (Hoboken) 2013;65(10): 1600–7.
108. Enga KF, Braekkan SK, Hansen-Krone IJ, et al. Cigarette smoking and the risk of venous thromboembolism: the Tromsø Study. J Thromb Haemost 2012;10(10): 2068–74.
109. Bernier MO, Mikaeloff Y, Hudson M, et al. Combined oral contraceptive use and the risk of systemic lupus erythematosus. Arthritis Rheum 2009;61(4):476–81.

Lessons from Cardiac and Vascular Biopsies from Patients with and without Inflammatory Rheumatic Diseases

Ivana Hollan, MD, PhD

KEYWORDS

- Rheumatic diseases • Cardiovascular disease • Immune system • Infections
- Inflammation

KEY POINTS

- Tissue specimens obtained during CABG and other surgeries can be useful for clinical and research purposes.
- Further studies are needed to determine if prevention and suppression of vascular (including that in deep vascular layers) and perivascular/epicardial inflammation could reduce the risk of development of atherosclerosis and aneurysms, and/or their destabilization (in particular in patients with IRD). These approaches might include, for example, drugs targeting the immune system or pathogens.
- Similarly, it is important to examine if the inhibition of proinflammatory factors overexpressed in the heart could reduce the risk of HF.
- Further studies are warranted to evaluate the role of microvascular impairment and characteristics of CV fat (eg, adventitial, perivascular, and epicardial), including its susceptibility to inflammation, in the pathogenesis of CV manifestations.

DISCLOSURES

The Feiring Heart Biopsy Study received research grants from the Norwegian Women's Public Health Association, Norwegian Rheumatism Association, South-Eastern Health Authorities, The Norwegian Association for People with Heart and Lung Diseases, The Norwegian Society of Rheumatology, Innlandet Hospital Trust, Eimar Munthes Memorial Fund, Alf and Aagot Helgesen's Fund, Nanki and Sigval Bergesen Fund, Roche Norway, Schering-Plough Norway, Sanofi-Aventis Norway, Wyeth Norway.

Department of Health Sciences, Norwegian University of Science and Technology Teknologivegen 22, 2815 Gjøvik, Norway
E-mail address: ivana.hollan@gmail.com

Rheum Dis Clin N Am 49 (2023) 129–150
https://doi.org/10.1016/j.rdc.2022.07.005
0889-857X/23/© 2022 Elsevier Inc. All rights reserved.

SUMMARY

Feiring Heart Biopsy Study (FHBS) utilizes clinical data and multiple types of tissue samples. Describing factors in tissues is a crucial step in elucidating pathophysiology and discovering new therapeutic targets and biomarkers.

FHBS indicates that subclinical vascular and cardiac inflammation occurs frequently in patients with coronary artery disease (CAD). In the aorta, inflammatory cell infiltrates (ICIs) occurred in all three vascular layers, with the highest frequency in the adventitia. The adventitial ICIs were more frequent and extensive in patients with IRDs, smokers, and in patients with a history of aortic aneurysm than in those without these characteristics. The occurrence of vascular ICIs paralleled the susceptibility of different types of vessels to atherosclerosis.

Patients with IRD had also higher occurrences of immunologic abnormalities, indicating microvascular impairment and inflammation in the myocardium.

It is possible that inflammation in the subintimal layers is involved in the formation of atherosclerotic lesions and/or aneurisms, facilitates their destabilization, and contributes to the increased cardiovascular (CV) risk in IRDs.

We found high occurrence of ICIs and fibrosis in the epicardium. As epicardial inflammation could influence the embedded coronary arteries, the role of the epicardium in CAD deserves further study.

Due to the therapeutic potential, we searched for immunologic factors and potential triggers of subintimal inflammation. The proportion of T-/B-cells was lower, expression of tumor necrosis factor (TNF), interleukin 33 and 18, and pentraxin 3 (PTX3) was higher, and mixed bacterial population significantly different in RA versus non-IRD. The subintimal layers also contained, for example, B-cell survival factors, calprotectin, C3, C3d, and citrullinated proteins. Thus, infections and/or autoimmunity might trigger or aggravate vascular inflammation.

Using microarrays, we detected, for example, differences in genes related to stress and D-vitamin receptor in the subintimal layers in rheumatoid arthritis (RA) versus non-IRD. The study enables also searching for noncoding RNAs in different compartments and circulating factors.

INCREASED CARDIOVASCULAR RISK IN INFLAMMATORY RHEUMATIC DISEASES

Atherosclerosis is the main cause of premature CV mortality in various IRDs, such as RA, spondyloarthritides, and systemic lupus erythematosus (SLE). The cause of accelerated atherosclerosis in IRDs has not been fully clarified yet. IRDs are also associated with other CV complications, including thromboembolism, arrhythmia, peri-, endo- and myocarditis, heart failure (HF), valvular disease, aneurysms, and vasculitis. Moreover, dysfunction of the autonomic nervous system may lead to abnormal CV reactivity in IRDs.[1]

Similar to atherosclerosis, vasculitis (in epicardial coronary arteries, in small intramural cardiac arteries, or in the aorta around the outlets of coronary arteries) can cause cardiac ischemia, but is considered to require different treatment (immunosuppressants).[2] However, opportunities to detect and thereby to treat vasculitis in vessels that supply the heart have been limited. Although new imaging modalities (eg, positron emission tomography-computed tomography) significantly improved the diagnostics of vasculitis, they have their restraints (such as limited resolution and specificity).[3] Histologic assessment represents the gold standard but is hard to attain in such locations as the heart and central vessels due to complication risk.

In studying atherosclerosis, there has been a great interest in circulating parameters, for example, inflammatory and metabolic markers, but much less focus on searching for clues directly in CV tissue. For vascular tissue assessment, endarterectomy specimens were often utilized – but these contain only the luminal part of the artery. Although autopsy specimens are of great importance,[4–8] their usefulness is limited by postmortal alterations.

FEIRING HEART BIOPSY STUDY

Therefore, in 2001 we established FHBS. We wanted to search for opportunities to detect inflammation in the supplying vessels of the heart, in patients with IRD and non-IRD, and to bring more insights into the potential pathomechanisms of atherosclerosis and other CV manifestations.[9]

We collected detailed demographic, lifestyle, and medical data, blood samples, and surgical specimens from 70 patients with IRDs and 53 age- and sex-matched patients without IRDs, undergoing coronary artery bypass grafting (CABG) due to CAD. In addition, we collected corresponding information and blood samples from 30 healthy individuals (HC) and 32 RA patients without CV disease (CVD); these groups were matched for sex and had the same age range as the CABG groups.[9]

The biobank included frozen and paraffin fixed specimens from tissue routinely removed during CABG, for example, a part of the ascendant aorta removed in connection with the establishment of the aortic part of the aortocoronary bypasses (a specimen containing the aortic adventitia covered by the aortic part of the epicardium, and specimens containing the intima and media); remnants of saphenous vein after the establishment of the graft; cardiac valves in those undergoing valvular surgery, and full-thickness aortic specimen in those undergoing repair of the ascendant aortic aneurysm at the time of CABG (**Fig. 1**). In addition, we collected small biopsies from surgical cuts (right atrium; internal mammary artery = IMA; rectus abdominis muscle; skin).[9,10]

FHBS was later expanded (Phase 2) by a cohort of 237 consecutive patients undergoing CABG, who were examined according to the same protocol as those included in Phase 1, except that several types of tissue specimens were collected. In this article, except for micro-RNA analyses, all the results are based on Phase 1.

For safety, the aortocoronary grafts are preferably connected to the aorta at places with the least pronounced atherosclerosis. Thus, the aortic specimens that we examined are expected to have less pronounced pathologies than the more diseased parts of the aorta.

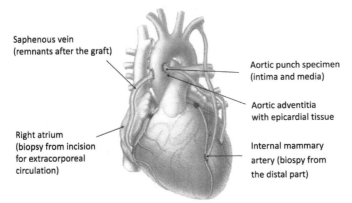

Saphenous vein
(remnants after the graft)

Aortic punch specimen
(intima and media)

Aortic adventitia
with epicardial tissue

Right atrium
(biopsy from incision
for extracorporeal
circulation)

Internal mammary
artery (biospy from
the distal part)

Fig. 1. Schematic illustration of sampling of some of the main tissue specimens during CABG in FHBS. (Courtesy of Rasmus Moer, MD, Feiring, Norway.)

In this article, I summarize some of the main results achieved so far, as well as hypotheses and questions that they evoke. I focus more on the aspects that have so far gotten less attention in mainstream medicine. I wish to illustrate both the complexity of the topic, but also opportunities of the study design.

VASCULAR INFLAMMATION IN CORONARY ARTERY DISEASE AND INFLAMMATORY RHEUMATIC DISEASES

Inflammatory Cell Infiltrates in Intima

Inflammation in plaques is known to contribute to their destabilization, and consequently to the initiation of acute coronary syndromes. We were, therefore, curious if patients with IRD had more inflammation in atherosclerotic lesions, which could possibly contribute to their increased rate of CV events. In FHBS, the rates of ICIs in atherosclerotic lesions were similar in IRD and non-IRD patients with CAD (6% vs 5%, $P = .69$). However, we cannot rule out type-2 error because of the low occurrence of atherosclerotic lesions (21% in IRD and 14% in non-IRD) due to the surgical technique.[10] Moreover, both patients with IRD and non-IRD had advanced CAD requiring CABG, which could contribute to the similar occurrences of plaque inflammation.

Other studies indicate that RA may predispose to increased plaque vulnerability.[7,11,12]

Inflammatory Cell Infiltrates and Neovascularization in Media

In the media, ICIs occurred only in patients with IRD (10%), and only in those who also had ICIs in the adventitia. They were present in all three patients with concomitant thoracic aneurysms. The medial ICIs were localized at sites with abnormal ingrowth of microvessels.[10]

Inflammatory Cell Infiltrates in Adventitia

FHBS demonstrated a surprisingly high occurrence of ICIs in the aortic adventitia of patients with CAD.[10] They contained mainly lymphocytes and were localized mostly between adipose cells and/or around vasa vasorum (VV) (**Fig. 2**). ICIs were more frequent in patients with IRD than in those without IRD (47% vs 20%; $P = .002$). Although patients without IRD were more likely to have smaller and fewer ICIs, some also had pronounced ICIs (see **Fig. 2**).

The occurrence and extent of ICIs were positively linked to current smoking and, in particular, to the history of aortic aneurysms (thoracic or abdominal, current or previous).[9,10]

Of note, smoking is known to have proinflammatory effects in different tissues including the respiratory system, joints, even vessels (Buerger's disease, inflammatory aortic aneurysms). In theory, its proatherosclerotic effects could be also partly underlain by its proinflammatory effects on vessels.

Inflammatory Cell Infiltrates in Epicardium

At the site whereby the aortic specimens were taken, the adventitia is covered by the aortic part of the epicardium. Because there is no clear anatomic border, we distinguished between these 2 compartments using an arbitrary approach[10] About 50% of patients with CAD had ICIs along the aortic epicardium (with similar rates in patients with IRD and non-IRD). The epicardial ICIs were often spreading into the adventitia (see **Fig. 2**).[10]

The occurrence of ICIs was even slightly higher (56% in IRD and 60% in non-IRD) in the cardiac epicardium compared to the aortic epicardium.[13]

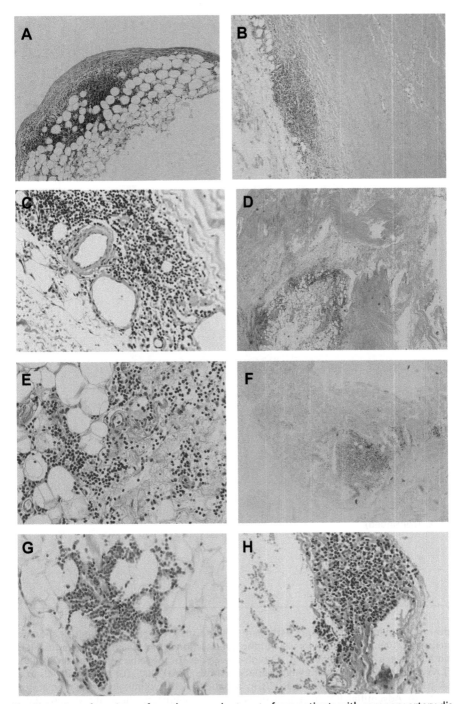

Fig. 2. Images of specimens from the ascendant aorta from patients with coronary artery disease (hematoxylin-eosin). (*A*) Pronounced inflammatory cell infiltrates (ICIs) along the aortic part of the epicardium and in the adventitia in a patient with rheumatoid arthritis (RA) and a concomitant thoracic aneurysm (x100). (*B*) ICIs along the border between the aortic

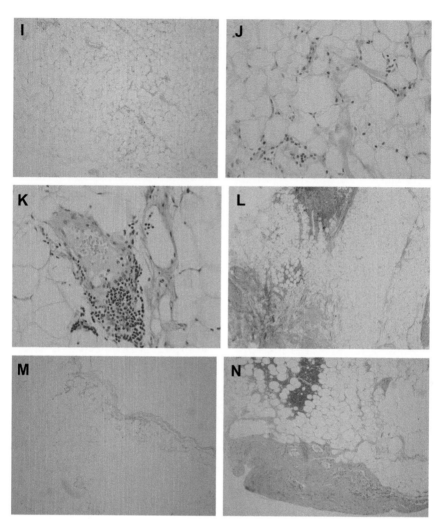

Fig. 2. (continued)

adventitia and media in a patient with giant cell arteritis (GCA) and a concomitant thoracic aneurysm (x100). (*C*) High-power view of the same section as in B (x400). (*D*) Adventitial ICIs and fibrosis in a GCA patient (x40). (*E*) High-power view of the same section as in D (x400). (*F*) Adventitial ICIs in a patient with psoriatic arthritis (PsA) (x100). (*G*) Adventitial ICIs in a PsA patient (x400). (*H*) Adventitial ICIs in a patient with systemic lupus erythematosus (x400). (*I*) Adventitial ICIs in a patient without inflammatory rheumatic disease (IRD) (x100). (*J*) High-power view of the same section as in H (x400). (*K*) Adventitial ICI in a patient without IRD (x400). (*L*) Pronounced adventitial ICIs in a non-IRD patient (x100). (*M*) ICIs along the epicardium of a patient with polymyalgia rheumatica (x100). (*N*) Pronounced fibrosis with ICIs in the epicardium of a patient with polymyalgia rheumatica (x100).

Fibrosis in Subintimal Layers

Fibrosis was observed both in the adventitia, and, in particular, along the epicardium, often accompanied by ICIs (see **Fig. 2**). Fibrosis in these layers was more pronounced in RA than patients than in those without IRDs.[14] Fibrosis occurred also in the cardiac part of the epicardium.

Subintimal Inflammation, Atherosclerosis, Aneurysms, and Hypertension

Because there has already been a substantial focus on inflammation in atherosclerotic lesions, and because we observed more inflammation in subintimal layers, we concentrate foremost on the later.

The clinical importance of the observed subintimal inflammation is still unclear and could be unrelated or secondary to atherosclerosis. However, based on the increasing body of evidence, it is plausible that subintimal inflammation could play a role in the development and/or destabilization of atherosclerotic lesions.[6,15,16] Furthermore, subintimal inflammation might contribute to the development of aortic aneurysms and/or their complications (disruption).[17,18] It is possible that the exaggerated subintimal inflammation in IRDs can at least partly underlie the increased risk of ischemic events and aneurysms in IRDs.

Interestingly, atherosclerosis and aneurysms are interrelated and share common risk factors. Atherosclerosis is often found in aortic aneurysms, while vulnerable plaques in coronary arteries are often accompanied by a segmental enlargement (aneurysm) of the affected artery.[6] Hence, it would be interesting to clarify if vascular inflammation can lead to either a stenotic lesion or aneurysm or both, depending on other modifying factors (eg, blood pressure, rheologic characteristics of blood, and alterations of extracellular matrix) during different stages of the inflammatory process.

Of note, also hypertension is linked to inflammation (including the infiltration of vessel walls by immune cells), and the relationship appears to be reciprocal.[19] Furthermore, there are indications that drugs reducing inflammation, such as TNFi, might ameliorate hypertension.[20] Thus, further research is needed to clarify if vascular inflammation is a common denominator in hypertension, atherosclerosis, and aneurysms, and if it shares some common causes.

In accordance with our results, a higher occurrence of subintimal inflammation in RA versus non-RA individuals was observed also in coronary arteries, in an autopsy study.[7]

Outside-in Progression

Our findings evoke a hypothesis that the medial inflammation might represent a more advanced stage of the vascular inflammation than the adventitial inflammation and are in line with the outside-in theory in atherosclerosis.[21,22] Vascular inflammation, accompanied by the proliferation of VV, may start in the outer part of the vessel (even in the perivascular tissue), and progress toward the lumen.

Aortitis or not?

We found massive ICIs and fibrosis in the aorta of some of patients with CAD (see **Fig. 2**). If some of these patients were examined on suspicion of aortitis, the histologic findings could be considered as confirmative of the diagnosis.

However, the diagnosis of aortitis is challenging. Although the presence of inflammatory cells in a vessel wall is one of the criteria of vasculitis, there is no clear cutoff for the number of inflammatory cells and their location in a vessel wall. For example, inflamed atherosclerotic lesions are usually not called vasculitis—although some voices advocate considering atherosclerosis a low-grade vasculitis.[23] In clinical settings, aortitis is usually diagnosed via a complex evaluation of the clinical picture and imaging and laboratory tests; clinicians should not have unrealistic expectations to histologic assessment only. Therefore, in FHBS we preferred to describe the pathologic changes rather than using the vasculitis label.

Clinicians should be aware of the relatively high frequency of vascular inflammation in asymptomatic patients. It is possible that this kind of findings underlie some of the cases of idiopathic aortitis diagnosed at the time of aortic surgery.[24]

Because of the limited diagnostic opportunities, the spontaneous course of vascular inflammation (including "idiopathic aortitis") and its optimal treatment are unclear. More research on this topic is, therefore, warranted. For example, it is important to search for additional prognostic markers and treatment targets for different types of vascular inflammation.

Inflammatory Cell Infiltrates in Vessels with Different Susceptibilities to Atherosclerosis

The rates of ICIs in the adventitia or media in the CAD population were highest in the aorta (35%), which is predisposed to atherosclerosis; lower in the saphenous vein (17%), and lowest in IMA (2%), which is known to be strongly protected from atherosclerosis, even when it is used as a graft. Of note, while we did not observe any atherosclerotic lesions in IMA, they were present in 3% of the venous specimens, although veins are usually considered to be more protected from atherosclerosis than arteries.[25]

Thus, in hypothesis, a susceptibility of a vessel to atherosclerosis might be dependent on its susceptibility to inflammation (that could be related to the local occurrence of antigens, immunologic milieu—such as the distribution of toll-like receptors, vascularization, biochemical and biophysical conditions, and so forth). The vascular microenvironment may also contribute to the fact that IMA grafts have superior patency to venous grafts.

Studying vessels with different resistances to atherosclerosis can help to uncover the pathomechanisms of this disease, and identify atheroprotective factors.

Epicardium and Coronary Arteries

In theory, pathologic changes in epicardial coronary arteries could induce reactive changes in the surrounding epicardial tissue. However, it is also plausible that pathologic changes in the epicardium could contribute to CAD, for example, through effects of proinflammatory mediators, impairment of vascular elasticity, or microcirculation.[2] Thus, the link between the epicardium and CAD is gaining increasing interest.[26,27] It should be examined if predisposition to pericarditis contributes to the increased CAD morbidity in RA.

Of note, patients with FHBS who had epicardial ICIs in the cardiac biopsies were on average 7 years younger at the time of CABG, but had a longer CAD duration.[13] Thus, these patients might have a more aggressive CAD, starting at a younger age and developing faster, and their CAD might be more strongly related to inflammation (epicardial). Nevertheless, as with other hypotheses generated by FHBS, also this one remains to be explored in future studies.

Search for Potential Treatment Targets

If inflammation plays a role in the pathogenesis of CV manifestations, its prevention or inhibition could reduce CV risk. Hence, it is important to identify its potential causes, and the involved pathophysiologic factors.

In theory, vascular and perivascular inflammation could have multiple causes including biophysical factors (eg, blood pressure, shear stress), metabolic factors and chemical substances (including harmful components from smoking or diet), hormonal disturbances, oxidative stress, hypoxia, systemic or local dysregulation of the immune system/autoimmunity, cellular abnormalities in the vasculature (eg, mitochondrial dysfunction), infections, and so forth (and there could be overlaps between some of these factors).[2,23,28] It is also possible that some of these factors play particularly important roles.

Microorganisms

Using 16S rRNA, we detected multiple bacteria (including environmental and oral bacteria) in the adventitial and epicardial layer in 27% of RA and 36% patients withoutIRDs undergoing CABG. Patients with RA had less diverse bacterial flora than patients without IRDs (9 vs 31 phylotypes). Methylobacterium oryzae (44% of the bacterial flora) and Stenotrophomonas sp. (32%) were predominant in RA, while Stenotrophomonas sp. (15%), Eubacterium (13%) and Haemophilus oral clone (13%) were predominant in non-IRD.[29]

Interestingly, some of our findings resemble those from a study of aortic aneurysms, that also uncovered a mixed bacterial population and presence of Stenotrophomonas and Methylobacterium sp.[30]

There has been increasing interest in the role of microbiota in health and disease. However, there is still low awareness of the fact that microorganisms (or at least their parts) may occur also in tissues that are usually considered sterile (if not suffering an infection), such as blood vessels.

Some of the observed bacteria in our study, such as Stenotrophomonas and Methylobacterium, are opportunistic pathogens that have been described to cause infections in the CV system, for example, endocarditis and central venous catheter infection.[31-34] However, none of the patients in FHBS who had these bacteria in their aortas had apparent infection signs.

It remains to be examined in future studies if the observed bacteria in the subintimal layers are innocent bystanders, if they accumulate there secondary to CVD, if they represent iatrogenic contamination (but the samples were taken and processed under sterile conditions), or if they are involved in CVD pathogenesis through their effects on the immune system or on the local tissue. Intriguingly, Stenotrophomonas maltophilia produces StmPr1 that breaks down fibrinogen, fibronectin, and collagen, which could contribute to vascular injury, and so forth.[35]

Although we do not know if the observed bacteria were viable (and therefore have planned new studies), it is plausible that even parts of dead bacteria could influence an immune reaction or other processes in the vessel wall.

The observed aberrations in RA versus non-IRD could be caused by alterations in the RA-related immune response, dysregulation of microbiota, and/or immunosuppressive treatment (which might enable opportunistic bacteria to become pathogenic). Furthermore, there is a need to determine if some of the observed bacteria could even play a role in RA pathogenesis. Interestingly, Stenotrophomonas and Methylobacterium sp. have been reported in joints (such as reactive and septic arthritis, temporomandibular disorders, prosthetic joints).[31,36-40]

In our study, Methylobacterium oryzae induced a robust proinflammatory response in human primary macrophages (including the upregulation of interleukin (IL)-1 alpha and beta, IL-6, and TNF), but no TLR4 stimulation and only a mild stimulation of TLR2-mediated NFκB signaling in transfected HEK-293 cells.[29]

Of note, these bacteria can represent a therapeutic challenge: for example, Stenotrophomonas is known for its resistance to antibiotics. Thus, other antibiotic regimens can be necessary to counteract these bacteria than those analyzed in previous studies examining the effects of antibiotics on CVD.

In FHBS, there was no difference in occurrences of serum antibodies to Chlamydia pneumoniae, Mycoplasma pneumoniae, Helicobacter pylori, Cytomegalovirus, Streptococcus pyogenes, Parvovirus B19, and Hepatitis B and C virus in CAD patients with IRDs, CAD patients without CAD, RA patients without CAD and in HC. Nor was there any positive relationship between these circulating antibodies and inflammation in the subintimal aortic layers. Thus, the findings do not support the notion that these infections contribute to atherogenesis in IRDs.[41]

Autoantigens

We detected 2 RA-related antigens in specimens containing the aortic adventitia and epicardium in both RA and non-IRD patients with CAD: heat shock protein 47 and citrullinated protein (CP).[23] Because citrullination can occur, for example, in response to inflammation and smoking, it might not be surprising that CP occurred in both groups. However, as most of the patients with RA have antibodies to CP, the autoimmune reaction in blood vessels might contribute to accelerating the atherosclerotic process.[42]

Taken together, our results support the hypotheses that infections and/or autoimmunity might trigger or aggravate vascular/epicardial inflammation and play a role in CVD pathogenesis.

Immune Factors in Subintimal Layers

A detailed characterization of factors involved in an inflammatory process is critical for the identification of therapeutic targets. In the subintimal layers, we identified, for example, neutrophils, T- and B-cells, and factors influencing the survival of B-cells (BAFF=B-cell activating factor; APRIL = A proliferation-inducing ligand). The accumulation of B-cells, BAFF, and APRIL was greater in the aorta than in the atheroresistant IMA, and the number of B-cells correlated positively to CP expression.[23,43] The proportion of B- to T-cells in ICIs was higher in RA than non-IRD patients .[44] Similarly, a previous study of 2 RA patients with CAD revealed a relatively high proportion of B-cells in ICIs in coronary arteries (in plaques and adventitia), although typical atherosclerosis-related ICIs consist predominantly of T-cells.[8] In theory, B-cells might have a particular role in accelerated CVD in RA, for example, due to the production of autoantibodies.

Expression of TNF, IL-18, and IL-33 in the aortic adventitial and epicardial layers was higher in RA than patients without IRDs. IL-33 expression occurred in most of the patients with CAD, was restricted to nuclei of endothelial cells (EC) of VV and was related to the number of swollen joints. Patients with RA had also higher levels of soluble ST2, a receptor for IL-33.[45] Interestingly, IL-33 is considered to be protective against CVD.[46]

PTX3 expression was higher in the aorta than IMA, and colocalized areas with ICIs and/or fibrosis.[44] We also detected higher circulating PTX3 levels in several IRDs compared with non-IRD individuals.[47] However, patients with SLE had relatively low PTX3 levels, as observed also by others; thus, PTX3 could parallel CRP, that tends to be decreased in SLE.[47,48] Increased serum PTX3 levels were also independently related to acute coronary syndrome and low alcohol intake.[47]

Of note, in another study (ANAT), we observed greater PTX3 expression in aneurysmal versus nondilated abdominal aortas. PTX3 colocalized ICIs, and was related to hypervascularization, hypoxia, and increased amount of collagen in the vessel wall.[17]

PTX3 is a pattern recognition molecule of the innate immune system, from the same protein family as C-reactive protein (CRP). In contrast to CRP, which is produced in liver after IL-6 stimulation, PTX3 is produced directly in the inflamed tissue as well as stored in neutrophils. PTX3 is a marker of CVD and its prognosis and seems to complement high-sensitivity CRP. Compared with CRP, it responds faster and might have a better ability to reflect local inflammation in CV system.[44,47,49,50] Interestingly, there are indications that PTX3 can play a protective role in CVD. In theory, this might be due to its regulating role on complement and inflammation. Moreover, PTX3 could even counteract causes of vascular inflammation, for example, by its antimicrobial actions or its role in the maintenance of immunologic tolerance (eg, by its contribution to clearance of apoptotic cells).[48,51] PTX3 exhibits also other functions, for example, participates in tissue repair and remodeling.[14,44,52,53]

Similar to PTX3, calprotectin is an antimicrobial factor and inflammatory marker that also originates from neutrophils, and that modulates inflammation (although these proteins have proinflammatory functions, they can also downregulate exaggerated inflammation). Moreover, calprotectin promotes apoptosis.[54] In FHBS, also calprotectin colocalized subintimal ICIs.[29] Taken together, calprotectin could have some similar functions in CVD as PTX3. In theory, also the roles of these proteins in apoptosis and efferocytosis could be of importance.[55]

Interestingly, there are indications that complement may be involved in the pathogenesis of CVD and contribute to the development of vascular stiffness, but this fact has not gained much attention yet.[23,56–58] In FHBS, patients with IRD with CAD had higher levels of circulating terminal complement complexes (TCC; a marker of complement activation) than CAD patients without IRDs and RA patients without CVD (but C3 levels in these groups were similar). Of note, the RA non-CVD and CAD non-IRD group had similar TCC levels, although the latter group had 13 years higher mean age and had advanced CAD requiring CABG. TCC levels were related to CRP.[57] In a small substudy examining aortic specimens in 3 SLE, 3 RA, and 3 non-IRD patients with CAD, C3 was present in a diffuse pattern in the media and adventitia, and C3d (C3 activation product) in the media of all samples. In the adventitia, C3d expression occurred only in patients with IRD - diffuse in all SLE and focal in one RA. Indeed, complement is known to play an important role in SLE, and systemic and vascular complement activation could accelerate CVD in SLE, and potentially also in RA as well as other conditions.[57]

It is possible that targeting some of the immunologic factors observed in the subintimal layers might reduce CV risk, in particular in individuals with the most pronounced subintimal inflammation.[55,59]

Importantly, some already available drugs target some of the observed factors and/or the related pathways (eg, B-cells, T-cells, B-cell survival factors, TNF, complement system), and others are under development (eg, therapies targeting IL-18 and IL-33/ST2 signaling).[19,46] Some anti-inflammatory drugs (such as methotrexate, TNFi, and T-cell targeting therapy) have been shown to reduce CVD morbidity in IRDs.[19,60] Also anti-CD20 therapy could have beneficial effects on vascular health.[61] Moreover, some anti-inflammatory drugs may have cardioprotective effect even in the general population.[62,63] Although this effect may be caused by the inhibition of systemic inflammation and other mechanisms,[64] it is also possible that suppression of inflammation in vessel walls (inside the plaques and beyond) and in perivascular tissue might be of particular importance. Currently, the cardioprotective effects of IL-1 (in particular IL-1β) inhibition have gained great interest.[62,63,65] It would be interesting to determine if this effect is mediated also through the inhibition of the subintimal inflammation.

Microarrays

We searched for differences in gene expression between RA (n = 8) and non-RA (n = 8) patients with CAD, analyzing total RNA from the aortic adventitial and epicardial layers by Affymetrix microarrays and evaluating the results by one-way ANOVA ($P < .05$; FC>1.1). RA group had higher levels of the stress-induced transcriptional regulator NUPR1 (z-score: 3.0). Nine target molecules of NUPR1 were identified, including GADD45 A, which was upregulated in RA ($P = .006$; FC = 1.474). In theory, the increased CV risk in RA might be related to the overexpression of NUPR1 (whereby vascular stress could play a role), with downstream overexpression of GADD45 A, which in turn promotes endothelial dysfunction.[66]

Vitamin D deficiency is linked to both IRDs and CVD, but the exact mechanisms are still unclear. Therefore, we searched for differences in the expression of genes related to vitamin D signaling. Of these, patients with RA had a higher expression of NCOR1 and the aforementioned GADD45 A, and a lower expression of PON2.[67]

Further studies are needed to determine the roles of the differentially expressed genes in CVD; for example, if any of them promote the acceleration of atherosclerosis in RA, or if they reflect an underlying proatherogenic pathology (such as vascular stress). In theory, the relative PON2 deficit in RA could contribute to accelerated atherogenesis, for example, via increased LDL oxidation and oxidative stress and inflammation in vessel walls.[67]

Circulating Factors in Inflammatory Rheumatic Diseases and Coronary Artery Disease

Better insights into circulating factors in IRDs and CAD can help to understand the pathogenesis of these conditions, and to identify new biomarkers and therapeutic targets. We have already discussed differences in PTX3 and TCC levels in FHBS.

Furthermore, among patients with CAD, those with IRD had higher plasma levels of vascular cell adhesion molecule-1 (VCAM-1), von Willebrand factor and osteoprotegerin (OPG), and lower levels of CCL21. OPG levels were positively related to acute coronary syndromes and to the extent of adventitial ICIs. The extent of adventitial ICIs was also related to plasma levels of von Willebrand factor (vWf). Levels of vWf and soluble TNF receptor-1 were higher in patients with adventitial ICIs than in those without.[68]

OPG, which is involved in bone metabolism, is also linked to atherosclerosis and aneurysms. In our aforementioned ANAT study, OPG was less expressed in aneurysmal versus nondilated aortas, which could support the suspected protective role of OPG in aneurysms.[17]

In adjusted analyses, lower plasma levels of 1,25(OH)2D3 were associated with adventitial ICIs.[69] It remains to be investigated if there is a causal relationship between this biologically active vitamin D metabolite and vascular inflammation.

Inflammation and Vascular Stiffness

Vascular stiffness is a predictor of CV risk, but the pathologic substrate has not been fully elucidated yet. Several factors seem to be involved, including atherosclerotic lesions and ECM characteristics. Also, vascular and perivascular inflammation, depositions of components of the complement system, and fibrosis (ie, end-result of an inflammatory process) might be important. In support of the inflammatory hypothesis, anti-inflammatory treatment has been shown to relatively rapidly reduce vascular stiffness.[10,23,57]

Inflammation and Microvascular Impairment in Heart - Potential Pathogenic Mechanisms in Cardiac Ischemia and Heart Failure

In cardiac biopsies from patients with CAD in FHBS, we observed a high occurrence of inflammatory cells and expression of all 3 HLA types (expressed on mononuclear cells, ECs, and cardiomyocytes), proinflammatory cytokines (TNF and IL-1β on mononuclear cells and cardiomyocytes; IL1α on mononuclear cells, cardiomyocytes, and ECs), and adhesion molecules (intercellular adhesion molecule-1 (ICAM-1) and VCAM-1).[70] The alterations indicative of inflammation and EC activation were more pronounced in patients with IRDs than in those without, and in the myocardium than in the skeletal muscle.[70] Patients with IRDs had also increased amount of collagen in their cardiac specimens than patients without IRD.[13]

The link between IRDs and cardiac inflammation and microvascular impairment is supported also by findings from imaging studies.[61,71] In theory, these disturbances could at least partly explain why RA is predisposed to cardiac dysfunction and HF which cannot be fully explained by the increased CAD occurrence. Furthermore, they can contribute to the fact that even patients with RA without significant stenoses in epicardial coronary arteries can experience cardiac ischemia.

Hence, it is important to clarify if the inhibition of cardiac inflammatory changes to limit cardiac damage could be particularly important in patients with IRDs. There are some indications that anti-inflammatory treatment might protect from HF in RA, but more research is needed. Of note, although TNFi have been suspected to increase HF risk in the general population, the treatment might be safe, and even beneficial, in RA.[61] In theory, besides its beneficial effects on vessels, inhibition of IL-1 (in particular IL-1β) might have beneficial effects also on the heart, especially in IRDs.[62,63,65] Of note, previous research already suggests that IL-1 blocking could protect from HF.[72]

High mobility Group Protein 1 in Heart

HMGB1 is a protein with multiple functions which vary with its location and posttranslational modifications.[73–75] As a chromatin protein, it regulates, for example, DNA transcription and repair. However, various triggers (including activation, stress, and death of cells) can induce HMGB1 translocation from the nuclei into the cytoplasm and further into the extracellular space. In the cytoplasm it regulates autophagy, and in the extracellular position, it turns into alarmin, promoting the production of proinflammatory cytokines such as TNF. It is also involved in tissue repair and remodeling. Extranuclear HMGB1 seems to be involved in the pathogenesis of IRDs and may be implicated also in cardiac and endothelial dysfunction and atherosclerosis.[76–78]

In an FHBS substudy, we characterized the expression of HMGB1 in cardiac biopsies from patients with CAD, using immunohistochemistry. HMGB1 expression in the cytosol of cardiomyocytes was detected in all 10 patients with IRD (6 strong and 4 weak), but only in 1 of 8 patients with non-IRD (weak). The total amount of HMGB1 in the cardiac specimens (measured by Western blot) was lower in IRD than non-IRD patients, which is compatible with increased release of HMGB1 from the heart into the circulation in the IRD group. All patients had 3 receptors for HMGB1, that is, receptor for advanced glycation end-products (RAGE), TLR2, and TLR-4, present in nuclei and cytosol of their cardiomyocytes (RAGE and TLR4 were more expressed than TLR2).[76]

Taken together, the enhanced translocation of HMGB1 could potentially contribute to inflammation, EC dysfunction, remodeling, and impaired contractility in the heart of patients with IRD. Furthermore, HMGB1 relocated into the circulation could exacerbate systemic inflammation. In theory, there could be a vicious cycle whereby cardiac

HMGB1 could be translocated due to inflammation or hypoxia, and in turn, it could contribute to the aggravation of inflammatory activity and CVD. In case, drugs targeting extracellular HMGB1 could be beneficial. Indeed, studies examining the effects of HMGB1 neutralization have shown promising results. Of note, both novel and repurposed drugs might be relevant.[75,79,80]

Subintimal and Cardiac Inflammation in Coronary Artery Disease – Common Phenomenon?

It is important to point out that we examined only one section per specimen. Moreover, the specimens were small, and their sampling was not aimed at pathologic changes. On the contrary, to avoid surgical complications, the aortic specimens were preferably taken from the macroscopically healthiest areas. Thus, vascular/perivascular and cardiac inflammation may be a widespread phenomenon in patients with CAD, in particular in those with IRDs.

In none of the examined patients, there was a clinical suspicion of inflammation in vessels or heart before CABG.

Microvascular Disease as a Cause of Macrovascular Disease?

In patients with CAD from FHBS, inflammation related to small vessels (mainly perivascular inflammatory cell infiltration) was found in multiple compartments including vessel walls, heart, skeletal muscle, and skin.[23] In theory, these manifestations can be related to a generalized EC activation/microvascular impairment, and that related to the CV system (heart and macrovessels) might play a special role in the pathogenesis of CV complications including atherosclerosis.[81–84] The microvascular injury could be a result of various triggers including local or systemic inflammation, diabetes, dyslipidemia, smoking, and other toxic substances, hypoxia, oxidative stress, hypertension, sheared stress alterations, exaggerated NET formation, characteristics of extracellular vesicles, dysautonomia, microorganisms, and mitochondrial or endoplasmic reticulum stress and abnormal cell senescence, and so forth.

Interestingly, in the ANAT study, we observed increased vascularization in aneurysmal versus non-dilated aortas. Vascularization correlated positively with expression of PTX3, hypoxia-inducible factor-1α (HIF-1α, a marker of hypoxia), ICIs, and aneurysm size.[17] It is notable that the hypervascularization did not seem to completely counteract the markers of hypoxia in the vessel wall. HIF-1α expression was related to ECM alterations compatible with decreased elasticity. One of the possible explanations for our findings is that hypoxia in the vessel wall promotes angiogenesis and inflammation, accompanied by ECM deterioration.

Under physiologic conditions, the inner part of the vessel wall is supplied by oxygen from the lumen, and the outer part via vasa vasorum. Thus, vessel wall hypoxia could have various causes such as reduced diffusion from the lumen (eg, due to hypertension and disturbances in blood viscoelasticity and flow), alterations in the vascular tissue limiting O2 transport (eg, due to ECM impairment), pathologies in VV (including inflammation, EC activation, and compression of VV), erythrocytes malfunctions and systemic hypoxia.[81,85]

On the other hand, besides hypoxia, also inflammation can trigger HIF-1α.[85]

Of note, small vessels are also involved in the development of some IRD manifestations, such as synovitis and rheumatoid nodules in RA, and large vessel vasculitides.[23]

Cardiovascular Fat in CVD

In FHBS, the adventitial and perivascular/epicardial ICIs were commonly located in adipose tissue.[10,13]

It is well-known that the impact of fat on CV health is dependent on its distribution; that is, visceral adiposity is more dangerous than subcutaneous adiposity. In hypothesis, visceral fat in the CV system might be particularly important for CVD risk.[22,86–88] Both the quality and quantity (ie, CV adiposity) could be important.[26] Indeed, there is emerging evidence that the amount of perivascular and epicardial fat is linked to CV prognosis. Further, there are indications that RA patients have alterations in body composition, including predisposition to visceral adiposity. Hence, alterations in CV fat could contribute to CVD excess in IRDs.[26,89]

CV fat could influence CVD risk, for example, by biophysical, metabolic, and proinflammatory effects. Inflammation in the adipose tissue might affect the adjacent structures of the vessels and heart either directly or through proinflammatory signals.[83,88]

Micro-RNA Analyses

Analyses of skin from diabetic and nondiabetic patients from FHBS-Phase 2 were part of comprehensive studies comprising also cellular, animal, and organoid models.[90,91] These studies indicate that microRNA-135a-3p is a crucial regulator of pathophysiological angiogenesis and tissue repair, through targeting a VEGF-HIP1-p38 K signaling axis. Therapeutic targeting of this axis could promote tissue repair.[90]

Furthermore, microRNA-615-5p has been shown to inhibit VEGF-AKT/eNOS–mediated EC angiogenic responses, and manipulating microRNA-615-5p expression could provide a new target for angiogenic therapy in response to tissue injury.[91]

METHODOLOGICAL CONSIDERATIONS ON FEIRING HEART BIOPSY STUDY

As other cross-sectional studies, FHBS is not able to affirm causal relationships, but can generate hypotheses, and prompt further research. Knowledge about factors present in tissues of interest is essential for designing adequate mechanistic studies.

One of the main advantages of FHBS is the well-characterized population, and the possibility to perform comprehensive evaluations of tissues from various compartments, blood analyses, and clinical parameters.

As FHBS stems from 2 nonacademic hospitals, the funding opportunities were limited. Hence, not all the intended studies have been completed yet (but some studies are going on). Because with current laboratory methods, tiny pieces of tissue can be sufficient for many analyses, the biobank gives possibilities for a lot of future research, and collaborative projects are welcome.

The possibility to perform multiple analyses on each subject can be considered not only as a strength but also as a limitation. Indeed, with the increasing number of tests, also the probability of false positive findings increases. On the other hand, researchers usually do not fully rely on results from a single study but require their confirmation by other studies (as findings can be influenced by biases, confounders, or chance). It is important to interpret any research findings with an eye on the study design.

Statistical corrections for multiple testing do not solve all challenges and have their limitations (eg, they increase the probability of false negative results, which can cause ignoring important leads).[92–94]

Obviously, one could limit the risk of false positive results in one study by performing some of the analyses in new studies instead. However, this approach would be costlier and less ethical. New patients would have to spend their time on the participation in a study and be exposed to invasive interventions, although the already collected data and samples could serve the purpose. In addition, it would not solve the problem as the probability of false positive findings increases not only with multiple tests in one study but also with multiple studies.

In spite of the limitations,exploratory research is essential in guiding other studies, and biobanks and data registries in a feasible and efficient way enable development of complex and numerous studies on the same patient population.

SUMMARY

FHBS can provide inspiration for comprehensive studies of various health disorders, using medical data and multiple types of tissue samples. Characterization of tissues is a cornerstone for studying pathomechanisms and searching for biomarkers and therapeutic targets. Furthermore, it is important to increase awareness regarding the possibility to sample specimens during CV surgery, for clinical and research purposes.

FHBS revealed a high occurrence of inflammatory signs in the aorta (in particular in the adventitia) and heart of patients with CAD. These changes were more pronounced in patients with IRDs. We also observed a high occurrence of alterations related to microvessels in different compartments, including vessel walls and heart. Thus, inflammation and microvascular impairment in the CV system (in the vasculature, inside and beyond atherosclerotic lesions, and in the heart) might be involved in the pathogenesis of atherosclerosis, aneurysms and/or HF, and contribute to the accelerated CVD in IRDs.

The subintimal aortic layers contained, for example, B- and T-cells (lower proportion of T- to B-cells in RA vs non-IRD), calprotectin, C3, and C3d. Expression of TNF, Il-33, IL-18, and pentraxin 3 was higher in RA versus non-IRD. In the heart, patients with IRD had a higher expression of all 3 HLA types, TNF and IL-1β, and adhesion molecules, and altered distribution of HMGB1. Using microarrays, we detected, for example, differences in genes related to stress and D-vitamin receptor in the subintimal aortic layers in RA versus non-IRD. The presence of bacteria (with differences between patients with RA and non-IRD) and autoantigens (including CP) in vessel walls point to their potential role in triggering or aggravation of vascular inflammation.

Of note, patients with CAD had a high occurrence of ICIs and fibrosis (end-result of inflammation) in the epicardium. As epicardial inflammation could affect the embedded coronary arteries, the role of epicardial inflammation in CAD deserves further study.

FHBS also provides clues for potential pathophysiologic roles of circulating factors and noncoding RNAs in different compartments.

In theory, therapies targeting some of the observed alterations, and their causes, could protect from some CV manifestations in IRDs, but possibly also in the general population.

The FHBS biobank gives opportunity for many future studies.

CLINICS CARE POINTS

- Aortic and cardiac inflammation are detectable using biopsies during CABG, a relatively frequent surgery.

- Inflammation, microvascular impairment, and alterations in adipose tissue of the CV system could be involved in the pathogenesis of CV manifestations and contribute to the increased CVD risk in IRDs. Inflammation in the CV system could be a result of various causes, such as biophysical and metabolic factors, immune dysregulation/autoimmune reactions, infections, hypoxia, stress, and cellular abnormalities in the local tissue.

ACKNOWLEDGMENTS

I would like to express gratitude to all the participants as well as collaborators in FHBS (including the staff at Lillehammer Hospital for Rheumatic Diseases, Lillehammer; Feiring Heart Clinic, Feiring; LHL Hospital Gardermoen, Jessheim, Norway; and all the external advisors and collaborating laboratories). I thank Helena Erlandsson Harris (Center for Molecular Medicine, Karolinska Institutet, Stockholm, Sweden), Barbara Bottazzi (Laboratory of Research in Immunology and Inflammation, Istituto Clinico Humanitas, IRCCS, Rozzano, Milan, Italy) and Morten Wang Fagerland Unit of Biostatistics and Epidemiology, Oslo University Hospital, Oslo, Norway, for their advice on this article. I am grateful to all the grants that enabled these studies.

REFERENCES

1. Ingegnoli F, Buoli M, Antonucci F, et al. The Link Between Autonomic Nervous System and Rheumatoid Arthritis: From Bench to Bedside. Front Med 2020;7.
2. Hollan I. Vascular Inflammation in Systemic Rheumatic Diseases. Curr Med Litterature - Rheumatol 2011;30(2):33–45.
3. Raynor WY, Park PSU, Borja AJ, et al. PET-Based Imaging with (18)F-FDG and (18)F-NaF to Assess Inflammation and Microcalcification in Atherosclerosis and Other Vascular and Thrombotic Disorders. Diagnostics (Basel, Switzerland) 2021;11(12).
4. Gravallese EM, Corson JM, Coblyn JS, et al. Rheumatoid aortitis: a rarely recognized but clinically significant entity. Medicine (Baltimore) 1989;68(2):95–106.
5. Bely M, Apathy A, Beke-Martos E. Cardiac changes in rheumatoid arthritis. Acta MorpholHung 1992;40(1–4):149–86.
6. Higuchi ML, Gutierrez PS, Bezerra HG, et al. Comparison between adventitial and intimal inflammation of ruptured and nonruptured atherosclerotic plaques in human coronary arteries. Arq BrasCardiol 2002;79(1):20–4.
7. Aubry MC, Maradit-Kremers H, Reinalda MS, et al. Differences in atherosclerotic coronary heart disease between subjects with and without rheumatoid arthritis. JRheumatol 2007;34(5):937–42.
8. Aubry MC, Riehle DL, Edwards WD, et al. B-Lymphocytes in plaque and adventitia of coronary arteries in two patients with rheumatoid arthritis and coronary atherosclerosis: preliminary observations. CardiovascPathol 2004;13(4):233–6.
9. Hollan I. Vascular inflammation in rheumatic and non-rheumatic patients: a controlled study of biopsy specimens obtained during coronary artery surgery (Feiring heart biopsy study). Oslo: University of Oslo; 2009. p. 2–48.
10. Hollan I, Scott H, Saatvedt K, et al. Inflammatory rheumatic disease and smoking are predictors of aortic inflammation: a controlled study of biopsy specimens obtained at coronary artery surgery. Arthritis Rheum 2007;56(6):2072–9.
11. Semb AG, Rollefstad S, Provan SA, et al. Carotid plaque characteristics and disease activity in rheumatoid arthritis. J Rheumatol 2013;40(4):359–68.
12. Karpouzas GA, Malpeso J, Choi TY, et al. Prevalence, extent and composition of coronary plaque in patients with rheumatoid arthritis without symptoms or prior diagnosis of coronary artery disease. Ann Rheum Dis 2014;73(10):1797–804.
13. Andersen JK, Oma I, Prayson RA, et al. Inflammatory cell infiltrates in the heart of patients with coronary artery disease with and without inflammatory rheumatic disease: a biopsy study. Arthritis Res Ther 2016;18(1):232.
14. Hollan I, Bottazzi B, Førre Ø, et al. Pentraxin 3 (PTX), a Novel Cardiovascular Biomarker, is Expressed in Vascular Specimens of Patients with Coronary Artery Disease (CAD). 7th International Congress on autoimmunity 2010.

15. Nakajima A, Sugiyama T, Araki M, et al. Plaque Rupture, Compared With Plaque Erosion, Is Associated With a Higher Level of Pancoronary Inflammation. JACC Cardiovascular imaging 2021.
16. Maiellaro K, Taylor WR. The role of the adventitia in vascular inflammation. CardiovascRes 2007;75(4):640–8.
17. Blassova T, Tonar Z, Tomasek P, et al. Inflammatory cell infiltrates, hypoxia, vascularization, pentraxin 3 and osteoprotegerin in abdominal aortic aneurysms - A quantitative histological study. PloS one 2019;14(11):e0224818.
18. Skotsimara G, Antonopoulos A, Oikonomou E, et al. Aortic Wall Inflammation in the Pathogenesis, Diagnosis and Treatment of Aortic Aneurysms. Inflammation 2022.
19. Hollan I, Dessein PH, Ronda N, et al. Prevention of cardiovascular disease in rheumatoid arthritis. Autoimmun Rev 2015;14(10):952–69.
20. Murray EC, Nosalski R, MacRitchie N, et al. Therapeutic targeting of inflammation in hypertension: from novel mechanisms to translational perspective. Cardiovasc Res 2021;117(13):2589–609.
21. Kawabe J-i, Hasebe N. Role of the Vasa Vasorum and Vascular Resident Stem Cells in Atherosclerosis. Biomed Research International 2014;2014:701571.
22. Kim HW, Shi H, Winkler MA, et al. Perivascular Adipose Tissue and Vascular Perturbation/Atherosclerosis. Arterioscler Thromb Vasc Biol 2020;40(11):2569–76.
23. Hollan I, Meroni PL, Ahearn JM, et al. Cardiovascular disease in autoimmune rheumatic diseases. Autoimmun Rev 2013;12(10):1004–15.
24. Rojo-Leyva F, Ratliff NB, Cosgrove DM III, et al. Study of 52 patients with idiopathic aortitis from a cohort of 1,204 surgical cases. Arthritis Rheum 2000; 43(4):901–7.
25. Hollan I, Prayson R, Saatvedt K, et al. Inflammatory cell infiltrates in vessels with different susceptibility to atherosclerosis in rheumatic and non-rheumatic patients. CircJ 2008;72(12):1986–92.
26. Karpouzas GA, Rezaeian P, Ormseth SR, et al. Epicardial Adipose Tissue Volume As a Marker of Subclinical Coronary Atherosclerosis in Rheumatoid Arthritis. Arthritis Rheumatol (Hoboken, NJ) 2021;73(8):1412–20.
27. Ito H, Wakatsuki T, Yamaguchi K, et al. Atherosclerotic Coronary Plaque Is Associated With Adventitial Vasa Vasorum and Local Inflammation in Adjacent Epicardial Adipose Tissue in Fresh Cadavers. Circ J 2020;84(5):769–75.
28. Pavillard LE, Marín-Aguilar F, Bullon P, et al. Cardiovascular diseases, NLRP3 inflammasome, and western dietary patterns. Pharmacol Res 2018;131:44–50.
29. Curran SA, Hollan I, Erridge C, et al. Bacteria in the Adventitia of Cardiovascular Disease Patients with and without Rheumatoid Arthritis. PLoSOne 2014;9(5):e98627.
30. Marques da SR, Caugant DA, Eribe ER, et al. Bacterial diversity in aortic aneurysms determined by 16S ribosomal RNA gene analysis. J Vascsurg 2006; 44(5):1055–60.
31. Adegoke AA, Stenström TA, Okoh AI. Stenotrophomonas maltophilia as an Emerging Ubiquitous Pathogen: Looking Beyond Contemporary Antibiotic Therapy. Front Microbiol 2017;8:2276.
32. Li L, Tarrand JJ, Han XY. Microbiological and clinical features of four cases of catheter-related infection by Methylobacterium radiotolerans. J Clin Microbiol 2015;53(4):1375–9.
33. Chen R, Qi X, Ma B, et al. First case of infective endocarditis caused by Methylobacterium radiotolerans. Eur J Clin Microbiol Infect Dis 2020;39(9):1785–8.

34. Ahlström MG, Knudsen JD, Hertz FB. Stenotrophomonas maltophilia bacteraemia: 61 cases in a tertiary hospital in Denmark. Infect Dis (Lond) 2022;54(1): 26–35.
35. Windhorst S, Frank E, Georgieva DN, et al. The major extracellular protease of the nosocomial pathogen Stenotrophomonas maltophilia: characterization of the protein and molecular cloning of the gene. J Biol Chem 2002;277(13):11042–9.
36. Muir P, Oldenhoff WE, Hudson AP, et al. Detection of DNA from a range of bacterial species in the knee joints of dogs with inflammatory knee arthritis and associated degenerative anterior cruciate ligament rupture. MicrobPathog 2007; 42(2–3):47–55.
37. Pinol I, Alier A, Hinarejos P, et al. Septic arthritis of the knee by Stenotrophomonas maltophilia. Revista espanola de quimioterapia : publicacion oficial de la Sociedad Espanola de Quimioterapia 2012;25(3):218–9.
38. Chiu LQ, Wang W. A case of unusual Gram-negative bacilli septic arthritis in an immunocompetent patient. Singapore Med J 2013;54(8):e164–8.
39. Siala M, Gdoura R, Fourati H, et al. Broad-range PCR, cloning and sequencing of the full 16S rRNA gene for detection of bacterial DNA in synovial fluid samples of Tunisian patients with reactive and undifferentiated arthritis. Arthritis ResTher 2009;11(4):R102.
40. Sun W, Dong L, Kaneyama K, et al. Bacterial diversity in synovial fluids of patients with TMD determined by cloning and sequencing analysis of the 16S ribosomal RNA gene. Oral Surg Oral Med Oral Pathol Oral Radiol Endod 2008;105(5): 566–71.
41. Grub C, Brunborg C, Hasseltvedt V, et al. Antibodies to common infectious agents in coronary artery disease patients with and without rheumatic conditions. Rheumatology(Oxford) 2011;51(4):679–85.
42. Fent G, Mankia K, Erhayiem B, et al. First cardiovascular MRI study in individuals at risk of rheumatoid arthritis detects abnormal aortic stiffness suggesting an anti-citrullinated peptide antibody-mediated role for accelerated atherosclerosis. Ann Rheum Dis 2019;78(8):1138–40.
43. Ahmed A, Hollan I, Mikkelsen K, et al. The aortic adventitia of coronary bypass patients with rheumatoid arthritis provides a survival niche, and antigen depot, for B cells. Annu Scientific Meet Am Coll Rheumatol 2009.
44. Hollan I, Nebuloni M, Bottazzi B, et al. Pentraxin 3, a novel cardiovascular biomarker, is expressed in aortic specimens of patients with coronary artery disease with and without rheumatoid arthritis. Cardiovasc Pathol : official J Soc Cardiovasc Pathol 2013;22(5):324–31.
45. Ahmed A, Hollan I, Curran SA, et al. Rheumatoid arthritis patients have a pro-atherogenic cytokine microenvironment in the aortic adventitia. Arthritis Rheumatol (Hoboken, NJ) 2016;68(6):1361–6.
46. Chen WY, Tsai TH, Yang JL, et al. Therapeutic Strategies for Targeting IL-33/ST2 Signalling for the Treatment of Inflammatory Diseases. Cell Physiol Biochem 2018;49(1):349–58.
47. Hollan I, Bottazzi B, Cuccovillo I, et al. Increased levels of serum pentraxin 3, a novel cardiovascular biomarker, in patients with inflammatory rheumatic disease. Arthritis Care Res(Hoboken). 2010;62(3):378–85.
48. Brilland B, Vinatier E, Subra JF, et al. Anti-Pentraxin Antibodies in Autoimmune Diseases: Bystanders or Pathophysiological Actors? Front Immunol 2020;11: 626343.

49. Ding K, Shi Z, Qian C, et al. Higher Plasma Pentraxin-3 Level Predicts Adverse Clinical Outcomes in Patients With Coronary Artery Disease: A Meta-Analysis of Cohort Studies. Front Cardiovasc Med 2021;8:726289.

50. Ristagno G, Fumagalli F, Bottazzi B, et al. Pentraxin 3 in Cardiovascular Disease. Front Immunol 2019;10:823.

51. Ortega-Hernandez OD, Bassi N, Shoenfeld Y, et al. The long pentraxin 3 and its role in autoimmunity. Semin Arthritis Rheum 2009;39(1):38–54.

52. Guo T, Ke L, Qi B, et al. PTX3 is located at the membrane of late apoptotic macrophages and mediates the phagocytosis of macrophages. J Clin Immunol 2012; 32(2):330–9.

53. Doni A, Musso T, Morone D, et al. An acidic microenvironment sets the humoral pattern recognition molecule PTX3 in a tissue repair mode. J Exp Med 2015; 212(6):905–25.

54. Wang S, Song R, Wang Z, et al. S100A8/A9 in Inflammation. Front Immunol 2018; 9:1298.

55. Engelen SE, Robinson AJB, Zurke YX, et al. Therapeutic strategies targeting inflammation and immunity in atherosclerosis: how to proceed? Nat Rev Cardiol 2022;1–21.

56. Shields KJ, Stolz D, Watkins SC, et al. Complement proteins C3 and C4 bind to collagen and elastin in the vascular wall: a potential role in vascular stiffness and atherosclerosis. ClinTranslSci 2011;4(3):146–52.

57. Shields KJ, Mollnes TE, Eidet JR, et al. Plasma complement and vascular complement deposition in patients with coronary artery disease with and without inflammatory rheumatic diseases. PloS one 2017;12(3):e0174577.

58. Copenhaver M, Yu CY, Hoffman RP. Complement Components, C3 and C4, and the Metabolic Syndrome. Curr Diabetes Rev 2019;15(1):44–8.

59. Porsch F, Binder CJ. Impact of B-Cell–Targeted Therapies on Cardiovascular Disease. Arteriosclerosis, Thrombosis, and Vascular Biology 2019;39(9):1705–14.

60. Jin Y, Kang EH, Brill G, et al. Cardiovascular (CV) Risk after Initiation of Abatacept versus TNF Inhibitors in Rheumatoid Arthritis Patients with and without Baseline CV Disease. J Rheumatol 2018;45(9):1240–8.

61. Blyszczuk P, Szekanecz Z. Pathogenesis of ischaemic and non-ischaemic heart diseases in rheumatoid arthritis. RMD Open 2020;6(1).

62. Boland J, Long C. Update on the Inflammatory Hypothesis of Coronary Artery Disease. Curr Cardiol Rep 2021;23(2):6.

63. Ridker PM, Everett BM, Thuren T, et al. Antiinflammatory Therapy with Canakinumab for Atherosclerotic Disease. N Engl J Med 2017;377(12):1119–31.

64. Ronda N, Greco D, Adorni MP, et al. New anti-atherosclerotic activity of methotrexate and adalimumab: Complementary effects on lipoprotein function and macrophage cholesterol metabolism. Arthritis Rheumatol (Hoboken, NJ) 2015; 67(5):1155–64.

65. Thompson PL, Nidorf SM. Colchicine: an affordable anti-inflammatory agent for atherosclerosis. Curr Opin Lipidol 2018;29(6):467–73.

66. Fostad I, Eidet JR, Lyberg T, et al. The Increased Risk of Cardiovascular Disease in Rheumatoid Arthritis May be Related to NUPR1 Activation. Ann Rheum Dis 2015;74(Suppl2):686.

67. Oma I, Olstad OK, Andersen JK, et al. Differential expression of vitamin D associated genes in the aorta of coronary artery disease patients with and without rheumatoid arthritis. PloS one 2018;13(8):e0202346.

68. Breland UM, Hollan I, Saatvedt K, et al. Inflammatory markers in patients with coronary artery disease with and without inflammatory rheumatic disease. Rheumatology 2010;keq005.

69. Oma I, Andersen JK, Lyberg T, et al. Plasma vitamin D levels and inflammation in the aortic wall of patients with coronary artery disease with and without inflammatory rheumatic disease. Scand J Rheumatol 2016;1–8.

70. Grundtman C, Hollan I, Forre OT, et al. Cardiovascular disease in patients with inflammatory rheumatic disease is associated with up-regulation of markers of inflammation in cardiac microvessels and cardiomyocytes. Arthritis Rheum 2010;62(3):667–73.

71. Malczuk E, Tłustochowicz W, Kramarz E, et al. Early Myocardial Changes in Patients with Rheumatoid Arthritis without Known Cardiovascular Diseases-A Comprehensive Cardiac Magnetic Resonance Study. Diagnostics (Basel, Switzerland) 2021;11(12).

72. Quagliariello V, Paccone A, Iovine M, et al. Interleukin-1 blocking agents as promising strategy for prevention of anticancer drug-induced cardiotoxicities: possible implications in cancer patients with COVID-19. Eur Rev Med Pharmacol Sci 2021; 25(21):6797–812.

73. Bianchi ME, Crippa MP, Manfredi AA, et al. High-mobility group box 1 protein orchestrates responses to tissue damage via inflammation, innate and adaptive immunity, and tissue repair. Immunol Rev 2017;280(1):74–82.

74. Foglio E, Pellegrini L, Russo MA, et al. HMGB1-Mediated Activation of the Inflammatory-Reparative Response Following Myocardial Infarction. Cells 2022; 11(2):216.

75. Andersson U, Yang H, Harris H. Extracellular HMGB1 as a therapeutic target in inflammatory diseases. Expert Opin Ther Targets 2018;22(3):263–77.

76. Bruton M, Hollan I, Xiao J, et al. Expression of High Mobility Group Protein B1 in Cardiac Tissue of Elderly Patients with Coronary Artery Disease with or without Inflammatory Rheumatic Disease. Gerontology 2017;63(4):337–49.

77. Singh GB, Zhang Y, Boini KM, et al. High Mobility Group Box 1 Mediates TMAO-Induced Endothelial Dysfunction. Int J Mol Sci 2019;20(14).

78. Wang HH, Lin M, Xiang GD. Serum HMGB1 levels and its association with endothelial dysfunction in patients with polycystic ovary syndrome. Physiol Res 2018; 67(6):911–9.

79. Yang H, Wang H, Andersson U. Targeting Inflammation Driven by HMGB1. Front Immunol 2020;11.

80. VanPatten S, Al-Abed Y. High Mobility Group Box-1 (HMGb1): Current Wisdom and Advancement as a Potential Drug Target. J Med Chem 2018;61(12): 5093–107.

81. Sedding DG, Boyle EC, Demandt JAF, et al. Vasa Vasorum Angiogenesis: Key Player in the Initiation and Progression of Atherosclerosis and Potential Target for the Treatment of Cardiovascular Disease. Front Immunol 2018;9:706.

82. Santilli SM, Fiegel VD, Knighton DR. Changes in the aortic wall oxygen tensions of hypertensive rabbits. Hypertension and aortic wall oxygen. Hypertension 1992; 19(1):33–9.

83. Mengozzi A, Pugliese NR, Taddei S, et al. Microvascular Inflammation and Cardiovascular Prevention: The Role of Microcirculation as Earlier Determinant of Cardiovascular Risk. High Blood Press Cardiovasc Prev 2022;29(1):41–8.

84. Tracy EP, Steilberg V, Rowe G, et al. State of the Field: Cellular Therapy Approaches in Microvascular Regeneration. Am J Physiol Heart Circ Physiol 2022; 322(4):H647-h680.

85. Tarbell J, Mahmoud M, Corti A, et al. The role of oxygen transport in atherosclerosis and vascular disease. J R Soc Interf 2020;17(165):20190732.
86. Rafeh R, Viveiros A, Oudit GY, et al. Targeting perivascular and epicardial adipose tissue inflammation: therapeutic opportunities for cardiovascular disease. Clin Sci (London, Engl : 1979) 2020;134(7):827–51.
87. Ahmadieh S, Kim HW, Weintraub NL. Potential role of perivascular adipose tissue in modulating atherosclerosis. Clin Sci (London, Engl: 1979) 2020;134(1):3–13.
88. Elkhatib MAW, Mroueh A, Rafeh RW, et al. Amelioration of perivascular adipose inflammation reverses vascular dysfunction in a model of nonobese prediabetic metabolic challenge: potential role of antidiabetic drugs. Transl Res 2019;214: 121–43.
89. Shields KJ, Barinas-Mitchell E, Gingo MR, et al. Perivascular adipose tissue of the descending thoracic aorta is associated with systemic lupus erythematosus and vascular calcification in women. Atherosclerosis 2013;231(1):129–35.
90. Icli B, Wu W, Ozdemir D, et al. MicroRNA-135a-3p regulates angiogenesis and tissue repair by targeting p38 signaling in endothelial cells. FASEB J 2019. fj201802063RR.
91. Icli B, Wu W, Ozdemir D, et al. MicroRNA-615-5p Regulates Angiogenesis and Tissue Repair by Targeting AKT/eNOS (Protein Kinase B/Endothelial Nitric Oxide Synthase) Signaling in Endothelial Cells. Arterioscler Thromb Vasc Biol 2019; 39(7):1458–74.
92. Rothman KJ. No Adjustments Are Needed for Multiple Comparisons. Epidemiology 1990;1(1):43–6.
93. Rothman KJ. Six persistent research misconceptions. J Gen Intern Med 2014; 29(7):1060–4.
94. Rothman KJ. Modern Epidemiology: 3rd (third). Eur J Epidemiol 1994;0(0):234–7.

Role of Lipoprotein Levels and Function in Atherosclerosis Associated with Autoimmune Rheumatic Diseases

Nicoletta Ronda, MD, PhD[a],*, Francesca Zimetti, PhD[a],
Maria Pia Adorni, PhD[b], Marcella Palumbo, ScD[a],
George A. Karpouzas, MD[c], Franco Bernini, PhD[a]

KEYWORDS

- Autoimmune rheumatic diseases • Atherosclerosis • Lipid metabolism
- Lipoproteins • LDL • HDL • Cell cholesterol content

KEY POINTS

- Lipid levels and functions are altered in autoimmune rheumatic diseases.
- Inflammation, oxidation, and immune system activation affect enzymes and transfer proteins regulating lipoprotein generation and remodeling, and also directly affect lipoprotein composition and function.
- Lipoprotein dysfunction leads to increased cholesterol content in macrophages, smooth muscle cells, and platelets, and to their proinflammatory activation, both effects resulting in the promotion of atherosclerosis and thrombosis.

INTRODUCTION

As in the general population, atherosclerosis (ATH) in autoimmune rheumatic diseases (ARDs) is due to the contribution of several factors including lifestyle, hypertension, local arterial flow, lipid and glucose metabolism disturbances, inflammation, infections, autoimmune phenomena, and drugs. The distinction between traditional and specific factors related to the autoimmune diseases on the initiation and progression of ATH is becoming increasingly blurred. For example, inflammatory and autoimmune processes are also important for plaque formation and progression in the general population.[1–4] On the other hand, the alterations of lipoproteins have a great impact not

[a] Department of Food and Drug, University of Parma, Parco Area delle Scienze, 27/A, Parma 43124, Italy; [b] Department of Medicine and Surgery, Unit of Neuroscience, University of Parma, Via Volturno 39/F, Parma 43125, Italy; [c] Division of Rheumatology, Harbor-UCLA Medical Center and the Lundquist Institute, Torrance, CA, USA
* Corresponding author. nicoletta.ronda@unipr.it
E-mail address: nicoletta.ronda@unipr.it

only on the atherosclerotic process but also on the activation of the immune system, for example, modifying cholesterol availability in immune cell lipid rafts and thus modulating the function of several receptors.[3,5]

In any case, defining the relative weight of each mechanism in ATH development in the single rheumatic disease is difficult. One of the most studied topics, trying to develop better prevention and treatment strategies for ATH in ARDs, is that of alteration in lipid levels and function. Lipid metabolism includes several pathways aimed to supply tissues with energy and structural molecules. Lipid metabolism begins with dietary lipid consumption; it is influenced by gut absorption, assembly in transporter elements (the lipoproteins) together with various other molecules, remodeling by circulating and tissue enzymes and transfer proteins, and liver activity and bile secretion; and it ends with gut elimination and reabsorption. Owing to the complex structure and variety of circulating lipoproteins, and because of the continuous exchange of their components, both levels and functions are dynamic, interrelated, and contribute to the atherosclerotic process.

Lipoproteins can be divided into chylomicrons and their remnants, very-low-density lipoproteins (VLDLs), intermediate-density lipoproteins (IDLs), low-density lipoproteins (LDLs), and high-density lipoproteins (HDLs) and have different size and composition. Furthermore, each of these lipoprotein classes includes subclasses of particles differing for their content in cholesterol, triglycerides (TGs), phospholipids, apolipoproteins, and carried molecules such as enzymes, hormones, and other elements with a variety of activities.[6] Thus, the overall effect on vessels is the result of total lipoprotein levels, class or subclass lipoprotein distribution, and also carried molecules. All these characteristics can be altered in ARDs.

The most important lipoprotein functions for the atherosclerotic process are those related to inflammation, oxidation, and cell cholesterol homeostasis, all affecting plaque formation and stability and also endothelial function, platelet activation, and thrombosis.

This review examines the main lipoprotein disturbances associated with ARDs, in terms of both plasma levels and function, and their contribution to ATH in these pathologic conditions.

High-Density Lipoproteins

In physiologic conditions, HDLs are anti-inflammatory and antioxidant[7] and promote cholesterol efflux from cells through various pathways,[8] thus opposing foam cell formation and limiting proinflammatory activation of vessel cells.

Overall, HDL activity depends on their composition in apolipoproteins, lipids, and other carried molecules, determining their shape, dimension, and interactions with other lipoproteins and cells.[9] It was recently reported that almost 1000 proteins have been found in HDL particles, able to influence innate immunity, inflammation, cell adhesion, hemostasis, protease regulation, and vitamin and metal binding. Apolipoprotein A-I (apoA-I), the major protein of HDLs, exerts antioxidant and anti-inflammatory activities, and promotes cell cholesterol efflux.[10] ApoA-I also modulates immune functions through reduction of cholesterol in the receptor-rich regions of cell membrane, the lipid rafts in macrophages,[11] and also in dendritic cells[12] and lymphocytes.[13] On the contrary, increase in apoA-II and apoC-III lipoproteins in HDL is associated with the development of ATH, due to displacement of the antioxidant enzyme paraoxonase-1 (PON1) and increased macrophage proinflammatory cytokine secretion.[14]

Indeed, native HDLs can prevent LDL oxidation by removing oxidized lipid species through PON1 and other enzymes. PON1, in particular, binds to and is activated by apoAI in HDLs, and it is a known antiatherogenic factor, not only through its antioxidant activity but also because it enhances endothelial NO production and cholesterol efflux from cells.[15] Among HDL-associated molecules, carried sphingosine-1-phosphate has an anti-inflammatory activity and contributes to endothelial-mediated vasodilation.[16] Increased serum amyloid A (SAA) content in HDLs causes HDL dysfunction, with a switch to proinflammatory activity and reduced ability to promote cell cholesterol efflux.[17,18]

The regulation of cell cholesterol content is the main effect of HDL particles. According to their degree of maturation and remodeling occurring in plasma after liver secretion of apoA-I, HDLs can promote cell cholesterol efflux through different mechanisms.[8] Free apoA-I and lipid-poor discoidal HDLs interact with the membrane cholesterol transporter ATP-binding cassette A1 (ABCA1). More mature, lipid-rich HDL interacts with the ATP-binding cassette G1 (ABCG1) and scavenger receptor class B type I (SR-BI). Mature HDL also accepts cholesterol effluxed through gradient-driven aqueous diffusion. Cholesterol is then carried to the liver for bile excretion, as the final step of the reverse cholesterol transport. The HDL maturation process is controlled by the activity of enzymes like lecithin-cholesterol acyltransferase (LCAT), transfer proteins such as cholesteryl ester transfer protein, and lipoprotein lipases, in the context of the complex dynamic equilibrium existing between the various lipoproteins and the exchange in their lipid components. Disturbances in these processes and modifications in HDL protein cargo both contribute to serum cholesterol efflux capacity (CEC) impairment in various conditions, including ARDs, and thus to increased ATH. Indeed, HDL CEC has been significantly associated with cardiovascular (CV) protection in several cross-sectional and longitudinal clinical trials, although the methods used for its measurement vary between studies.[19]

HDLs are important also to prevent acute CV events. In fact, on the one hand, they contribute to plaque stabilization, thanks to the associated antiproteases preventing degradation of extracellular matrix and smooth muscle cell apoptosis.[9] On the other hand, HDLs prevent thrombosis through the regulation of platelet and erythrocyte cholesterol content.[20,21]

Low-Density Lipoproteins

LDLs are the most important cholesterol donors to cells, which internalize cholesterol from native LDL through LDL receptors and from modified LDLs, for example, oxidized particles (oxLDL), through scavenger receptors. In the latter case, intracellular cholesterol content does not limit receptor expression so that the uptake proceeds in an uncontrolled way. This process largely contributes to foam cell formation from macrophages and smooth muscle cells.[22] Oxidation of lipoproteins also occurs in the vessel wall. Particular arterial locations, such as bifurcations, are prone to endothelial activation/damage and may allow intimal deposition of apolipoprotein B (apoB)-containing lipoproteins (LDLs, VLDLs, IDLs, and chylomicron remnants) that can be oxidized, decomposed, aggregated by local proteases or lipases, and finally taken up by macrophages and smooth muscle cells.[3,23,24] Serum levels of lipoprotein (a) (Lp(a)), an LDL particle bound to a glycoprotein apo(a), are associated with CV events at any LDL serum concentration. Lp(a) proatherogenic activity is mostly due to its content in oxidized phospholipids, affecting the function of monocytes, macrophages, and endothelial and smooth muscle cells.[25]

Autoantibodies produced both in rheumatologic and in general patients, such as anti-oxLDL IgG (but not IgM) and anti-b2GPI IgG, can increase cell cholesterol uptake, favoring unregulated modified LDL interaction with cell scavenger receptors and Fc-γ receptor 1.[26]

Cell Cholesterol Homeostasis

In physiologic conditions, a balance exists between proinflammatory and pro-oxidant effects of non-HLD particles and opposite activities of HDLs. When this balance is impaired, cell cholesterol supply and removal are also disturbed. Cell cholesterol homeostasis results from cell cholesterol synthesis, uptake, and efflux.[8] Excess free cholesterol is strictly controlled by intracellular esterification, because free cholesterol may be harmful for the cell. During initial plaque development, macrophage cholesterol increases in its esterified form, stored in cytoplasmic lipid droplets, but when the lesion evolves, free cholesterol accumulates in other compartments, such as lysosomes and plasma membrane. Membrane free cholesterol affects, among others, signaling pathways involved in regulating macrophage motility and organization of the actin cytoskeleton.[27,28] Cell cholesterol content increase is also important in smooth muscle cells, which accounts for up to 50% of foam cell formation in plaques, and affects endothelial function.[29] Increased cholesterol content in platelets induces their activation and adhesion to endothelium and aggregation and is associated with CV risk.[20]

Thus, an overall increased capacity of circulating lipoproteins to upload cells with cholesterol has a great impact on ATH, both in terms of chronic plaque progression and acute events. An in vitro measure of this function is serum cholesterol loading capacity (CLC), evaluated on human monocyte-derived macrophages.[30] Serum CLC has been reported to be increased in pathologic conditions associated with high CV risk.[31–33]

LIPID LEVELS AND FUNCTIONS IN AUTOIMMUNE RHEUMATIC DISEASES

It is currently recognized that lipid levels and functions are strictly interrelated and both should to be taken into account to properly assess atherosclerotic disease burden in patients. Indeed, standard lipid profile measurement alone is not a sufficient tool to define CV risk, particularly in ARDs.[34] Additional markers are being looked at, in an attempt to identify the actual proatherogenic lipid disturbances present in an index patient. In addition, a clearer view of lipid metabolism and functions would allow development of better treatment protocols. However, at present the tools to evaluate lipoprotein function are time consuming, expensive, and sometimes not sufficiently standardized. Although implementation of such tests in routine clinical care is still not possible, they do provide substantial information on the ATH process.

In ARDs, many disturbances of serum lipid profile and lipoprotein functions have been described, depending on the particular disease, and also on disease activity and medications used. Many aspects are common to various conditions, for example, those induced by acute-phase molecules and cytokines, and others are more specific. The largest body of data is available for systemic lupus erythematosus (SLE) and rheumatoid arthritis (RA). A schematic representation of lipid-related atherogenic mechanisms in ARDs is provided in **Fig. 1**.

Systemic Lupus Erythematosus

SLE is associated with increased CV risk[35] and with a proatherogenic serum lipid profile characterized by high TG and Lp(a) levels, and reduced HDL-cholesterol (HDL-C) levels. Serum LDL-cholesterol (LDL-C) and total cholesterol levels are often increased, but may be within normal range. Modifications in TG metabolism have been reported in SLE, mainly due to impairment of the activity of lipoprotein lipase[36] due to cytokine activity and antilipoprotein lipase autoantibodies.[37] Hypertriglyceridemia is proatherogenic through several mechanisms, involving uncontrolled uptake of TG-rich particles by macrophages, damage to endothelial cells and reactive oxygen species (ROS) generation, proinflammatory activity of TG-rich HDL, and procoagulant activity.[38,39] Secondary to TG increase, small dense LDL, particularly proatherogenic, are produced in excess by the liver in patients with SLE.[40]

Inflammation stimulates liver apo(a) production and indeed the proatherogenic Lp(a) is increased in SLE.[41] Small dense LDL and Lp(a) are particularly prone to oxidation, and oxLDL as well as oxLDL immune complexes are increased in SLE and associate with ATH.[42,43]

In SLE, due to the increase in acute-phase proteins, such as SAA and secretory Phospolipase A2, apoA-I is displaced from HDL and undergoes increased catabolism in the liver and kidney.[5] As a consequence, lower levels of HDL are generated, as dysfunctional particles. The increased neutrophil-dependent production of ROS,[44] activation of oxidative enzymes during neutrophil extracellular traps formation in

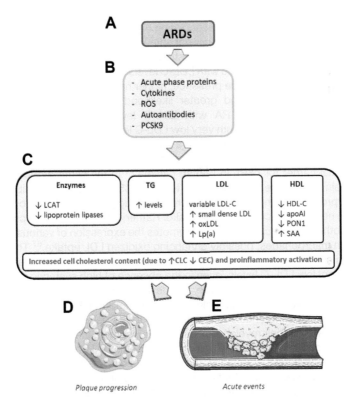

Fig. 1. Schematic representation of lipid-related atherogenic mechanisms in ARDs. Immune and inflammatory mediators in ARDs induce (A) modification in the activity of enzymes pivotal for lipid metabolism, (B) increase in TG levels, (C) disturbances in HDL maturation and in TG and lipid exchange between LDL and HDL, (D) alteration of LDL and HDL composition, and (E) increase in lipid oxidation. As a consequence, lipoprotein dysfunction, through increased CLC and decreased CEC, causes intracellular cholesterol accumulation in macrophages, smooth muscle cells, and platelets. Increased cholesterol cell content and other mechanisms of lipoprotein dysfunction also induce cell proinflammatory activation. Overall, both plaque progression and acute cardiovascular events are promoted. ↓, Decrease; ↑, increase; PCSK9, proprotein convertase subtilisin/kexin type 9; ROS, reactive oxygen species; SAA, serum amyloid A.

SLE,[45] as well as the reduction in PON1 contribute to increased lipid oxidation and HDL dysfunction. Indeed, HDL dysfunction in patients with SLE has been demonstrated as a reduction in their antioxidant activity[46] as well as CEC, through both ABCA1 and ABCG1 pathways, indicating a global HDL function impairment.[47] In a recent study, HDL CEC was inversely and independently associated with the presence of carotid plaques in patients with SLE.[48]

Rheumatoid Arthritis

The serum lipid profile in patients with RA is characterized by reduced HDL-C levels and is inversely associated with disease activity and inflammation.[49,50] Serum TG levels tend to be increased in patients with RA,[51] but the most typical finding is the high serum concentration of small dense LDL[52] and Lp(a).[53] LDL-C instead can vary between subjects and also according to the disease activity. In particular, LDL-C level may be very low in case of flare in certain patients. The RA "lipid paradox" is a finding that, in contrast to the general population, patients with very low LDL levels have an increased CV risk, with a U-shaped association between the 2 variables.[54] The mechanisms underlying this phenomenon are not entirely understood. Recently, we demonstrated for the first time that, in a population of patients with RA with low disease activity and inflammation, subjects with LDL-C levels less than 1.8 mmol/L had greater coronary ATH, obstructive plaque presence, higher number of segments with plaque, increased stenotic severity, and greater likelihood of high-risk plaque presence compared with patients with RA with LDL-C levels greater than or equal to 1.8 mmol/L.[55] Patients with RA with very low LDL-C levels in our study also had higher oxidized phospholipids (oxPL)-apoB100 (a measure of oxLDL) and anti-oxLDL antibody levels, associated with higher Lp(a), consistently with the concept that Lp(a) is the preferential carrier for oxPL in human plasma.[56] In the same group of patients, the proprotein convertase subtilisin/kexin type 9 (PCSK9), the major inhibitor of LDL receptor expression in the liver, was increased, suggesting that the low levels of LDL-C were not due to increased liver uptake. Rather, alternative clearance pathways may be hypothesized, because PCSK9 promotes the expression of various scavenger receptors on macrophages, possibly enhancing oxidized LDL uptake.[57] Thus, CV risk stratification and prevention strategies in RA should consider the potential risk associated with very low LDL-C levels, even in the absence of high systemic inflammation and disease activity. At the same time, the development of therapies to inhibit LDL oxidation may be warranted; this looks particularly important also considering that, as in SLE, in RA also the antioxidant activity of HDL is decreased,[58] at least in part due to the increase in their myeloperoxidase (MPO) content and decrease in PON1.[59]

Data on HDL capacity to promote cell cholesterol efflux in RA compared with control subjects are controversial.[60] Actually, the main problem with CEC determination and comparison between studies is that measurement protocols profoundly differ in terms of cell models, acceptors used, and also quantification methods. As explained in the introduction, HDLs are a family of lipoproteins including various subclasses substantially differing in size and composition and promoting cholesterol efflux through at least 4 mechanisms: aqueous diffusion, ABCA1, ABCG1, and SR-BI mediated. Beyond the general effects of a reduction of intracellular cholesterol on the cell, specific intracellular transduction signals may be activated by each of these pathways of cholesterol efflux, resulting in different functional consequences.[61,62]

Most of the methods applied so far to study CEC in patients with RA do not distinguish between the pathways of cholesterol efflux and are a mixed measure with unknown relative contribution of the various types of HDL; this might explain the different results reported in literature. We demonstrated in a small number of patients with RA that, in contrast to SLE, only ABCG1-mediated CEC was impaired and that its values inversely correlated with the disease activity score DAS28.[47] Interestingly, ABCG1-mediated cholesterol efflux is the pathway that more than others modulates macrophage inflammatory response by affecting the lipid composition of plasma membrane lipid rafts.[61] ABCG1 CEC is predominantly due to the activity of mature HDL. As aforementioned, apoAI secretion and HDL formation and remodeling occur through the activity of various enzymes. This process is altered in RA, because LCAT activity is reduced, thus limiting HDL maturation.[63] An impairment of HDL maturation seems typical of inflammatory conditions.[18]

The potential impact of lipoprotein alterations described so far in RA, both in terms of cell cholesterol content and of clinical outcome, is confirmed by a previous report[64] and by recent findings from the authors' group. In fact, in the authors' RA cohort, oxPL-apoB100, anti-oxLDL IgG, and PCSK9 positively associated with serum CLC on macrophages, independently of LDL-C levels.[65] Dual seropositivity and C-reactive Protein levels moderated the impact of oxLDL on CLC, consistent with the notion that RA-specific autoantibodies and low-grade inflammation are proatherogenic factors.[66,67] The authors also demonstrated a strong independent association of CLC with high-risk plaque burden in biologic Disease Modifying Anti-Rheumatic Drugs (bDMARDs)-naive patients with RA and long-term CV risk with a mitigating effect of bDMARD treatment, after adjusting for ASCVD score and for statin use.[65]

ANTIRHEUMATIC DRUGS EFFECTS ON LIPOPROTEIN LEVELS AND FUNCTION AND IMPACT ON ATHEROSCLEROSIS

The study of lipid levels and function in ARDs should take into account the effects of antirheumatic pharmacologic treatment, because anti-inflammatory drugs and DMARDs modify lipid metabolism with various mechanisms. In general, antirheumatic treatment ameliorates lipid profile and function, and is associated with CV protection.[68–70] Lipid modifications upon ARD treatment have a positive, atheroprotective effect, despite the increase in LDL-C levels that may occur, particularly in patients with RA showing reduced low LDL-C levels during active phases of the disease.[68,71]

Hydroxychloroquine (HCQ) increases HDL levels[72] and reduces non-HDL lipoproteins and TG.[73] HCQ also seems to ameliorate HDL's capacity to accept cholesterol.[74]

Generally, the quality and function of both HDL and LDL particles recover upon antirheumatic treatment. For example, various DMARD combinations improved HDL composition, increasing PON1 and reducing haptoglobin and MPO content, thus improving antioxidant activity.[75] Adalimumab, abatacept, and rituximab were associated with similar improvements in HDL quality.[76,77] In a study on global HDL CEC, tocilizumab induced the most significant CEC increase, followed by infliximab and rituximab, whereas methotrexate (MTX) did not associate with CEC modifications.[78] However, testing individual CEC pathways, we found that MTX treatment alone induced an increase in ABCG1- and SR-BI-mediated HDL CEC.[79] In the same study, adalimumab associated with serum HDL-C level increase together with transient modifications of SRBI-mediated CEC (increased) and ABCA1-mediated CEC (decreased), consistent with a maturation shift of HDL particles. The improvement of CEC mediated by mature HDL particles both for MTX and adalimumab may reflect the restoration of HDL maturation, which is impaired in inflammatory conditions.[18]

In a pilot study by the authors on patients with RA treated with conventional synthetic DMARDs, tocilizumab induced an improvement in ABCG1- and SR-BI-mediated CEC, despite HDL-C stability. Tocilizumab was also associated with better LDL quality, as indicated by a reduction of CLC:LDL-C ratio.[30]

Besides having effects on lipoprotein levels and function, DMARDs can also act directly on macrophage expression of cholesterol transporters, like reported for MTX[80] and inflix-imab.[81] In addition, adalimumab can reduce macrophage cholesterol uptake by binding to membrane-expressed tumor necrosis factor and inducing reverse signaling.[79]

CLINICS CARE POINTS

- Alterations in lipid level and function associated with ARDs are highly proatherogenic.
- Patients with ARDs should be carefully evaluated for CV risk, through a multidisciplinary approach including an expert in lipid metabolism.
- At present, no specific lipid function markers are sufficiently standardized or streamlined for broad use in routine clinical practice.
- Several European and American society guidelines for CV risk stratification and management acknowledge the increased risk incurred by patients with ARDs. Although the general framework is present and available for general patients, there is no sufficient clarity, agreement, or evidence rigor as to how should those be specifically applied and/or adapted for patients with ARDs; this includes specific disease states, frequency and timing of cardiac risk factor evaluation, specificity, and/or adaptation of therapeutic targets. Therefore, expert opinion on the management of certain such risk factors, such as lipid control in ARDs, maybe helpful.[82]
- Antirheumatic drugs, despite inducing an increase in non-HDL levels in some cases, positively affect lipid quality and functions resulting in a net atheroprotective effect.

DISCLOSURE

None of the authors has any disclosure on commercial or financial conflicts of interest and funding sources.

REFERENCES

1. Hansson GK, Holm J, Jonasson L. Detection of activated T lymphocytes in the human atherosclerotic plaque. Am J Pathol 1989;135(1):169–75.
2. Almanzar G, Öllinger R, Leuenberger J, et al. Autoreactive HSP60 epitope-specific T-cells in early human atherosclerotic lesions. J Autoimmun 2012;39(4):441–50.
3. Lorey MB, Öörni K, Kovanen PT. Modified Lipoproteins Induce Arterial Wall Inflammation During Atherogenesis. Front Cardiovasc Med 2022;9:841545.
4. Stemme S, Faber B, Holm J, et al. T lymphocytes from human atherosclerotic plaques recognize oxidized low density lipoprotein. Proc Natl Acad Sci U S A 1995;92(9):3893–7.
5. Catapano AL, Pirillo A, Bonacina F, et al. HDL in innate and adaptive immunity. Cardiovasc Res 2014;103(3):372–83.
6. Deng S, Xu Y, Zheng L. HDL Structure. Adv Exp Med Biol 2022;1377:1–11.
7. Zhang Q, Jiang Z, Xu Y. HDL and Oxidation. Adv Exp Med Biol 2022;1377:63–77.
8. Adorni MP, Ronda N, Bernini F, et al. High Density Lipoprotein Cholesterol Efflux Capacity and Atherosclerosis in Cardiovascular Disease: Pathophysiological Aspects and Pharmacological Perspectives. Cells 2021;10(3).
9. Davidson WS, Shah AS, Sexmith H, et al. The HDL Proteome Watch: Compilation of studies leads to new insights on HDL function. Biochim Biophys Acta Mol Cell Biol Lipids 2022;1867(2):159072.

10. Brites F, Martin M, Guillas I, et al. Antioxidative activity of high-density lipoprotein (HDL): Mechanistic insights into potential clinical benefit. BBA Clin 2017;8:66–77.
11. Yin K, Chen W-J, Zhou Z-G, et al. Apolipoprotein A-I inhibits CD40 proinflammatory signaling via ATP-binding cassette transporter A1-mediated modulation of lipid raft in macrophages. J Atheroscler Thromb 2012;19(9):823–36.
12. Perrin-Cocon L, Diaz O, Carreras M, et al. High-density lipoprotein phospholipids interfere with dendritic cell Th1 functional maturation. Immunobiology 2012; 217(1):91–9.
13. Wilhelm AJ, Zabalawi M, Grayson JM, et al. Apolipoprotein A-I and its role in lymphocyte cholesterol homeostasis and autoimmunity. Arterioscler Thromb Vasc Biol 2009;29(6):843–9.
14. Zewinger S, Reiser J, Jankowski V, et al. Apolipoprotein C3 induces inflammation and organ damage by alternative inflammasome activation. Nat Immunol 2020; 21(1):30–41.
15. Gugliucci A, Menini T. Paraoxonase 1 and HDL maturation. Clin Chim Acta 2015; 439:5–13.
16. Chen Z, Hu M. The apoM-S1P axis in hepatic diseases. Clin Chim Acta 2020;511: 235–42.
17. Webb NR. High-Density Lipoproteins and Serum Amyloid A (SAA). Curr Atheroscler Rep 2021;23(2):7.
18. Zimetti F, De Vuono S, Gomaraschi M, et al. Plasma cholesterol homeostasis, HDL remodeling and function during the acute phase reaction. J Lipid Res 2017; 58(10):2051–60.
19. Soria-Florido MT, Schröder H, Grau M, et al. High density lipoprotein functionality and cardiovascular events and mortality: A systematic review and meta-analysis. Atherosclerosis 2020;302:36–42.
20. Ravindran R, Krishnan LK. Increased platelet cholesterol and decreased percentage volume of platelets as a secondary risk factor for coronary artery disease. Pathophysiol Haemost Thromb 2007;36(1):45–51.
21. Tziakas DN, Kaski JC, Chalikias GK, et al. Total cholesterol content of erythrocyte membranes is increased in patients with acute coronary syndrome: a new marker of clinical instability? J Am Coll Cardiol 2007;49(21):2081–9.
22. Allahverdian S, Chehroudi AC, McManus BM, et al. Contribution of intimal smooth muscle cells to cholesterol accumulation and macrophage-like cells in human atherosclerosis. Circulation 2014;129(15):1551–9.
23. Borén J, Chapman MJ, Krauss RM, et al. Low-density lipoproteins cause atherosclerotic cardiovascular disease: pathophysiological, genetic, and therapeutic insights: a consensus statement from the European Atherosclerosis Society Consensus Panel. Eur Heart J 2020;41(24):2313–30.
24. Skålén K, Gustafsson M, Rydberg EK, et al. Subendothelial retention of atherogenic lipoproteins in early atherosclerosis. Nature 2002;417(6890):750–4.
25. Koschinsky ML, Boffa MB. Oxidized phospholipid modification of lipoprotein(a): Epidemiology, biochemistry and pathophysiology. Atherosclerosis 2022;349: 92–100.
26. Iseme RA, McEvoy M, Kelly B, et al. A role for autoantibodies in atherogenesis. Cardiovasc Res 2017;113(10):1102–12.
27. Qin C, Nagao T, Grosheva I, et al. Elevated plasma membrane cholesterol content alters macrophage signaling and function. Arterioscler Thromb Vasc Biol 2006;26(2):372–8.

28. Adorni MP, Favari E, Ronda N, et al. Free cholesterol alters macrophage morphology and mobility by an ABCA1 dependent mechanism. Atherosclerosis 2011;215(1):70–6.
29. Liu Y-X, Yuan P-Z, Wu J-H, et al. Lipid accumulation and novel insight into vascular smooth muscle cells in atherosclerosis. J Mol Med (Berl) 2021;99(11): 1511–26.
30. Greco D, Gualtierotti R, Agosti P, et al. Anti-atherogenic Modification of Serum Lipoprotein Function in Patients with Rheumatoid Arthritis after Tocilizumab Treatment, a Pilot Study. J Clin Med 2020;9(7). https://doi.org/10.3390/jcm9072157.
31. Adorni MP, Zimetti F, Cangiano B, et al. High-Density Lipoprotein Function Is Reduced in Patients Affected by Genetic or Idiopathic Hypogonadism. J Clin Endocrinol Metab 2019;104(8):3097–107.
32. Stefanutti C, Pisciotta L, Favari E, et al. Lipoprotein(a) concentration, genetic variants, apo(a) isoform size, and cellular cholesterol efflux in patients with elevated Lp(a) and coronary heart disease submitted or not to lipoprotein apheresis: An Italian case-control multicenter study on Lp(a). J Clin Lipidol 2020;14(4): 487–97.e1.
33. Di Costanzo A, Ronca A, D'Erasmo L, et al. HDL-Mediated Cholesterol Efflux and Plasma Loading Capacities Are Altered in Subjects with Metabolically- but Not Genetically Driven Non-Alcoholic Fatty Liver Disease (NAFLD). Biomedicines 2020;8(12). https://doi.org/10.3390/biomedicines8120625.
34. Ciurtin C, Robinson GA, Pineda-Torra I, et al. Challenges in Implementing Cardiovascular Risk Scores for Assessment of Young People With Childhood-Onset Autoimmune Rheumatic Conditions. Front Med 2022;9:814905.
35. Shoenfeld Y, Gerli R, Doria A, et al. Accelerated atherosclerosis in autoimmune rheumatic diseases. Circulation 2005;112(21):3337–47.
36. Quevedo-Abeledo JC, Martín-González C, Ferrer-Moure C, et al. Key Molecules of Triglycerides Pathway Metabolism Are Disturbed in Patients With Systemic Lupus Erythematosus. Front Immunol 2022;13:827355.
37. Reichlin M, Fesmire J, Quintero-Del-Rio AI, et al. Autoantibodies to lipoprotein lipase and dyslipidemia in systemic lupus erythematosus. Arthritis Rheum 2002;46(11):2957–63.
38. Peng J, Luo F, Ruan G, et al. Hypertriglyceridemia and atherosclerosis. Lipids Health Dis 2017;16(1):233.
39. Chapman MJ, Ginsberg HN, Amarenco P, et al. Triglyceride-rich lipoproteins and high-density lipoprotein cholesterol in patients at high risk of cardiovascular disease: evidence and guidance for management. Eur Heart J 2011;32(11): 1345–61.
40. Feingold KR, Grunfeld C. In: Feingold KR, Anawalt B, Boyce A, et al, editors. The effect of inflammation and infection on lipids and lipoproteins. 2000.
41. Borba EF, Santos RD, Bonfa E, et al. Lipoprotein(a) levels in systemic lupus erythematosus. J Rheumatol 1994;21(2):220–3.
42. Ahmad HM, Sarhan EM, Komber U. Higher circulating levels of OxLDL % of LDL are associated with subclinical atherosclerosis in female patients with systemic lupus erythematosus. Rheumatol Int 2014;34(5):617–23.
43. Oates JC, Ramakrishnan V, Nietert PJ, et al. Associations between accelerated atherosclerosis, oxidized ldl immune complexes, and in vitro endothelial dysfunction in systemic lupus erythematosus. Trans Am Clin Climatol Assoc 2020;131: 157–77.

44. Ferreira HB, Pereira AM, Melo T, et al. Lipidomics in autoimmune diseases with main focus on systemic lupus erythematosus. J Pharm Biomed Anal 2019;174: 386–95.

45. Smith CK, Vivekanandan-Giri A, Tang C, et al. Neutrophil extracellular trap-derived enzymes oxidize high-density lipoprotein: an additional proatherogenic mechanism in systemic lupus erythematosus. Arthritis Rheumatol (Hoboken, Nj) 2014;66(9):2532–44.

46. McMahon M, Grossman J, FitzGerald J, et al. Proinflammatory high-density lipo-protein as a biomarker for atherosclerosis in patients with systemic lupus erythe-matosus and rheumatoid arthritis. Arthritis Rheum 2006;54(8):2541–9.

47. Ronda N, Favari E, Borghi MO, et al. Impaired serum cholesterol efflux capacity in rheumatoid arthritis and systemic lupus erythematosus. Ann Rheum Dis 2014; 73(3):609–15.

48. Sánchez-Pérez H, Quevedo-Abeledo JC, de Armas-Rillo L, et al. Impaired HDL cholesterol efflux capacity in systemic lupus erythematosus patients is related to subclinical carotid atherosclerosis. Rheumatology (Oxford) 2020;59(10): 2847–56.

49. Choi HK, Seeger JD. Lipid profiles among US elderly with untreated rheumatoid arthritis–the Third National Health and Nutrition Examination Survey. J Rheumatol 2005;32(12):2311–6.

50. Georgiadis AN, Papavasiliou EC, Lourida ES, et al. Atherogenic lipid profile is a feature characteristic of patients with early rheumatoid arthritis: effect of early treatment–a prospective, controlled study. Arthritis Res Ther 2006;8(3):R82.

51. Steiner G, Urowitz MB. Lipid profiles in patients with rheumatoid arthritis: mech-anisms and the impact of treatment. Semin Arthritis Rheum 2009;38(5):372–81.

52. Schulte DM, Paulsen K, Türk K, et al. Small dense LDL cholesterol in human sub-jects with different chronic inflammatory diseases. Nutr Metab Cardiovasc Dis 2018;28(11):1100–5.

53. Dursunoğlu D, Evrengül H, Polat B, et al. Lp(a) lipoprotein and lipids in patients with rheumatoid arthritis: serum levels and relationship to inflammation. Rheuma-tol Int 2005;25(4):241–5.

54. Myasoedova E, Crowson CS, Kremers HM, et al. Lipid paradox in rheumatoid arthritis: the impact of serum lipid measures and systemic inflammation on the risk of cardiovascular disease. Ann Rheum Dis 2011;70(3):482–7.

55. Karpouzas GA, Ormseth SR, Ronda N, et al. Lipoprotein oxidation may underlie the paradoxical association of low cholesterol with coronary atherosclerotic risk in rheumatoid arthritis. J Autoimmun 2022;129:102815.

56. Bergmark C, Dewan A, Orsoni A, et al. A novel function of lipoprotein [a] as a preferential carrier of oxidized phospholipids in human plasma. J Lipid Res 2008;49(10):2230–9.

57. Ruscica M, Tokgözoğlu L, Corsini A, et al. PCSK9 inhibition and inflammation: A narrative review. Atherosclerosis 2019;288:146–55.

58. Charles-Schoeman C, Watanabe J, Lee YY, et al. Abnormal function of high-density lipoprotein is associated with poor disease control and an altered protein cargo in rheumatoid arthritis. Arthritis Rheum 2009;60(10):2870–9.

59. Tanimoto N, Kumon Y, Suehiro T, et al. Serum paraoxonase activity decreases in rheumatoid arthritis. Life Sci 2003;72(25):2877–85.

60. Xie B, He J, Liu Y, et al. A meta-analysis of HDL cholesterol efflux capacity and concentration in patients with rheumatoid arthritis. Lipids Health Dis 2021; 20(1):18.

61. Yvan-Charvet L, Wang N, Tall AR. Role of HDL, ABCA1, and ABCG1 transporters in cholesterol efflux and immune responses. Arterioscler Thromb Vasc Biol 2010; 30(2):139–43.

62. Prosser HC, Ng MKC, Bursill CA. The role of cholesterol efflux in mechanisms of endothelial protection by HDL 2012;23(3):182–9.

63. de Armas-Rillo L, Quevedo-Abeledo JC, Hernández-Hernández V, et al. The angiopoietin-like protein 4, apolipoprotein C3, and lipoprotein lipase axis is disrupted in patients with rheumatoid arthritis. Arthritis Res Ther 2022;24(1):99.

64. Voloshyna I, Modayil S, Littlefield MJ, et al. Plasma from rheumatoid arthritis patients promotes pro-atherogenic cholesterol transport gene expression in THP-1 human macrophages. Exp Biol Med (Maywood) 2013;238(10):1192–7.

65. Karpouzas GA, Papotti B, Ormseth SR, et al. Serum cholesterol loading capacity on macrophages is regulated by seropositivity and C-reactive protein in rheumatoid arthritis patients, Rheumatology. (Oxford) 2022;keac394.

66. Cambridge G, Acharya J, Cooper JA, et al. Antibodies to citrullinated peptides and risk of coronary heart disease. Atherosclerosis 2013;228(1):243–6.

67. Fu Y, Wu Y, Liu E. C-reactive protein and cardiovascular disease: From animal studies to the clinic (Review). Exp Ther Med 2020;20(2):1211–9.

68. Behl T, Kaur I, Sehgal A, et al. The Lipid Paradox as a Metabolic Checkpoint and Its Therapeutic Significance in Ameliorating the Associated Cardiovascular Risks in Rheumatoid Arthritis Patients. Int J Mol Sci 2020;21(24). https://doi.org/10.3390/ijms21249505.

69. Naerr GW, Rein P, Saely CH, et al. Effects of synthetic and biological disease modifying antirheumatic drugs on lipid and lipoprotein parameters in patients with rheumatoid arthritis. Vascul Pharmacol 2016;81:22–30.

70. Charles-Schoeman C, Gonzalez-Gay MA, Kaplan I, et al. Effects of tofacitinib and other DMARDs on lipid profiles in rheumatoid arthritis: implications for the rheumatologist. Semin Arthritis Rheum 2016;46(1):71–80.

71. Karpouzas GA, Ormseth SR, Hernandez E, et al. Biologics May Prevent Cardiovascular Events in Rheumatoid Arthritis by Inhibiting Coronary Plaque Formation and Stabilizing High-Risk Lesions. Arthritis Rheumatol (Hoboken, Nj) 2020;72(9): 1467–75.

72. Morris SJ, Wasko MCM, Antohe JL, et al. Hydroxychloroquine use associated with improvement in lipid profiles in rheumatoid arthritis patients. Arthritis Care Res (Hoboken) 2011;63(4):530–4.

73. Wallace DJ, Metzger AL, Stecher VJ, et al. Cholesterol-lowering effect of hydroxychloroquine in patients with rheumatic disease: reversal of deleterious effects of steroids on lipids. Am J Med 1990;89(3):322–6.

74. Lang MG, Vinagre CG, Bonfa E, et al. Hydroxychloroquine increased cholesterol transfer to high-density lipoprotein in systemic lupus erythematosus: A possible mechanism for the reversal of atherosclerosis in the disease. Lupus 2022; 31(6):659–65.

75. Charles-Schoeman C, Yin Lee Y, Shahbazian A, et al. Improvement of High-Density Lipoprotein Function in Patients With Early Rheumatoid Arthritis Treated With Methotrexate Monotherapy or Combination Therapies in a Randomized Controlled Trial. Arthritis Rheumatol (Hoboken, Nj) 2017;69(1):46–57.

76. Charles-Schoeman C, Gugiu GB, Ge H, et al. Remodeling of the HDL proteome with treatment response to abatacept or adalimumab in the AMPLE trial of patients with rheumatoid arthritis. Atherosclerosis 2018;275:107–14.

77. Raterman HG, Levels H, Voskuyl AE, et al. HDL protein composition alters from proatherogenic into less atherogenic and proinflammatory in rheumatoid arthritis patients responding to rituximab. Ann Rheum Dis 2013;72(4):560–5.
78. Cacciapaglia F, Perniola S, Venerito V, et al. The Impact of Biologic Drugs on High-Density Lipoprotein Cholesterol Efflux Capacity in Rheumatoid Arthritis Patients. J Clin Rheumatol Pract Reports Rheum Musculoskelet Dis 2022;28(1): e145–9.
79. Ronda N, Greco D, Adorni MP, et al. Newly identified antiatherosclerotic activity of methotrexate and adalimumab: complementary effects on lipoprotein function and macrophage cholesterol metabolism. Arthritis Rheumatol (Hoboken, Nj) 2015;67(5):1155–64.
80. Reiss AB, Carsons SE, Anwar K, et al. Atheroprotective effects of methotrexate on reverse cholesterol transport proteins and foam cell transformation in human THP-1 monocyte/macrophages. Arthritis Rheum 2008;58(12):3675–83.
81. Voloshyna I, Seshadri S, Anwar K, et al. Infliximab reverses suppression of cholesterol efflux proteins by TNF-α: a possible mechanism for modulation of atherogenesis. Biomed Res Int 2014;2014:312647.
82. Hollan I, Ronda N, Dessein P, et al. Lipid management in rheumatoid arthritis: a position paper of the Working Group on Cardiovascular Pharmacotherapy of the European Society of Cardiology. Eur Hear Journal Cardiovasc Pharmacother 2020;6(2):104–14.

Evidence for Biologic Drug Modifying Anti-Rheumatoid Drugs and Association with Cardiovascular Disease Risk Mitigation in Inflammatory Arthritis

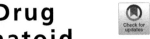

Brittany Weber, MD, PhD[a,b,*], Katherine P. Liao, MD, MPH[c]

KEYWORDS

- Disease-modifying antirheumatic drug (DMARD) • Cardiovascular • Inflammation
- Rheumatoid arthritis • Spondylarthritis • Psoriatic arthritis

KEY POINTS

- Overall current evidence suggests that bDMARDs mitigate CV risk in inflammatory arthritis.
- RA is the most well-studied but emerging evidence for SpA and PsA suggest similar findings.
- The role of JAK inhibition on CV Risk mitigation is inconclusive.

INTRODUCTION

Systemic inflammatory arthritides are associated with increased risk of atherosclerosis and ultimately cardiovascular (CV) risk.[1–8] Key inflammatory cytokines prominent in these conditions also play a major role in atherosclerosis development and endothelial dysfunction. Endothelial dysfunction is an early event in the development of atherosclerosis and can be detected before structural changes in vessels on angiography.[9] In the heart, endothelial dysfunction can manifest as coronary vascular dysfunction, associated with both systemic inflammation and may precede or coexist

[a] Department of Medicine, Division of Cardiovascular Medicine, Brigham and Women's Hospital, Harvard Medical School, 75 Francis Street, Boston, MA 02115, USA; [b] Cardiovascular Imaging Program, Department of Radiology, Brigham and Women's Hospital, Harvard Medical School, Boston, MA, USA; [c] Division of Rheumatology, Inflammation, and Immunity, Brigham and Women's Hospital, Harvard Medical School, Boston, MA, USA
* Corresponding author. Brigham and Women's Hospital, 75 Francis Street, Boston, MA 02115.
E-mail address: bweber@bwh.harvard.edu

Rheum Dis Clin N Am 49 (2023) 165–178
https://doi.org/10.1016/j.rdc.2022.08.005
0889-857X/23/© 2022 Elsevier Inc. All rights reserved.

with high-risk coronary atherosclerosis. The endothelium, serving as a major regulator of vascular homeostasis, provides a permeability barrier for the vasculature, maintains a nonthrombogenic surface, regulates vascular tone and tissue flow, and inhibits vascular smooth muscle cell growth. In the presence of inflammatory cytokines, endothelial cells are activated which facilitates leukocyte adhesion and migration into the vessel wall, production of prothrombotic substances, and vasoconstriction, thereby creating a proatherogenic and procoagulant environment.[10,11] At the individual patient level, this proatherogenic and procoagulant environment promote the development of acute thrombi that can cause a myocardial infarction (MI). Consequently, inflammation is a key mediator of a constellation of abnormalities that initiate and accelerate the progression of atherosclerosis.[12-14]

A complex interplay exists between underlying systemic inflammation and classic cardiovascular risk factors, such as obesity, diabetes mellitus (DM), hypertension (HTN), and dyslipidemia in patients with inflammatory arthritis. The increased CV mortality attributed to inflammation, observed in patients with inflammatory arthritis is independent of traditional CV risk factors.[15-25] Over the last 3 decades, biologic disease-modifying drugs (bDMARDs) and more recently, small molecules that target specific pathways involved in the pathogenesis of these conditions enable tight control of disease activity and in some cases remission. We will focus our review on the inflammatory arthritides, namely rheumatoid arthritis (RA), psoriatic arthritis (PsA), and spondyloarthritis (SpA). Across these conditions, the pathways targeted include, CD20, interleukin (IL)-1, IL-6, IL-17, IL-12/IL-23, TNFα, the T-cell costimulatory pathway through CD80/86, and more recently inhibition through the Janus kinases (JAK).

While nuances remain in the decision of overall therapy for each disease and the individual patient, these therapies are well tolerated and safe with regards to infection with regular monitoring.[26,27] However, the data on CV risk, including both benefit and possible harm, remain an area of active investigation. Rheumatoid arthritis (RA) has the most robust data on the bDMARDs and modulation of CV risk compared to the other inflammatory arthritides, PsA and SpA. For psoriatic conditions, the majority of the data on CV risk mitigation comes from the psoriasis literature among which 25–30% have concurrent joint involvement. The aim of this review is to provide an overview of the data on CV risk modulation within each class of bDMARDs with a focus on studies that address the impact on surrogate markers of CVD and cardiovascular outcomes.

TNFα INHIBITORS

TNFα is one of the key pathologic cytokines implicated in the pathogenesis of increased CV risk within systemic inflammatory arthritides. TNFα and related proinflammatory cytokines, implicated in the initial insult of endothelial dysfunction and injury to the vascular endothelium, is considered one of the earliest events in atherosclerosis. TNFα inhibitors (TNFi) are commonly used throughout the inflammatory arthritides of which 5 options are available in this class, adalimumab, certolizumab, etanercept, golimumab, and infliximab (Table 1). In RA, epidemiological evidence suggests that treatment with TNFi is largely associated with a reduction in the incidence of cardiovascular disease compared to subjects on nonbiologic DMARDs (nbDMARDs) such as methotrexate and sulfasalazine.[28,29] One of the earlier large-scale studies examining the effect of TNFi on cardiovascular mortality in patients with RA found TNFi use led to a reduction of CV mortality by 35% compared to a standard treatment regimen.[30] A large British registry of patients with RA treated with TNFi compared to

Table 1
Evidence of CV risk mitigation across bDMARDs and small molecules for the treatment of inflammatory arthritis

Pathway	Therapies	RA	SpA	PsA
CD20/B-cell depletion	Rituximab	D		
CTLA4	Abatacept	C		D
IL-1	Anakinra	C		
IL-6	Sarilumab, tocilizumab	C		
IL-17A	Ixekizumab, secukinumab		D	C
IL-12/23	Ustekinumab			D
IL23	Guselkumab			D
JAK	Baricitinib, tofacitinib, upadacitinib	B		B (FDA approved for tofacitinib only)
TNF-a	Adalimumab, certolizumab, etanercept, golimumab, infliximab	A	C	B

A, multiple robust large observational studies; B, moderate observational data of varying sizes; C, few small studies; D, limited or awaiting data.
Gray box = treatment not FDA approved for condition.

bDMARD-naïve patients on nbDMARDs were examined over time for incident MI. A total of 252 verified first MIs were analyzed and among these, there were 58/3058 patients receiving nbDMARD and 194/11200 patients receiving TNFi (median follow-up per person was 3.5 years and 5.3 years, respectively). This was associated with a reduced risk of MI among subjects on TNFi compared to nonbiologic nbDMARD therapy, adjusted hazard ratio for MI of 0.61 (95% CI 0.41 to 0.89) TNFi vs nbDMARD. There was not a statistically significant difference observed between mortality[29] and in the same cohort, assessment of ischemic stroke did not reveal a difference in the occurrence between TNFi-treated patients compared to conventional therapy.[31] The QUEST-RA cross-sectional study examined over 4000 patients on a range of DMARD therapies and observed that prolonged exposure to TNFi was associated with a lower risk of CV events, with a greater relative risk reduction compared to other nbDMARDs.[32]

Data on the impact of bDMARDs on CV risk among SpA are sparse. Patients with ankylosing spondylitis (AS) AS, as part of a cohort including RA and PsA, from 2001 to 2015 in an Australian-based rheumatic disease cohort were included to evaluate the risk of CV events and the association with TNFi.[33] A small percentage of patients were on other non-TNF biologics (among the patients on biologics, 5.2% on non-TNF versus 94.8% on TNFi), and 36.8% were biologic-naïve at enrollment; 55.6% of the participants were on methotrexate at study enrollment and 39% on prednisone. TNFi was associated with a reduction in major CV events, (HR 0.85, 95% CI 0.76–0.95) which was abrogated in those who stopped therapy (HR 0.96, 95% CI 0.83–1.11). No differences in CV event rate were observed between the inflammatory conditions after statistical adjustment.[33]

Due to the relatively low prevalence of inflammatory arthritides compared to other conditions such as HTN, obtaining sufficient numbers of hard clinical endpoints is one of the challenges in studying CV risk in rheumatic conditions. Thus, surrogate CV endpoints are typically used for studies in the inflammatory arthritides to understand associations between bDMARDs with CV risk. As described previously, endothelial dysfunction is a key early event in the development of atherosclerosis. In two small short-duration mechanistic studies, infliximab was demonstrated to improve flow-mediated vasodilation in patients with RA [n = 11][34] and patients with AS (n = 12)[35] after 12 weeks of therapy. Conversely, another study that examined pulse wave velocity (PWV), a surrogate measure of arterial stiffness, was not shown to be significantly improved in patients with AS after 24 weeks[36] or after 6 and 12 months[37] of TNFi therapy. In PsA, TNFi compared to other nbDMARDs led to a greater reduction in the development of carotid atherosclerotic plaques after 4 years of treatment, 40.4% of those on TNFi vs 15.8% on nbDMARD.[38] A single-center observational study examined whether TNFi had any effect of coronary artery plaque formation or progression via the evaluation of coronary atherosclerosis by coronary computed tomographic angiography (CCTA) in patients with RA. TNFi therapy was associated with lower CV risk in patients who had evidence of high-risk plaque features at baseline but not in patients without and was associated with the transition to more stable plaque features (OR 4.0 [95% CI 1.015–15.32]). Furthermore, TNFi therapy was associated with low-attenuation plaque regression/loss. These results suggest that TNFi use may alter coronary plaque features and reduce the risk of new coronary plaque in patients with the evidence of atherosclerosis at baseline.[39] Lastly, although some controversy exists, given the association of adverse outcomes in patients with heart failure and TNFi in the general population, TNFi is not currently recommended in patients with inflammatory arthritis with a known history of Class III or Class IV heart failure.[40]

INTERLEUKIN-1 AND INTERLEUKIN-6 INHIBITION

IL-1 and IL-6 are pivotal cytokines in innate immunity and over the past 10 years, increasing evidence have demonstrated an important role for IL-1 and IL-6 in CVD for the general population.[41–44] IL-6 signaling is implicated in plaque initiation and destabilization as well as adverse outcomes in acute coronary syndrome.[45] Tocilizumab is a humanized monoclonal antibody to the soluble IL-6 receptor and is the most commonly prescribed agent with the most data for CV effects. However, additional options such as sarilumab a fully human monoclonal antibody to the IL-6 receptor are also now approved.[46] Both agents are approved bDMARDs utilized in RA predominantly after inadequate response to TNFi.[47] Both IL-1 and IL-6 blockade are not FDA approved agents utilized in the SpA or PsA. Thus, the data on CV risk reduction regarding IL-6 are focused on RA.

Lipid parameters are known to be altered by IL-6 inhibition. The AMBITION study was a randomized clinical trial that examined the efficacy and safety of tocilizumab monotherapy versus methotrexate in patients with active RA. In patients undergoing tocilizumab therapy, total cholesterol, LDL, HDL, and triglycerides increased within the first 24 weeks when compared to methotrexate. However, after week 24 these levels returned to their baseline. Additionally, the ratio of LDL to HDL cholesterol was also unchanged, suggesting that these transient changes in lipid parameters did not result in a more proatherogenic profile.[48,49] Another small study that examined the fractional catabolic rate of LDL in 11 patients with severe RA undergoing tocilizumab therapy found that lower LDL levels were due to the hypercatabolism of LDL particles and IL-6 inhibition reversed this catabolism; these data suggest that hepatic IL-6 signaling plays a role in these lipid alterations.[50] In fact, some data may suggest that IL-6 inhibition provides greater CV risk reduction than TNFi. A meta-analysis examined the comparative effects of TNFi compared to non-TNFi bDMARDS and nbDMARDs on CV risk in patients with RA. Interestingly, tocilizumab was associated with a decreased risk of major adverse CV events (MACE) (OR 0.59 [95% CI 0.34–1.00]) compared to patients on TNFi, although rates of stroke were similar (OR 0.98 [95% CI 0.59–1.61]).[51]

Few studies directly compare bDMARDs and CV risk reduction and existing data on this topic are predominantly in RA. In one systematic review and meta-analysis, a comparison was made between bDMARDs by drug class and overall MACE. In this study, tocilizumab was associated with a reduced risk of MACE compared to TNFi as a group (OR 0.59). In these studies, this protective effect was observed predominantly among patients with pre-existing CVD.[51]

Data on IL-1 inhibition in RA are limited although there are data to support its salutary effect on CV risk in the general population.[41] In a cross-over trial of 80 patients with RA randomized to anakinra or placebo, and after 48 hours to the other treatment, investigators found that IL-1 inhibition was associated with improved coronary flow reserve assessed by doppler flow of the left anterior descending artery (LAD). Data from the general population demonstrated inflammation as an independent risk factor for CVD and that reducing inflammation via IL-1 inhibition, reduced CV risk. The Canakinumab Anti-Inflammatory Thrombosis Outcomes Study (CANTOS) trial was the first large-scale cardiovascular study to show that blocking interleukin-1β prospectively reduced incident CV events without modifying other CV risk markers, e.g. lipid levels.[41] Further, subgroup analyses demonstrated that the magnitude of clinical benefit was directly related to the degree of reduction in IL-6 levels achieved by individual trial participants.[52] These data suggest that IL-6 may be the primary target and has been further supported by recent data from the RESCUE trial showing that ziltivekimab, a novel IL-6 inhibitor, reduced biomarkers of systemic inflammation and thrombosis central to atherosclerosis in patients with chronic kidney disease (CKD) and elevated hsCRP.[53] Based on these results there is now a large double-blinded randomized control trial, Ziltivekimab Cardiovascular Outcomes Study (ZEUS), which will formally test whether reducing circulating IL-6 leads to a reduction in CV event rates with ziltvekiumab compared to placebo in patients with chronic kidney disease and elevated hsCRP.[54]

ABATACEPT

Abatacept is a recombinant fusion CTLA4 protein that inhibits the CD80/CD86 costimulation important in T-cell activation. Similar to tocilizumab and anakinra, abatacept is often used after patients have an inadequate response to TNFi and other nbDMARDS. Limited data exist on the effects of abatacept on CV risk or surrogate markers of CV risk. In the AMPLE study, comparing patients with RA initiating abatacept versus TNFi therapy, HDL function was observed to improve with both treatments.[55] In one comparative effectiveness study of Medicare participants abatacept treatment initiators served as the reference group to compare the incidence of MI. In this study, TNFi initiators had a similar risk of incident MI (adjusted HR 1.3 95% CI 1.0, 1.6) compared to abatacept, and tocilizumab initiators had a lower risk (adjusted HR 0.64 95% CI 0.41, 0.99).[56]

RITUXIMAB

Rituximab is currently only FDA approved for RA and not for other systemic arthritides. It is a chimeric monoclonal antibody specific for B-cell specific cell-surface marker, CD20, and thus depletes B-cells. Given the mechanism and long half-life, it is typically dosed every 6 to 12 months. Limited data exist on the cardiovascular benefit of B-cell depleting therapy. In a small analysis, 6 patients with RA who were refractory to TNFi therapy, rituximab was able to improve endothelial function detected by flow-mediated dilation.[57] Larger studies on B-cell inhibition are needed; B cells are also known to play atheroprotective roles and it is thus plausible that CV risk modulation could be neutral or increased.[58]

INTERLEUKIN-17 AND IL12/23 INHIBITION

Recent data have emerged on the pathogenic role of the Th17/IL17 axis in psoriatic disease and spondyloarthropathies. Although high levels of IL-17A and Th17 cells have been reported in RA, the response to therapy has been mixed and thus are not approved agents for RA. Several anti-IL-17 inhibitors have been developed and are approved for psoriatic arthritis and spondyloarthropathies. These include anti-IL-17A monoclonal antibodies, secukinumab and ixekizumab. IL-12/23 inhibition also blocks the Th17 response and is achieved through targeting p40, a subunit shared by IL-12 and IL-23.[59] IL-12/23, e.g. ustekinumab, and IL-23 inhibitors, e.g. geselkumab, are only approved for psoriatic disease as secondary endpoints were not met for spondylarthritis. Thus far, the data on IL-17 and IL-23 inhibition and cardiovascular benefit have been reported in psoriatic disease and not for PsA specifically or for SpA.

While psoriasis was not a focus of this review, we will briefly cover data on bDMARD studies in psoriasis, for treatments also approved for PsA, examining cardiac imaging data as a surrogate marker of CV risk. Two randomized double-blind placebo-controlled trials examined changes in aortic inflammation as measured using FDG PET of the aorta before and after treatment with the IL-12/23 blocker, ustekinumab, the Vascular Inflammation in Psoriasis (VIP)-U study and another with IL-17A blocker, secukinumab, VIP-S; all subjects had moderate to severe psoriasis. Treatment with ustekinumab in the VIP-U study resulted in a reduction in aortic inflammation measured by FDG PET at 12 weeks (6.6% versus 12.1% in placebo, p = 0.001) yet differences were not seen at 52 weeks; similarly, no differences were observed with secukinumab therapy at 52 weeks,[60,61] suggesting the effects of these treatments on CV risk may be neutral.

Similar to the theme of CV biomarkers, another prospective study examined the role of ustekinumab (IL-12/23 inhibitor) in comparison with TNFα inhibition or cyclosporine therapy in 150 subjects with moderate psoriasis and measured their effects on left ventricular remodeling, the coronary microcirculation (coronary flow reserve (CFR) by LAD doppler echocardiography), arterial stiffness, and biomarkers of oxidative stress and inflammation. There was successful resolution of psoriasis skin disease among all therapies; interestingly, IL-12/23 inhibition displayed a greater improvement in left ventricular strain, arterial stiffness and Doppler assessed LAD CFR.[62] In addition to potential benefit, safety concerns have also been raised predominantly in psoriasis but are relevant in this discussion. An IL-12/23 inhibitor, briakinumab (an IL-12/23 inhibitor) which has the same mechanism of action as guselkumab and ustekinumab approved for PsA, was halted due to safety concerns after one of the 4 clinical trials reported an increase in MACE events.[63,64] In phases II and III placebo-controlled studies for ustekinumab, a total of 5 MACE events occurred all in the ustekinumab arm and these events occurred in patients with at least three cardiovascular risk factors. Unfortunately, the lack of a control group will preclude definitive assessment with long-term follow-up.[65,66] Furthermore, in a recent nationwide cohort study of patients with PsA, a total of 9510 new users of bDMARDs were included and the risk of MACE was assessed from 2015 to 2019. The majority of patients initiated a TNFi (7,289) compared to IL12/23 (1,058), IL-17 (1163), and apremilast (1885) users with a total of 51 (0.4%) MACE events captured. After propensity score weighting, the risk of

MACE was greater in patients with IL12/23 (HR 2.0, 95%CI 1.3–3.0) and IL17 (HR 1.9, 95%CI 1.2–3.0) inhibitors compared to TNFi, with no significant increased risk with apremilast.[67] On the other hand, a meta-analysis encompassing these studies has been performed that incorporates nine independent double-blind, randomized, clinical trials to further assess an association of MACE with psoriatic treatment which did not reveal any significantly observed differences.[68,69]

It is clear that further data are required to clarify the role of these agents in CV risk mitigation. In atherogenic mouse models, IL-17 has been shown to be proatherogenic and functional blockade of IL-17A reduced plaque vulnerability and inflammatory cellular infiltration and cytokine expression.[70–72] Conversely, IL-17 has also been proposed in other models to have antiatherogenic roles.[73–75] These results highlight the context dependence and further highlight that we should exhibit caution in the extrapolation of data to a specific inflammatory disease.[76]

JANUS KINASE INHIBITORS

Janus kinase (JAK) is a family of nonreceptor tyrosine kinases and includes JAK1, JAK2, JAK3, and TYK2 (tyrosine kinase 2) which transmits signals through the signal transducer and activator of transcription (STAT). There are 3 JAK inhibitors approved for use in autoimmune diseases: tofacitinib, baricitinib, and upadacitinib and all are oral small molecules. The JAK-STAT kinase system is implicated as an important pathway for RA, PsA, and SpA and functions upstream of the cytokine cascade.[77]Tofacitinib is currently approved in RA and PsA, and is a nonspecific JAKi, targeting JAK 1, 2, and 3. Baricitinib targets JAK1 and 2. The selective JAK1 inhibitor, upadacitinib, is approved in RA and is currently being evaluated in PsA.[78] Currently, data regarding the cardiovascular safety of JAKi in these inflammatory conditions remain inconclusive. On one hand, there have been six phase III studies and two open-label long-term extension studies of tofacitinib in patients with RA which have shown overall low incidence of cardiovascular events.[79] A meta-analysis of 26 RCTs did not demonstrate significant differences in CV events rate in RA patients treated with JAK inhibitors.[82] Tofacitinib is associated with increases in the lipid parameters; yet the relevance of this on cardiovascular risk is less clear. A small mechanistic prospective demonstrated that tofacitinib could positively affect atherosclerosis by regression of carotid intima media thickness in patients who had elevated levels of baseline.[84] However, more recently, the FDA issued a black box warning of all JAK inhibitors which have added ambiguity after the results of the ORAL-Surveillance study was released.[84] The black box warning is specifically for increased risk of adverse cardiovascular events, malignancy, thrombosis and death in RA. ORAL Surveillance was a prospective, phase 3b/4 randomized, open- label, non-inferiority, study that compared tofacitinib and TNFi, which was mandated by the FDA as part of a post-marketing safety study. This trial enrolled RA patients with inadequate response to MTX, age>50, and at least one cardiovascular risk factor (cigarette smoking, hypertension, hyperlipidemia, DM, family history of premature CAD, prior history of CAD, or extra-articular disease associated with RA). The primary analysis demonstrated increased incidence rates for VTE and MACE when compared with the TNFi group and reached the threshold for a safety signal. This in turn, led to the FDA issuing a black box warning for tofacitinib for the treatment of RA. Increased risk of MACE was higher among patients >65 years, those who had ever smoked or aspirin users. Malignancy rates were also numerically higher compared to the TNF inhibitor group. Whether these results are specific to tofacitinib or specific to RA remains unclear. A meta-analysis that included ORAL-Surveillance analyzed a total of 66 RCTs across inflammatory conditions found that JAK inhibitors had a numerically higher rate of VTE when compared with controls (OR: 1.65; 95% CI: 0.97-2.79) and primarily driven by the studies which had follow-up of greater than 12 months. The increased risk of VTE was observed when compared with active comparators but not with placebo. The results of MACE were similar but did not reach statistical significance.[85] In a study using real-world data comparing tofacitinib vs TNFi with similar parameters as ORAL-Surveillance, no increased CV risk was observed in the overall population; a non-significant trend toward increased CV risk was observed among RA patients initiating tofacitinib with CV risk factors, similar to ORAL-Surveillance.[86] Thus, future clinical trials and mechanistic investigations are needed to understand the role of JAK inhibition in promoting or mitigating cardiovascular disease.

SUMMARY

Overall, the current evidence suggests that the use of bDMARDs mitigate CV risk in patients with inflammatory arthritis; however, the benefit may not be true for all bDMARDs and small molecules. The mixed findings are likely the result of the sample study, the difference in surrogate endpoints and MACE definitions, and heterogeneity of the patient population, and the different pathways targeted. Patients with systemic arthritides and established CV risk factors or known CVD are likely a different patient population compared to systemic arthritis patients without established CV risk factor. As more patients are prescribed these newer therapies, more data will allow us to decipher how to select the best therapy for the individual patient. The emergence of noninvasive cardiovascular imaging modalities that are linked to CV outcomes, such as cardiac PET may serve as important tools that can be employed to help address some of these questions. The integration of a care model with both cardio-rheumatology, a growing field, embedded within routine rheumatologic care will allow a patient-centered approach with risk counseling and individualization of therapy.[8,80,81,83] The rapid expansion of bDMARDs and small molecules for the treatment of inflammatory arthritis has provided a growing armamentarium for the rheumatologist. Along with new CV imaging tools, the specificity of each inflammatory pathway and the effect on coronary vascular health and cardiovascular risk can now be addressed.

FUNDING

B. Weber is funded, in part, by an NIH K23 HL159276-01 and American Heart Association, United States Career Development Grant (Dallas, TX) 21CDA851511. K.P. Liao reports grants from NIH, United States R01 HL127118, Harold and DuVal Bowen Fund.

COMPLIANCE WITH ETHICAL STANDARDS
Conflict of Interest

B. Weber has nothing to disclose. K.P. Liao has nothing to disclose.

HUMAN AND ANIMAL RIGHTS AND INFORMED CONSENT

All procedures performed by the authors of this review in studies involving human participants were in accordance with the ethical standards of the institutional and/or national research committee and with the 1964 Helsinki Declaration and its later amendments or comparable ethical standards.

CLINICS CARE POINTS

- Biologic dMARDS are highy efficacious to control disease activity in inflammatory arthrits.
- The translation of bDMARD to migitation of CV risk is overall favorable although currently mixed findings suggest that not all bdMARDs and small molecules benefit CV risk mitigation equally.

REFERENCES

1. Agca R, Heslinga SC, van Halm VP, et al. Atherosclerotic cardiovascular disease in patients with chronic inflammatory joint disorders. Heart 2016;102:790–5.
2. Gelfand JM, Troxel AB, Lewis JD, et al. The risk of mortality in patients with psoriasis: results from a population-based study. Arch Dermatol 2007;143:1493–9.
3. Urowitz MB, Gladman D, Ibañez D, et al. Atherosclerotic vascular events in a multinational inception cohort of systemic lupus erythematosus. Arthritis Care Res (Hoboken) 2010;62:881–7.
4. Avina-Zubieta JA, Thomas J, Sadatsafavi M, et al. Risk of incident cardiovascular events in patients with rheumatoid arthritis: a meta-analysis of observational studies. Ann Rheum Dis 2012;71:1524–9.
5. England BR, Thiele GM, Anderson DR, et al. Increased cardiovascular risk in rheumatoid arthritis: mechanisms and implications. BMJ 2018;361:k1036.
6. Liew JW, Ramiro S, Gensler LS. Cardiovascular morbidity and mortality in ankylosing spondylitis and psoriatic arthritis. Best Pract Res Clin Rheumatol 2018;32: 369–89.
7. Teague H, Mehta NN. The link between inflammatory disorders and coronary heart disease: a look at recent studies and novel drugs in development. Curr Atheroscler Rep 2016;18:3.
8. Weber B, Liao KP, DiCarli M, et al. Cardiovascular disease prevention in individuals with underlying chronic inflammatory disease. Curr Opin Cardiol 2021;36: 549–55.
9. Davignon J, Ganz P. Role of endothelial dysfunction in atherosclerosis. Circulation 2004;109:III-27.
10. Cahill PA, Redmond EM. Vascular endothelium – Gatekeeper of vessel health. Atherosclerosis 2016;248:97–109.
11. Boulanger CM. Endothelium. Arterioscler Thromb Vasc Biol 2016;36:e26–31.
12. Hansson GK, Robertson A-KL, Söderberg-Nauclér C. Inflammation and atherosclerosis. Annu Rev Pathol 2006;1:297–329.
13. Libby P. Inflammation in atherosclerosis. Arterioscler Thromb Vasc Biol 2012;32: 2045–51.
14. Libby P, Buring JE, Badimon L, et al. Atherosclerosis. Nat Rev Dis Primers 2019; 5:56.
15. Abuabara K, Azfar RS, Shin DB, et al. Cause-specific mortality in patients with severe psoriasis: a population-based cohort study in the United Kingdom. Br J Dermatol 2010;163:586–92.
16. Kaye JA, Li L, Jick SS. Incidence of risk factors for myocardial infarction and other vascular diseases in patients with psoriasis. Br J Dermatol 2008;159: 895–902.
17. Shah K, Mellars L, Changolkar A, et al. Real-world burden of comorbidities in US patients with psoriasis. J Am Acad Dermatol 2017;77:287–92.e4.

18. Sommer DM, Jenisch S, Suchan M, et al. Increased prevalence of the metabolic syndrome in patients with moderate to severe psoriasis. Arch Dermatol Res 2006; 298:321–8.

19. Raychaudhuri SK, Chatterjee S, Nguyen C, et al. Increased Prevalence of the Metabolic Syndrome in Patients with Psoriatic Arthritis. Metab Syndr Relat Disord 2010;8:331–4.

20. Azfar RS, Seminara NM, Shin DB, et al. Increased risk of diabetes mellitus and likelihood of receiving diabetes mellitus treatment in patients with psoriasis. Arch Dermatol 2012;148:995–1000.

21. Kimhi O, Caspi D, Bornstein NM, et al. Prevalence and risk factors of atherosclerosis in patients with psoriatic arthritis. Semin Arthritis Rheum 2007;36:203–9.

22. del Rincón I, Polak JF, O'Leary DH, et al. Systemic inflammation and cardiovascular risk factors predict rapid progression of atherosclerosis in rheumatoid arthritis. Ann Rheum Dis 2015;74:1118–23.

23. Navarro-Millán I, Yang S, DuVall SL, et al. Association of hyperlipidaemia, inflammation and serological status and coronary heart disease among patients with rheumatoid arthritis: data from the National Veterans Health Administration. Ann Rheum Dis 2016;75:341–7.

24. Solomon DH, Kremer J, Curtis JR, et al. Explaining the cardiovascular risk associated with rheumatoid arthritis: traditional risk factors versus markers of rheumatoid arthritis severity. Ann Rheum Dis 2010;69:1920–5.

25. Liao KP, Liu J, Lu B, et al. Association between lipid levels and major adverse cardiovascular events in rheumatoid arthritis compared to non–rheumatoid arthritis patients. Arthritis Rheum 2015;67:2004–10.

26. Yiu ZZN, Exton LS, Jabbar-Lopez Z, et al. Risk of serious infections in patients with psoriasis on biologic therapies: a systematic review and meta-analysis. J Invest Dermatol 2016;136:1584–91.

27. Jani M, Barton A, Hyrich K. Prediction of infection risk in rheumatoid arthritis patients treated with biologics: are we any closer to risk stratification? Curr Opin Rheumatol 2019;31:285–92.

28. Barnabe C, Martin B-J, Ghali WA. Systematic review and meta-analysis: anti-tumor necrosis factor α therapy and cardiovascular events in rheumatoid arthritis. Arthritis Care Res (Hoboken) 2011;63:522–9.

29. Low ASL, Symmons DPM, Lunt M, et al. Relationship between exposure to tumour necrosis factor inhibitor therapy and incidence and severity of myocardial infarction in patients with rheumatoid arthritis. Ann Rheum Dis 2017;76:654–60.

30. Jacobsson LTH, Turesson C, Nilsson J-A, et al. Treatment with TNF blockers and mortality risk in patients with rheumatoid arthritis. Ann Rheum Dis 2007;66:670–5.

31. Low ASL, Lunt M, Mercer LK, et al. Association between ischemic stroke and tumor necrosis factor inhibitor therapy in patients with rheumatoid arthritis. Arthritis Rheum 2016;68:1337–45.

32. Naranjo A, Sokka T, Descalzo MA, et al. Cardiovascular disease in patients with rheumatoid arthritis: results from the QUEST-RA study. Arthritis Res Ther 2008; 10:R30.

33. Lee JL, Sinnathurai P, Buchbinder R, et al. Biologics and cardiovascular events in inflammatory arthritis: a prospective national cohort study. Arthritis Res Ther 2018;20:171.

34. Hürlimann D, Forster A, Noll G, et al. Anti-tumor necrosis factor-alpha treatment improves endothelial function in patients with rheumatoid arthritis. Circulation 2002;106:2184–7.

35. Syngle A, Vohra K, Sharma A, et al. Endothelial dysfunction in ankylosing spondylitis improves after tumor necrosis factor-alpha blockade. Clin Rheumatol 2010; 29:763–70.
36. Capkin E, Karkucak M, Kiris A, et al. Anti-TNF-α therapy may not improve arterial stiffness in patients with AS: a 24-week follow-up. Rheumatology (Oxford) 2012; 51:910–4.
37. Mathieu S, Pereira B, Couderc M, et al. No significant changes in arterial stiffness in patients with ankylosing spondylitis after tumour necrosis factor alpha blockade treatment for 6 and 12 months. Rheumatology (Oxford) 2013;52:204–9.
38. Di Minno MND, Iervolino S, Peluso R, et al, CaRRDs study group. Carotid intima-media thickness in psoriatic arthritis: differences between tumor necrosis factor-α blockers and traditional disease-modifying antirheumatic drugs. Arterioscler Thromb Vasc Biol 2011;31:705–12.
39. Karpouzas GA, Ormseth SR, Hernandez E, et al. Biologics May Prevent Cardiovascular Events in Rheumatoid Arthritis by Inhibiting Coronary Plaque Formation and Stabilizing High-Risk Lesions. Arthritis Rheum 2020;72:1467–75.
40. Elmets CA, Leonardi CL, Davis DMR, et al. Joint AAD-NPF guidelines of care for the management and treatment of psoriasis with awareness and attention to comorbidities. J Am Acad Dermatol 2019;80:1073–113.
41. Ridker PM, Everett BM, Thuren T, et al. Antiinflammatory therapy with canakinumab for atherosclerotic disease. N Engl J Med 2017;377:1119–31.
42. Ridker PM. From CRP to IL-6 to IL-1: moving upstream to identify novel targets for atheroprotection. Circ Res 2016;118:145–56.
43. Ridker PM, Rane M. Interleukin-6 signaling and anti-interleukin-6 therapeutics in cardiovascular disease. Circ Res 2021;128:1728–46.
44. Ridker PM, MacFadyen JG, Glynn RJ, et al. Comparison of interleukin-6, C-reactive protein, and low-density lipoprotein cholesterol as biomarkers of residual risk in contemporary practice: secondary analyses from the Cardiovascular Inflammation Reduction Trial. Eur Heart J. Available at: https://academic.oup.com/eurheartj/advance-article/doi/10.1093/eurheartj/ehaa160/5813080. Accessed April 6, 2020.
45. Lindmark E, Diderholm E, Wallentin L, et al. Relationship between interleukin 6 and mortality in patients with unstable coronary artery disease: effects of an early invasive or noninvasive strategy. JAMA 2001;286:2107–13.
46. Lamb YN, Deeks ED. Sarilumab: A Review in Moderate to Severe Rheumatoid Arthritis. Drugs 2018;78:929–40.
47. Smolen JS, Landewé RBM, Bijlsma JWJ, et al. EULAR recommendations for the management of rheumatoid arthritis with synthetic and biological disease-modifying antirheumatic drugs: 2019 update. Ann Rheum Dis 2020;79:685–99.
48. Cacciapaglia F, Anelli MG, Rinaldi A, et al. Lipids and Atherogenic Indices Fluctuation in Rheumatoid Arthritis Patients on Long-Term Tocilizumab Treatment. Mediators Inflamm 2018;2018:2453265.
49. Jones G, Sebba A, Gu J, et al. Comparison of tocilizumab monotherapy versus methotrexate monotherapy in patients with moderate to severe rheumatoid arthritis: the AMBITION study. Ann Rheum Dis 2010;69:88–96.
50. Robertson J, Porter D, Sattar N, et al. Interleukin-6 blockade raises LDL via reduced catabolism rather than via increased synthesis: a cytokine-specific mechanism for cholesterol changes in rheumatoid arthritis. Ann Rheum Dis 2017;76:1949–52.
51. Singh S, Fumery M, Singh AG, et al. Comparative Risk of Cardiovascular Events With Biologic and Synthetic Disease-Modifying Antirheumatic Drugs in Patients

With Rheumatoid Arthritis: A Systematic Review and Meta-Analysis. Arthritis Care Res 2020;72:561–76.

52. Ridker PM, Libby P, MacFadyen JG, et al. Modulation of the interleukin-6 signalling pathway and incidence rates of atherosclerotic events and all-cause mortality: analyses from the Canakinumab Anti-Inflammatory Thrombosis Outcomes Study (CANTOS). Eur Heart J 2018;39:3499–507.

53. Ridker PM, Devalaraja M, Baeres FMM, et al. IL-6 inhibition with ziltivekimab in patients at high atherosclerotic risk (RESCUE): a double-blind, randomised, placebo-controlled, phase 2 trial. The Lancet 2021;397:2060–9.

54. Ridker PM. From RESCUE to ZEUS: will interleukin-6 inhibition with ziltivekimab prove effective for cardiovascular event reduction? Cardiovasc Res 2021;117: e138–40.

55. Charles-Schoeman C, Gugiu GB, Ge H, et al. Remodeling of the HDL proteome with treatment response to abatacept or adalimumab in the AMPLE trial of patients with rheumatoid arthritis. Atherosclerosis 2018;275:107–14.

56. Zhang J, Xie F, Yun H, et al. Comparative effects of biologics on cardiovascular risk among older patients with rheumatoid arthritis. Ann Rheum Dis 2016;75: 1813–8.

57. Gonzalez-Juanatey C, Vazquez-Rodriguez TR, Miranda-Filloy JA, et al. The high prevalence of subclinical atherosclerosis in patients with ankylosing spondylitis without clinically evident cardiovascular disease. Medicine (Baltimore) 2009;88: 358–65.

58. Kyaw T, Tipping P, Bobik A, et al. Opposing roles of B lymphocyte subsets in atherosclerosis. Autoimmunity 2017;50:52–6.

59. Stritesky GL, Yeh N, Kaplan MH. IL-23 promotes maintenance but not commitment to the Th17 lineage. J Immunol 2008;181:5948–55.

60. Gelfand JM, Shin DB, Alavi A, et al. A Phase IV, Randomized, double-blind, placebo-controlled crossover study of the effects of ustekinumab on vascular inflammation in psoriasis (the VIP-U Trial). J Invest Dermatol 2020;140:85–93.e2.

61. Gelfand JM, Shin DB, Duffin KC, et al. A Randomized Placebo-Controlled Trial of Secukinumab on Aortic Vascular Inflammation in Moderate-to-Severe Plaque Psoriasis (VIP-S). J Invest Dermatol 2020;140:1784–93.e2.

62. Ignatios I, Evangelia P, George M, et al. Lowering interleukin-12 activity improves myocardial and vascular function compared with tumor necrosis factor-a antagonism or cyclosporine in psoriasis. Circ Cardiovasc Imaging 2017;10:e006283.

63. Gordon KB, Langley RG, Gottlieb AB, et al. A phase III, randomized, controlled trial of the fully human IL-12/23 mAb briakinumab in moderate-to-severe psoriasis. J Invest Dermatol 2012;132:304–14.

64. Tzellos T, Kyrgidis A, Trigoni A, et al. Association of ustekinumab and briakinumab with major adverse cardiovascular events. Dermatoendocrinol 2012;4: 320–3.

65. Reich K, Langley RG, Lebwohl M, et al. Cardiovascular safety of ustekinumab in patients with moderate to severe psoriasis: results of integrated analyses of data from phase II and III clinical studies. Br J Dermatol 2011;164:862–72.

66. Reich K, Papp KA, Griffiths CEM, et al. An update on the long-term safety experience of ustekinumab: results from the psoriasis clinical development program with up to four years of follow-up. J Drugs Dermatol 2012;11:300–12.

67. Pina Vegas L, Le Corvoisier P, Penso L, et al. Risk of major adverse cardiovascular events in patients initiating biologics/apremilast for psoriatic arthritis: a nationwide cohort study. Rheumatology. 2021. Available at: https://doi.org/10.1093/rheumatology/keab522. Accessed July 22, 2021.

68. Ryan C, Leonardi CL, Krueger JG, et al. Association between biologic therapies for chronic plaque psoriasis and cardiovascular events: a meta-analysis of randomized controlled trials. JAMA 2011;306:864–71.

69. Tzellos T, Kyrgidis A, Zouboulis CC. Re-evaluation of the risk for major adverse cardiovascular events in patients treated with anti-IL-12/23 biological agents for chronic plaque psoriasis: a meta-analysis of randomized controlled trials. J Eur Acad Dermatol Venereol 2013;27:622–7.

70. Erbel C, Akhavanpoor M, Okuyucu D, et al. IL-17A influences essential functions of the monocyte/macrophage lineage and is involved in advanced murine and human atherosclerosis. J Immunol 2014;193:4344–55.

71. Karbach S, Croxford AL, Oelze M, et al. Interleukin 17 drives vascular inflammation, endothelial dysfunction, and arterial hypertension in psoriasis-like skin disease. Arterioscler Thromb Vasc Biol 2014;34:2658–68.

72. Butcher MJ, Gjurich BN, Phillips T, et al. The IL-17A/IL-17RA axis plays a proatherogenic role via the regulation of aortic myeloid cell recruitment. Circ Res 2012;110:675–87.

73. Taleb S, Tedgui A, Mallat Z. IL-17 and Th17 cells in atherosclerosis: subtle and contextual roles. Arterioscler Thromb Vasc Biol 2015;35:258–64.

74. Gagliani N, Amezcua Vesely MC, Iseppon A, et al. Th17 cells transdifferentiate into regulatory T cells during resolution of inflammation. Nature 2015;523:221–5.

75. Brauner S, Jiang X, Thorlacius GE, et al. Augmented Th17 differentiation in Trim21 deficiency promotes a stable phenotype of atherosclerotic plaques with high collagen content. Cardiovasc Res 2018;114:158–67.

76. Lockshin B, Balagula Y, Merola JF. Interleukin 17, inflammation, and cardiovascular risk in patients with psoriasis. J Am Acad Dermatol 2018;79:345–52.

77. Gao W, McGarry T, Orr C, et al. Tofacitinib regulates synovial inflammation in psoriatic arthritis, inhibiting STAT activation and induction of negative feedback inhibitors. Ann Rheum Dis 2016;75:311–5.

78. D'Urso DF, Chiricozzi A, Pirro F, et al. New JAK inhibitors for the treatment of psoriasis and psoriatic arthritis. G Ital Dermatol Venereol 2020;155:411–20.

79. Charles-Schoeman C, Wicker P, Gonzalez-Gay MA, et al. Cardiovascular safety findings in patients with rheumatoid arthritis treated with tofacitinib, an oral Janus kinase inhibitor. Semin Arthritis Rheum 2016;46(3):261–71.

80. Yoo BW. Embarking on a Career in Cardio-Rheumatology. J Am Coll Cardiol 2020; 75:1488–92.

81. Anon A. Collaborative cardio-rheumatology clinic for primary prevention of cardiovascular diseases - a descriptive study. ACR Meeting Abstracts. Available at: https://acrabstracts.org/abstract/a-collaborative-cardio-rheumatology-clinic-for-primary-prevention-of-cardiovascular-diseases-a-descriptive-study/. Accessed February 17, 2021.

82. Xie W, Huang Y, Xiao S, et al. Impact of Janus kinase inhibitors on risk of cardiovascular events in patients with rheumatoid arthritis: systematic review and meta-analysis of randomised controlled trials. Meta-Analysis Ann Rheum Dis 2019; 78(8):1048–54.

83. Kume K, Amano K, Yamada S, et al. Tofacitinib improves atherosclerosis despite up-regulating serum cholesterol in patients with active rheumatoid arthritis: a cohort study. Rheumatology international 2017;37:2079–85.

84. Ytterberg SR, Bhatt DL, Mikuls TR, et al. Cardiovascular and Cancer Risk with Tofacitinib in Rheumatoid Arthritis. Randomized Controlled Trial N Engl J Med 2022; 386(4):316–26.

85. Maqsood MH, Weber BN, Haberman RH, et al. Cardiovascular and Venous Thromboembolic Risk With Janus Kinase Inhibitors in Immune-Mediated Inflammatory Diseases: A Systematic Review and Meta-Analysis of Randomized Trials. ACR Open Rheumatology 2022. https://doi.org/10.1002/acr2.11479.
86. Khosrow-Khavar F, Kim SC, Lee H, et al. Tofacitinib and risk of cardiovascular outcomes: results from the Safety of TofAcitinib in Routine care patients with Rheumatoid Arthritis (STAR-RA) study. Ann Rheum Dis 2022;81:798–804.

Recommendations for the Use of Nonsteroidal Anti-inflammatory Drugs and Cardiovascular Disease Risk

Decades Later, Any New Lessons Learned?

Deeba Minhas, MD[a],*, Anjali Nidhaan, MD[b],
M. Elaine Husni, MD, MPH[b]

KEYWORDS

- Nonsteroidal anti-inflammatory drugs • NSAIDs • Cardiovascular risk • Coxibs
- Nonselective

KEY POINTS

- Nonsteroidal anti-inflammatory drugs (NSAIDs) are among the most prescribed pharmacologic therapeutics worldwide.
- All NSAIDs, including both traditional and cyclo-oxygenase 2 (COX-2) selective, increase the risk of a cardiovascular adverse event.
- It is important to assess the benefit versus the risk of treatment before initiating NSAID treatment in each patient.
- Use the lowest dose of NSAIDs for the shortest amount of time.

INTRODUCTION

Nonsteroidal anti-inflammatory drugs (NSAIDs) are among the most widely prescribed medicines in the world due to their anti-inflammatory, analgesic, and pyretic effect properties (**Fig. 1**). Their therapeutic benefits result from the reduction of prostaglandin synthesis by their inhibition of the cyclo-oxygenase (COX) enzyme. Initial safety concerns were focused on the COX-1-dependent gastrointestinal toxicity of NSAIDs. Since the advent of selective cyclo-oxygenase 2 (COX-2) inhibitors (also known as coxibs), non-GI toxicities were highlighted such as the cardiovascular (CV) risk profile of NSAIDs.

Practical advise on NSAID use for PCPs.
[a] Department of Internal Medicine, Division of Rheumatology, University of Michigan, 300 North Ingalls Building, Ann Arbor, MI 48109-5422, USA; [b] Cleveland Clinic, Cleveland, 9500 Euclid Ave, Cleveland, Ohio 44195, USA
* Corresponding author.
E-mail address: minhasde@med.umich.edu

Rheum Dis Clin N Am 49 (2023) 179–191
https://doi.org/10.1016/j.rdc.2022.08.006
0889-857X/23/© 2022 Elsevier Inc. All rights reserved.

Table 1
Cardiovascular outcomes in select NSAID trials

Trial, Year	Patients	NSAID	Study Duration	Results	Limitations
PRECISION, 2016	Patients ages > 18 y with OA or RA and established or high risk of CV disease (N = 24,081)	Celecoxib 200 mg (OA) Celecoxib 400 mg (RA) vs Ibuprofen Ave dose 2045 mg vs Naproxen Ave dose 852 mg	20.3 ± 16.0 mo; total 34.1 ± 13.4 mo follow-up	ITT Celecoxib vs ibuprofen HR 0.85; 95% CI 0.7–1.04 Celecoxib vs naproxen HR 0.93; 95% CI 0.76–1.04 On treatment Celecoxib vs ibuprofen HR 0.81%; 95% CI 0.65–1.02 Celecoxib vs naproxen HR 0.90%; 95% CI 0.71–1.15 Low overall event rate celecoxib 2.3%; naproxen 2.5%; ibuprofen 2.7%	70% Drug discontinuation rate Unable to increase celecoxib dosing is OA group
SCOT, 2017	Patients ages >60 y with RA or OA (N = 7297)	Celecoxib vs nonselective NSAIDs	Median follow-up 3 y	MACE (per 100 PY) 1.14 vs 1.10 h, 1.04; 95% CI 0.81–1.33	Withdrawal from treatment: 48.2% vs 31.5%
MEDAL, 2006	Patients ages >50 y with RA or OA (N = 34,701)	Etoricoxib 60 mg (OA) Etoricoxib 90 mg (RA) vs diclofenac 150 mg	18 mo	Composite of any thrombotic CV events[a] Etoricoxib vs diclofenac HR 0.90%; 95% CI 0.81–1.11 Event rate (per 100 PY) Etoricoxib 1.24%; diclofenac 1.3%	Etoricoxib dosages differences not included in analysis

Study	Population	Intervention	Duration	Results	Comments
TARGET, 2004		Ibuprofen 800 mg TID vs lumiracoxib 400 mg/d	X52 wk	High-risk using ASA MACE 0.25% vs 2.14% (HR 9.08) High-risk NOT using ASA MACE 0.80% vs 0.92% (HR 0.91)	Post hoc analysis; not placebo controlled, 43% drug discontinuation
		Naproxen 500 mg BID vs lumiracoxib 400 mg/d		High-risk using ASA MACE 1.48% vs 1.58% (HR, 1.07) High-risk NOT using ASA MACE 1.57% vs 0% (HR, N/A)	
APPROVe, 2008	Patients with colorectal adenoma (N = 2586)	Rofecoxib 25 mg/d vs placebo X3 y	X3 y	Thrombotic event 1.50 vs 0.78 (HR 2.32) Cardiac events 1.01 vs 0.36 (HR 2.32) CVA events 0.49 vs 0.21 (HR 2.32)	Withdrawal from treatment: 31.9% vs 24.6%
Danish Registry	Patients > 30 y with first-time MI (N = 83,675)	Any NSAID	Variable	Risk for death or recurrent MI (>90 d tx) All NSAIDs: HR 1.55 Diclofenac: HR 1.92 Rofecoxib: HR 1.72 Celecoxib: HR 1.65 Ibuprofen: HR 1.53 Naproxen: HR 1.50 Other NSAIDs: HR 1.44	Observational design; informational bias

Abbreviations: ASA, aspirin; Ave, average; CI, confidence interval; CV, cardiovascular; HR, hazard ratio; ITT, intention to treat; MACE, major adverse cardiac events; MI, myocardial infarction; OA, osteoarthritis; PY, patient years; RA, rheumatoid arthritis; TID, three times a day.
[a] Composite of any thrombotic CV events, defined as sudden or unexplained death, MI, unstable angina pectoris, resuscitated cardiac arrest, thrombotic stroke, cerebrovascular thrombosis, transient ischemic attack, peripheral venous thrombosis, pulmonary embolism, and peripheral arterial thrombosis, evaluated for noninferiority.

All NSAIDs, including both traditional nonselective NSAIDs (nsNSAIDs) and COX-2 selective NSAIDs, increase the risk of a CV adverse event including increased risks of atherothrombotic events, myocardial infarction (MI), and cerebrovascular events (CVA) along with heart failure (HF) elevated blood pressure (BP), arrhythmias, and cardiac arrest.

In particular, patients with systemic rheumatic conditions may be more vulnerable as their conditions are lifelong requiring more chronic use. Rheumatologic diseases are associated with increased mortality compared with the general population with a major part of the excess mortality attributed to increased CV risk regardless of medications.[1] Balancing the need for pain relief with adverse effects of therapeutics is challenging and made even more so by the opiate epidemic and lack of analgesic options in the pharmaceutical pipeline. Educating clinicians on proper risk stratification of patients based on comorbidities to their choice of NSAIDs will be imperative to provide patients with the greatest pain relief while reducing side effects. In this review, we summarize the current evidence on the CV safety of NSAIDs and present an approach for their use in the context of rheumatologic chronic pain management.

Mechanisms of Cyclo-oxygenase

NSAIDs reduce inflammation by inhibiting the production of COX, which is involved in prostaglandin synthesis. There are 2 major isoforms of the COX enzyme: COX-1 and COX-2. The COX-1 is the "constitutive" isoform, ubiquitously expressed throughout the body all the time, and involved in hemostatic functions. COX-2 is the more "inducible" isoform expressed in response to inflammatory stimuli.

Platelets, which are involved in CV hemostasis including vascular and cardiac remodeling, express only COX-1, whereas endothelial cells express both COX-1 and COX-2. Both isozymes catalyze the conversion of arachidonic acid, via intermediates, to thromboxane A2 (TXA2), which promotes platelet aggregation and acts as a vasoconstrictor (prothrombotic), and prostacyclin (PGI2), an inhibitor of platelet aggregation and a vasodilator (antithrombotic) that also promotes renal sodium excretion.[2-4]

Aspirin (ASA) irreversibly binds to COX-1 leading to long-lasting suppression of TXA2, a vasoconstrictor and potent platelet activator, leading to ASA's antithrombotic properties. A proposed mechanism of increased thrombosis with NSAIDs occurs when COX-2 is inhibited relative to COX-1. The prothrombotic/antithrombotic balance on the endothelial surface shifts in favor of thrombosis by suppressing PGI2, while COX-1-dependent TXA2 is unopposed.[2,3]

Other mechanisms of NSAID-related CV toxicity involve inhibition of the biosynthesis of prostanoids involved in the maintenance of renal blood flow, especially Prostaglandin E2 and PGI2.[4] This may promote sodium and fluid retention, increase BP, and worsen HF[5,6] as detailed in **Fig. 1**.

NSAIDs are generally divided into nonselective, including naproxen, ibuprofen, diclofenac, meloxicam, and many others, and selective COX-2 inhibitors, such as celecoxib, rofecoxib, and etoricoxib. Importantly COX-selectivity is relative, rather than absolute.

Etoricoxib and rofecoxib have around 300-fold greater inhibitory activity against COX-2 than against COX-1 (IC_{50} ratio), while celecoxib (a selective COX-2 inhibitor) has a much lower activity (IC_{50} ratio 30) and is actually similar to diclofenac (a traditional NSAID commonly cited to have an IC_{50} ratio of 29). Naproxen and ibuprofen are relatively COX-1 selective.[7-9]

The first coxib, celecoxib (Celebrex), received Food and Drug Administration (FDA) approval in 1998 and was followed soon by rofecoxib (Vioxx) in 1999 along with several others. Without COX-1 inhibition, coxibs were expected to provide analgesic and anti-inflammatory therapy with lower incidence of severe GI side effects.

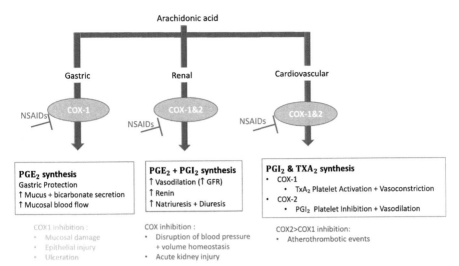

Fig. 1. Mechanisms of NSAID cardiovascular toxicity.

Did Coxibs Create Cardiovascular Hazards?

The coxibs were meant to prevent GI issues; however, a signal of potential CV hazards was also noted. The Vioxx Gastrointestinal Outcomes Research (VIGOR) trial[10] aimed to study the incidence of upper GI events in 8000 patients with rheumatoid arthritis (RA) or osteoarthritis (OA) taking either rofecoxib or naproxen.

While the trial showed a 53% decrease in the risk of upper GI toxicity, it unexpectedly discovered a fivefold increase in the risk of MI for rofecoxib compared with naproxen. This was surprising; however, notably the actual number of events was small (0.4 vs 0.1%), the duration of follow-up was short, and there was no placebo group.[10]

A new safety label was added to Vioxx in April 2002 after these results were discussed at a February 2001 Arthritis Advisory Committee. Merck planned to conduct trials to collect longer-term data on CV events with chronic use of Vioxx.

In September 2004, Merck voluntarily withdrew rofecoxib from the market, based on data from the Adenomatous Polyp PRevention On Vioxx (APPROVe) trial. This trial, assessing the efficacy of rofecoxib in prevention of colon polyp recurrence, was terminated early due to CV events. Twice the incidence of thromboembolic events, MI, and CVA (relative risk 1.92, 95% confidence interval [CI] 1.19–3.11, $P = .008$) were noted after 18 months in the rofecoxib arm when compared with placebo.[11] There was also increase in the composite of congestive heart failure, pulmonary edema, cardiac failure (hazard ratio [HR] 4.61, 95% CI 1.50–18.81), and hypertension (HR 2.02, 95% CI 1.71–2.38) which occurred much earlier in the study.[11] Additionally, a post hoc decision analysis of VIGOR in 2005 reported a longer projected life expectancy for the average RA patient taking naproxen than for the patient taking rofecoxib.[12]

In 2006, Kearney and colleagues published a meta-analysis of randomized controlled trials (RCTs) of NSAIDs and CV safety that reported that along with coxibs, ibuprofen and diclofenac might also enhance atherothrombotic risk, but these might depend on the degree and duration of suppression of platelet COX-1.[13] High-dose naproxen, unique among NSAIDs in that it is able to induce near-complete suppression of platelet TXA2 biosynthesis throughout the 12-hour dosing interval, did not appear to increase the risk.[13]

Other studies around this time did not find the same CV signal with coxibs. The Celecoxib Long-term Arthritis Safety Study (CLASS), a GI safety study, found no differences in the risk of CV events between celecoxib and 2 widely used traditional NSAIDs, ibuprofen and diclofenac, in patients with RA or OA.[14] The Multinational Etoricoxib and Diclofenac Arthritis Long-term (MEDAL) program showed no difference between etoricoxib and high-dose diclofenac for CV events.[15] These results should be interpreted with caution, as CLASS was underpowered with only 15 CVA events and 21 MI in total,[14] and the comparator group in MEDAL with diclofenac had higher COX-2 selectivity than other tNSAIDs.[15] Ultimately, in 2005, the FDA asked manufacturers to revise labeling for all NSAIDs to include black box warning on the increased risk of CV events and GI bleeding associated with their use.

The sponsors of the coxib trials provided data to assemble a database of all published and unpublished trials involving coxibs and NSAIDs to further characterize CV risk of NSAIDs among different patient subtypes, especially those at increased risk of CV disease. This resulted in the 2013 Coxib and traditional NSAID Trialists' (CNT) collaboration, a meta-analysis of 297 trials that published results supporting Kearney and colleagues's findings.[13] CV risks among the tNSAIDs versus placebo were highest with high-dose diclofenac (HR 1.41, 1.12-1.78) and ibuprofen (HR 1.44, 0.89-2.33) but were comparable to those with coxibs. Naproxen 500-mg twice daily dosing was associated with less CV risk than other NSAIDs (HR 0.93, 0.69-1.27).[16]

Following the publication of the CNT meta-analysis, the European Medicines Agency and FDA mandated 2 large safety trials, the Standard care vs. Celecoxib Outcome Trial (SCOT) trial[17] and Prospective Randomized Evaluation of Celecoxib Integrated Safety versus Ibuprofen or Naproxen (PRECISION) trial.[18]

The SCOT trial[17] assessed patients without established CV disease and currently on nsNSAIDs who were randomized to switch to celecoxib or continue their nsNSAID; no difference in CV events was found between both groups.[17] Notably, despite the improved GI profile with celecoxib, more patients in this arm discontinued treatment (48.2% vs 31.5%) mainly due to lack of efficacy.[17]

The PRECISION trial randomized 24,081 patients with OA (90%) or RA and elevated CV risk and reported celecoxib noninferiority to ibuprofen and naproxen with regard to primary CV outcomes after 3 years.[18] This contrasted with studies that previously had acknowledged potential CV safety advantage of naproxen.

The PRECISION trial was unique in that this was a very large *prospective* study using a "noninferiority" trial design. The trial was event-driven, requiring 762 events of the primary endpoint (a composite of death from CV causes, including hemorrhagic death, nonfatal MI, or nonfatal CVA) to provide 90% power to demonstrate noninferiority. However, the observed event rate was lower (1%) than expected, 69% of patients discontinued the study drug, and 27% were lost to follow-up. These factors along with slow recruitment resulted in lowering the power and level considered to be noninferior.[18] Additionally, among the OA patients using celecoxib, the dose was limited by FDA-labeling resulting in the comparatively weaker efficacy documented by pain score and may be associated with lowering rate of GI adverse effects. PRECISION provides insights into CV safety in tNSAIDs and coxibs, overall noting that celecoxib was noninferior to naproxen and ibuprofen in terms of CV risk. Most interesting is the very low rates of CV events with any of the NSAIDs overall[18]

Danish Registries

A series of Danish cohort studies has been published regarding the CV risks of NSAIDs, using data from a nationwide health care and prescription registry established in 1995. They have particularly been able to highlight the CV risks of diclo-fenac, the most widely prescribed NSAID in their database.

Gislason and colleagues reported that in patients with previous MI, there was an increased risk of death associated with any use of both the nsNSAIDs and coxibs, which was dose-dependent.[19] Notably, diclofenac had a similar risk of death (HR 2.40%, 95% CI 2.09–2.80) as rofecoxib (HR 2.80%, 95% CI 2.41–3.25) and celecoxib (HR 2.57%, 95% CI 2.15–3.08), higher than that of both ibuprofen (HR 1.50%, 95% CI 1.36–1.67) and other NSAIDs (HR 1.29%, 95% CI 1.16–1.43).[19]

Another study found diclofenac initiators were at increased risk of major adverse CV events (MACEs)—compared with no NSAID initiation, initiation of paracetamol as an analgesic alternative to NSAIDs, as well as initiation of other traditional NSAIDs.[7] They went on to show that the increased risk was already seen within the first 30 days, specifically in the first week with diclofenac (HR 3.52, 2.93–4.20), the second week with rofecoxib (HR 2.57, 1.91–3.46) and ibuprofen (HR 1.57, 1.27–1.94), and the third week with celecoxib (HR 2.33, 1.79–3.02).[20] After MI, the risk of reinfarction and death decreased over time although the increased risks with NSAID treatment overall persisted for at least 5 years.[21]

Similarly in patients with HF on NSAIDs after hospital discharge, the risk of death was dose-dependent and highest in coxibs and diclofenac: diclofenac (HR 2.08), celecoxib (HR 1.75) rofecoxib (HR 1.70), ibuprofen (HR 1.31), naproxen (HR 1.22). The risk of hospitalization for MI or HF also increased.[22]

Among healthy individuals with no signs of CV diseases (n = 1,028,437), the same group found dose-dependent and similarly increased risks of death or MI with rofecoxib (12.5–25 mg), celecoxib (200 mg), and diclofenac ($\geq$100 mg) but not with low-dose ibuprofen or naproxen regardless of the dose.[23]

A study assessing intermittent use of rofecoxib, celecoxib, and diclofenac (48%, 0–14 days; 25%, 15–30 days), as would be expected in the real world for pain control, again found rofecoxib, celecoxib, and diclofenac to have increased CV risk compared to ibuprofen and naproxen. Increased risks were also seen with low doses.[24]

An series of emulated monthly trials (n = 252) assessed MACEs at 30-day follow-up for patients who initiated diclofenac compared with other tNSAIDs, paracetamol, or no initiation.[7] Diclofenac initiators were at increased risk of MACE, including atrial fibrillation or flutter, CVA, HF, acute MI, and cardiac death, compared with no NSAID initiation (Incidence rate ratio [IRR] 1.5, 95% CI 1.4–1.7), paracetamol initiation, and tNSAIDs initiation within 30 days, in both genders and also for low doses of diclofenac in dose- and CV-risk-dependent manner.[7]

Diclofenac (odds ratio [OR] 1.5, 95% CI 1.23–1.82) and ibuprofen (OR 1.31, 95% CI 1.14–1.51) were associated with significantly increased risk of out-of-hospital cardiac arrest (OHCA).[25] While rofecoxib and celecoxib were not significantly associated with OHCA, these groups were characterized by few events.[25]

The use of diclofenac as part of tNSAIDs with naproxen and ibuprofen as a reference group in comparative trials, for example, CLASS, MEDAL, and SCOT, represents a potential flaw in safety trials given its CV risks and high COX-2 selectivity. All the nsNSAIDs were grouped together, including diclofenac, which is characterized by a degree of COX-2 selectivity and a CV hazard comparable with COX-2 inhibitors.

Naproxen continues to appear to have CV safety advantage. However, a recent large-population-based study found that all NSAIDs—including naproxen—were associated with increased risk of MI.[26] What was concerning is that any NSAID at any dose could dramatically increase the risk of MI in both patients with and without a history of CV disease.[26] Table 1 displays select trials discussing CV risk in NSAIDs.

Concomitant Nonsteroidal Anti-Inflammatory Drug + Aspirin Use

Concomitant use of NSAIDs and ASA also raises important CV risk-benefit ratios. In vitro studies suggest that NSAIDs may decrease the antiplatelet efficacy of ASA via competitive inhibition of prostanoid synthesis and by blocking ASA's ability to inhibit COX-1, which is required for platelet inhibition.[27] However, clinical data assessing the modification of NSAIDs' risk profiles by concomitant ASA use were lacking. The PRECISION Aspirin sub-study prespecified an analysis stratified by ASA to examine and address this issue. The addition of ASA attenuated celecoxib's safety advantage over naproxen and ibuprofen. However, even with ASA coadministration, celecoxib still retained an equal or better safety profile relative to both agents largely driven by fewer GI events (P = .004).[28]

Concomitant Nonsteroidal Anti-Inflammatory Drug + Proton Pump Inhibitor (PPI) Use

The general clinical practice, as seen in APPROVe, is a combination of PPIs with tNSAIDs for GI side effect reduction. However, results of the recent celecoxib versus omeprazole and diclofenac in patients with osteoarthritis and rheumatoid arthritis (CONDOR) trial supported switching patients to a COX-2 inhibitor such as celecoxib over using the combination of PPIs with tNSAIDs.[29]

Concomitant Nonsteroidal Anti-Inflammatory Drug + DMARD/Biologic Use

Many rheumatologic diseases are associated with increased CV risk when compared to the general population due in part to the continued low-grade inflammation. The exact mechanism for this is still not fully elucidated. While disease-modifying antirheumatic drugs (DMARDs) and biologics decrease inflammation and thus theoretically reduce CV risk, several of the drugs can aggravate traditional CV and thrombotic risk factors.[30] Methotrexate, a cornerstone in RA treatment, has repeatedly shown to have cardioprotective effectives on lipids and endothelium, 60% reduction in all-cause mortality and 70% reduction in CV-related mortality,[31] and protective effect on occurrence of type 2 diabetes mellitus in a separate meta-analysis.[32] Leflunomide has been associated with elevated BP. A meta-analysis showed that tumor necrosis factor (TNF) inhibitors in inflammatory arthritis have similarly been associated with 30% reduction on CV events.[33] Janus kinase inhibitors have a new black box warning regarding a numerically higher number of MACEs, malignancy, thrombosis, and death when compared with TNF inhibitors, largely based on tofacitinib data from the oral rheumatoid arthritis trial surveillance data.[34] Thus, simply decreasing inflammation by using various DMARDs in inflammatory arthritis may help but not necessarily eradicate the overall inflammatory burden in these patients. There may still be unintended consequences of biologic DMARDs that may increase certain CV risks in some patients. The ability to risk stratify these inflammatory arthritis patients has been an ongoing research discussion.

DISCUSSION AND RECOMMENDATIONS

Currently, evidence supports all NSAIDs are associated with an increased risk of adverse CV events. The SCOT and PRECISION trials are the largest trials to date evaluating this association. While they both similarly report that there are no differences in CV risks between coxibs and tNSAIDs, significant methodologic challenges exist in both trials. Other meta-analyses and large observation registries describe the increased rates of CV events with diclofenac similar to levels with coxibs, but without the decreased GI toxicity. Given both the CV and GI risks of diclofenac, initiating treatment with other tNSAIDs, either naproxen or low-dose ibuprofen, is likely preferable over diclofenac. Topical NSAIDs significantly reduce systemic exposure, minimizing the harmful side effects, and may be a good option for localized pain relief.

Oral NSAIDs are a better option for subsets of rheumatology patients who require more chronic use of analgesics than opiates with appropriate monitoring. The Strategies for Prescribing Analgesics Comparative Effectiveness (SPACE) RCT reported that opioids and nonopioid medications including NSAIDs had comparable pain-related function over 12 months with pain intensity, but the nonopioid arm had significantly lower adverse events.[35] In addition to the dependence issues and risk of overdose which have garnered more attention, opiate use has also been associated with increased incidence of coronary artery disease, stroke, and arrhythmias[36]; cardiac opioid receptors have also been identified.[37]

Several important questions remain regarding the long-term safety of NSAIDs. It is difficult to extrapolate precautions to the much lower prescription doses patients often take for a brief time to manage occasional pain exacerbations. In **Box 1**, we offer rheumatologists a simplified approach to choosing an appropriate NSAID for pain management along with additional recommendations for pain management using a whole-person approach.

Future Directions and Summary

Future studies focusing on the interindividual variability in the drug responses may lend to a precision medicine approach for better outcomes with NSAID use such that NSAID choice could depend on the individual ratio of the potential benefits to side effects, pharmacogenetics, and the comorbidities of a particular patient.

Studies have identified relevant medication-gene interactions in NSAIDs. While there is no direct shift in therapeutic efficacy, a relationship between *CYP2C9* polymorphism genotypes and increased risk of important side effects such as GI bleeding or CV events has been noted.[38]

Hypertension, HF, renal failure, and an increased tendency for thrombosis are some of the proposed biological mechanisms of the increased CV risk associated with the use of most NSAIDs. More thorough mechanistic investigations are needed to understand better how to mitigate the increased risks.

One such mitigation strategy currently being explored is the use of newer technology for modification of pharmacologic toxicity. Studies use the density functional theory and molecular docking simulations to evaluate the interaction of boron nitride nanotube with celecoxib and its inhibitor effect on proinflammatory cytokines TNF-α and IL-1A proteins. These calculations could be used to design a novel carrier for the celecoxib drug delivery system to manage CV risk in patients.[39]

Emerging factors, including biomarkers of COX inhibition and newer technologies, may assist clinicians in the rational selection of appropriate NSAID dose for individual patients in the future. This overview of CV risk and NSAIDs highlights the importance of balancing the benefit versus the risk of treatment before initiating NSAID treatment in each patient. In terms of CV risk, it may be critical to ascertain the CV risk factors and address the modifiable risk factors before long-term NSAID use. Because we do not know ahead of time how patients may respond to NSAIDs, it may be important to monitor patients closely after initiating an NSAID. For example, after 1 week of using a chronic NSAID, one may monitor BP and ask about symptoms. And in 2 to 4 weeks of chronic use, one may consider checking blood work to monitor any potential side effects and consider NSAID dose adjustment.

Box 1
Clinical guide to NSAID use in patients with consideration of cardiovascular risk using a whole patient approach

Use the lowest effective NSAID dose for the shortest period of time.

Depending on the site and intensity of the pain, a topical NSAID might be helpful.

Given that the onset of risk of acute MI occurred in the first week and appeared greatest in the first month of treatment with higher doses, prescribers should engage in shared decision-making with patients and consider weighing the risks and benefits of NSAIDs before instituting treatment, particularly for higher doses.

If concomitant use of corticosteroids is needed, use the lowest glucocorticoid dose (ideally <7.5 mg of prednisone or equivalent for the shortest possible time while continuing to control disease activity).[30]

This discussion should also include weighing the risks of NSAIDs versus the benefits of improved pain control providing increased functional mobility, which will in turn provide other health benefits. Untreated pain can lead patients to avoid physical activity and affects the quality of life in the context of physical function, pain, energy, emotional, social, and mental functions.[40]

Create a pain management toolkit for patients, with NSAIDs being 1 tool in their toolbelt. Incorporate nonpharmacologic therapies, transcutaneous electrical nerve stimulation (TENS) units, physical therapy, occupational therapy, myofascial release, and mindfulness, all providing additive effects for pain control.

As routine assessment of pain score is a difficult metric for assessment and monitoring, monitoring pain-related interference and creation of functional goals can be effective therapeutic targets.

Keep a patient pain/effect diary or apps and regularly review this at patient visits.

Regularly monitor for drug adverse events, including initial BP check 1 week after initiation of NSAIDs, with BP checks at every visit and blood counts and renal function assessed at least yearly.[41]

In patients with some type of CV risk,
• Consider starting with naproxen + PPI or ibuprofen + PPI
• Celecoxib 200 mg daily may be a good alternative; higher doses and twice daily regimens are not recommended
• In patients taking aspirin, recommend naproxen + PPI 2 hours after taking aspirin, or celecoxib 200 mg + PPI.
• Avoid the use of diclofenac

CLINICS CARE POINTS

• future studies focused on factors to interindividual variability in drug responses are needed for a more precision approach to NSAID use.

• Use the lowest effective NSAID dose for the shortest period of time.

• Diclofenac use should be avoided in patients with CV risk.

• Naproxen or ibuprofen may be good options for starting in patients with CV risk.

• Monitoring for adverse drug events including BO checks, and labs should occur regularly.

DISCLOSURE

The authors have nothing to disclose.

REFERENCES

1. Turesson C, Jacobsson LTH, Matteson EL. Cardiovascular co-morbidity in rheumatic diseases. Vasc Health Risk Manag 2008;4(3):605–14.
2. Marcus AJ, Broekman MJ, Pinsky DJ. COX inhibitors and thromboregulation. N Engl J Med 2002;347(13):1025–6. https://doi.org/10.1056/NEJMcibr021805. Available at:.
3. Yan C, AS C, Bianca R, et al. Role of Prostacyclin in the Cardiovascular Response to Thromboxane A2. Science (80-) 2002;296(5567):539–41. https://doi.org/10.1126/science.1068711. Available at:.
4. Kim GH. Renal effects of prostaglandins and cyclooxygenase-2 inhibitors. Electrolyte Blood Press 2008;6(1):35–41.
5. Houston MC. Nonsteroidal anti-inflammatory drugs and antihypertensives. Am J Med 1991;90(5):S42–7.
6. Fisher NDL, Hurwitz S, Ferri C, et al. Altered adrenal sensitivity to angiotensin II in low-renin essential hypertension. Hypertension 1999;34(3):388–94.
7. Schmidt M, Sørensen HT, Pedersen L. Diclofenac use and cardiovascular risks: Series of nationwide cohort studies. BMJ 2018;362.
8. Patrono C, Patrignani P, Rodríguez LAG. Cyclooxygenase-selective inhibition of prostanoid formation: transducing biochemical selectivity into clinical read-outs. J Clin Invest 2001;108(1):7–13.
9. Sciulli MG, Capone ML, Tacconelli S, et al. The future of traditional nonsteroidal antiinflammatory drugs and cyclooxygenase-2 inhibitors in the treatment of inflammation and pain. Pharmacol Rep 2005;57:66.
10. BOMBARDIER C, LAINE L, REICIN A, et al. Comparison of upper gastrointestinal toxicity of rofecoxib and naproxen in patients with rheumatoid arthritis. N Engl J Med 2000;343:1520–8.
11. Baron JA, Sandler RS, Bresalier RS, et al. Cardiovascular events associated with rofecoxib: final analysis of the APPROVe trial. Lancet 2008;372(9651):1756–64. https://doi.org/10.1016/S0140-6736(08)61490-7. Available at:.
12. Choi H, Seeger J, Kuntz K. Effects of rofecoxib and naproxen on life expectancy among patients with rheumatoid arthritis: a decision analysis. Am J Med 2004;116(9):621–9.
13. Kearney PM, Baigent C, Godwin J, et al. Do selective cyclo-oxygenase-2 inhibitors and traditional non-steroidal anti-inflammatory drugs increase the risk of atherothrombosis? Meta-analysis of randomised trials. Br Med J 2006;332(7553):1302–5.
14. Silverstein F, Faich G, Goldstein JL, et al. Gastrointestinal Toxicity With Celecoxib vs Nonsteroidal Anti-inflammatory Drugs for Osteoarthritis and Rheumatoid Arthritis The CLASS Study: A Randomized Controlled Trial. JAMA 2000;284(10):1247–55.
15. Cannon CP, Curtis SP, FitzGerald GA, et al. Cardiovascular outcomes with etoricoxib and diclofenac in patients with osteoarthritis and rheumatoid arthritis in the Multinational Etoricoxib and Diclofenac Arthritis Long-term (MEDAL) programme: a randomised comparison. Lancet 2006;368(9549):1771–81.
16. Bhala N, Emberson J, Merhi A, et al. Vascular and upper gastrointestinal effects of non-steroidal anti-inflammatory drugs: meta-analyses of individual participant data from randomised trials. Lancet (London, England) 2013;382(9894):769–79.
17. Macdonald TM, Hawkey CJ, Ford I, et al. Randomized trial of switching from prescribed non-selective non-steroidal anti-inflammatory drugs to prescribed

celecoxib: The Standard care vs. Celecoxib Outcome Trial (SCOT). Eur Heart J 2017;38(23):1843–50.

18. Nissen SE, Yeomans ND, Solomon DH, et al. Cardiovascular Safety of Celecoxib, Naproxen, or Ibuprofen for Arthritis. N Engl J Med 2016;375(26):2519–29.

19. Gislason GH, Jacobsen S, Rasmussen JN, et al. Risk of death or reinfarction associated with the use of selective cyclooxygenase-2 inhibitors and nonselective nonsteroidal antiinflammatory drugs after acute myocardial infarction. Circulation 2006;113(25):2906–13.

20. Schjerning Olsen A-M, Fosbøl EL, Lindhardsen J, et al. Duration of treatment with nonsteroidal anti-inflammatory drugs and impact on risk of death and recurrent myocardial infarction in patients with prior myocardial infarction: a nationwide cohort study. Circulation 2011;123(20):2226–35.

21. Olsen A-MS, Fosbøl EL, Lindhardsen J, et al. Long-term cardiovascular risk of nonsteroidal anti-inflammatory drug use according to time passed after first-time myocardial infarction: a nationwide cohort study. Circulation 2012;126(16):1955–63.

22. Gislason GH, Rasmussen JN, Abildstrom SZ, et al. Increased mortality and cardiovascular morbidity associated with use of nonsteroidal anti-inflammatory drugs in chronic heart failure. Arch Intern Med 2009;169(2):141–9.

23. Fosbøl EL, Gislason GH, Jacobsen S, et al. Risk of myocardial infarction and death associated with the use of nonsteroidal anti-inflammatory drugs (NSAIDs) among healthy individuals: a nationwide cohort study. Clin Pharmacol Ther 2009;85(2):190–7.

24. Barcella CA, Lamberts M, McGettigan P, et al. Differences in cardiovascular safety with non-steroidal anti-inflammatory drug therapy—A nationwide study in patients with osteoarthritis. Basic Clin Pharmacol Toxicol 2019;124(5):629–41.

25. Sondergaard KB, Weeke P, Wissenberg M, et al. Non-steroidal anti-inflammatory drug use is associated with increased risk of out-of-hospital cardiac arrest: a nationwide case-time-control study. Eur Hear Journal Cardiovasc Pharmacother 2017;3(2):100–7.

26. Bally M, Dendukuri N, Rich B, et al. Risk of acute myocardial infarction with NSAIDs in real world use: Bayesian meta-analysis of individual patient data. BMJ 2017;357.

27. Gladding PA, Webster MWI, Farrell HB, et al. The Antiplatelet Effect of Six Non-Steroidal Anti-Inflammatory Drugs and Their Pharmacodynamic Interaction With Aspirin in Healthy Volunteers. Am J Cardiol 2008;101(7):1060–3.

28. Reed GW, Abdallah MS, Shao M, et al. Effect of Aspirin Coadministration on the Safety of Celecoxib, Naproxen, or Ibuprofen. J Am Coll Cardiol 2018;71(16):1741–51.

29. Chan FKL, Lanas A, Scheiman J, et al. Celecoxib versus omeprazole and diclofenac in patients with osteoarthritis and rheumatoid arthritis (CONDOR): a randomised trial. Lancet (London, England) 2010;376(9736):173–9.

30. Atzeni F, Rodríguez-Carrio J, Popa CD, et al. Cardiovascular effects of approved drugs for rheumatoid arthritis. Nat Rev Rheumatol 2021;17(5):270–90.

31. Choi HK, Hernán MA, Seeger JD, et al. Methotrexate and mortality in patients with rheumatoid arthritis: A prospective study. Lancet 2002;359(9313):1173–7.

32. Xie W, Yang X, Ji LL, et al. Incident diabetes associated with hydroxychloroquine, methotrexate, biologics and glucocorticoids in rheumatoid arthritis: A systematic review and meta-analysis. Semin Arthritis Rheum 2020;50(4):598–607.

33. Roubille C, Richer V, Starnino T, et al. The effects of tumour necrosis factor inhibitors, methotrexate, non-steroidal anti-inflammatory drugs and corticosteroids on

cardiovascular events in rheumatoid arthritis, psoriasis and psoriatic arthritis: A systematic review and meta-analysis. Ann Rheum Dis 2015;74(3):480–9.

34. US Food and Drug Administration. FDA requires warnings about increased risk of serious heart-related events, cancer, blood clots, and death for JAK inhibitors that treat certain chronic inflammatory conditions [Internet]. 2021. Available at: https://www.fda.gov/drugs/drug-safety-and-availability/fda-requires-warnings-about-increased-risk-serious-heart-related-events-cancer-blood-clots-and-death.

35. Krebs EE, Gravely A, Nugent S, et al. Effect of opioid vs nonopioid medications on pain-related function in patients with chronic back pain or hip or knee osteoarthritis pain the SPACE randomized clinical trial. JAMA 2018;319(9):872–82.

36. Singleton JH, Abner EL, Akpunonu PD, et al. Association of nonacute opioid use and cardiovascular diseases: a scoping review of the literature. J Am Heart Assoc 2021;10(13):e021260.

37. Feng Y, He X, Yang Y, et al. Current research on opioid receptor function. Curr Drug Targets 2012;13(2):230–46.

38. Zobdeh F, Eremenko II, Akan MA, et al. Pharmacogenetics and Pain Treatment with a Focus on Non-Steroidal Anti-Inflammatory Drugs (NSAIDs) and Antidepressants: A Systematic Review. Pharmaceutics 2022;14(6):1190.

39. Cao Y, Noori M, Nazari M, et al. Molecular docking evaluation of celecoxib on the boron nitride nanostructures for alleviation of cardiovascular risk and inflammatory. Arab J Chem 2022;15(1):103521. https://doi.org/10.1016/j.arabjc.2021.103521. Available at:.

40. Öztürk İB, Garip Y, Sivas F, et al. Kinesiophobia in rheumatoid arthritis patients: Relationship with quadriceps muscle strength, fear of falling, functional status, disease activity, and quality of life. Arch Rheumatol 2021;36(3):427–34.

41. Ho KY, Cardosa MS, Chaiamnuay S, et al. Practice advisory on the appropriate use of NSAIDs in primary care. J Pain Res 2020;13:1925–39.